THE EPIDEMIC

ALSO BY JONATHAN ENGEL

Doctors and Reformers:
Discussion and Debate over Health Policy 1925–1950

Poor People's Medicine:
Medicaid and American Charity Care Since 1965

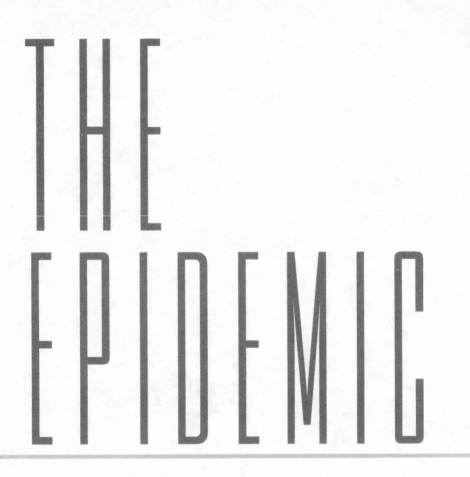

THE EPIDEMIC

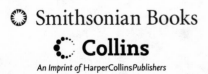

Smithsonian Books

Collins

An Imprint of HarperCollins*Publishers*

[A GLOBAL HISTORY OF AIDS]

JONATHAN ENGEL

FOR MY CHILDREN:

EZRA, RUTH, MIRIAM, AND JUDAH

Published 2006 in the United States of America by Smithsonian Books
In association with HarperCollins Publishers.

Designed by Lovedog Studio

Library-of-Congress Cataloging-in-Publication Data

Engel, Jonathan.
     The epidemic : a global history of AIDS / Jonathan Engel.
          p. cm.
     Includes bibliographical references and index.
     ISBN-13: 978-0-06-114488-2
     ISBN-10: 0-06-114488-6
     1. AIDS (Disease)—History. I. Title.

  RA643.8.E54 2006
  614.5'99392—dc22   2006044285

06   07   08   09   WBC/RRD   10   9   8   7   6   5   4   3   2   1

[CONTENTS]

PROLOGUE

Sometime in the 1930s, most probably 1931, a small bit of ribonucleic acid (RNA), one of two types of genetic material found in the world, spontaneously mutated.[1] This bit of RNA was the carrier of all genetic information for an insignificant virus now known as simian immuno-deficiency virus, which had lived in the bodies of various types of African monkeys and apes for several hundred thousand years. The virus lived parasitically in the apes, hindering them modestly without killing them, and thus enabled its hosts to live and incubate more viruses, generation after generation.

The mutation that occurred in 1931 was hardly unique. Genetic material—both DNA and RNA—mutates frequently, and such muta-tions are the basic engine of evolutionary change. This particular muta-tion, however, would prove to be extraordinarily consequential for the world, as it allowed the virus, which could previously live only in its ape hosts, to live in human beings.

Once the mutation occurred, random chance dictated that the virus would eventually find a human host. Whether by an African hunter eating an infected monkey, or a chance contamination of an open human sore with monkey blood, the virus would come to roost in a human host, and from there spread to any other humans with whom the primary host shared any of his or her bodily fluids that could harbor the pathogen.[2]

Such transmission from monkey to human probably occurred multiple times over the ensuing four decades, but for reasons specific to this particular virus, the range of contamination remained limited.[3] For one, the virus was unusually weak, unable to survive in air, and often unable to penetrate the skin, epithelial tissue, and the mucosal linings of its host's sexual partners. For another, lack of good roads or commercial air routes into infected areas of Africa prevented the virus from spreading beyond small, isolated tribal groups. And third, the absence of hypodermic syringes in these areas prevented its spread through contaminated needle pricks.[4]

The virus did spread sporadically, however. At least 19 times between 1950 and 1972 it managed to travel by car, boat, or plane, to infect an isolated individual in a far part of the globe. In 1959, for example, David Carr was admitted to the Manchester (England) Royal Infirmary with a variety of inexplicable symptoms including inflamed nostrils and gums, skin lesions, and severe fever and weight loss. Moreover, his immune system seemed to have wholly ceased functioning. And upon his death, 20 weeks later, an autopsy revealed that he had suffered from a rare form of pneumonia, *Pneumocystis carinii* (PCP), which was associated almost exclusively with elderly men of Mediterranean or Ashkenazic Jewish extraction.[5] That same year, a Bantu man died in Leopoldville, Belgian Congo, after having suffered similar symptoms.[6]

Other cases retroactively identified in those early years include that of Robert R., a Saint Louis teenager who died mysteriously in 1969 after having been found to suffer from odd swelling of the legs, torso, and genitalia, and whose autopsied body proved to be riddled with a rare skin cancer known as *Kaposi's sarcoma* (KS);[7] a Danish surgeon in 1977 who several years previously had been working in a rural surgical ward in Zaire;[8] and a Canadian woman who had once been a nun who left her order in 1972 to rehabilitate prostitutes in Port-au-Prince, Haiti, and who died in Canada in 1981.[9]

Toward the late 1970s, these early cases, all identified as resultant of similar pathogenic infections, began to appear more frequently. Between 1973 and 1979 at least 5 New York men contracted the mysterious illness,[10] as did at least a dozen others in Western Europe, the United States, and Israel.[11] But it was from Africa, particularly central Africa, that the preponderance of early cases emanated. Although medical records are scarce for many of the rural populations of that part of Africa, retrospective tests on collected sera conducted one to two decades later showed presence of the mysterious virus in the blood of decedents in Zaire from the early to mid 1970s, in over 50 cases.[12] By 1982, Zaire, alone, had produced 18 identifiable victims of the strange new disease, all of whom had sought care in Belgium.[13]

Years later, after the mutated pathogen had been identified, mapped, charted, described, explored, and blamed for the death of tens of millions of people, scientists would debate how and when the bit of RNA had jumped species. Was it definitely in Africa, or was this merely another example of a Eurocentric establishment blaming their ills on the dark continent? And if it had been in Africa, could the cause have been rooted in human actions? One tenacious author seized on the explanation that the virus, or at least one iteration of it, while of monkey origins, had actually been inadvertently included in batches of oral polio vaccine that were administered to patients in the Belgian Congo in the late 1950s.[14] The thesis, while compelling, and perhaps even titilating, couldn't stand up to rigorous investigation. As cases became known that predated the vaccine administration, and as genetic researchers confidently dated the primary mutation to two decades prior, the thesis was dismissed.[15]

The truth, it turned out, was more mundane. The troublesome pathogen was one of several that had mutated more toxic qualities during the course of the 20th century, and lodged in human hosts. Others, such as Ebola and Marburg, had arisen as rapidly and mysteriously. This one, however, had spontaneously stumbled upon the sublime trick of slow pathogenesis. While other fatal viruses killed so rapidly that they scarcely gave their hosts time enough to transmit the virus before dying, this one killed slowly. In the decade or so that it took the virus to wholly immobilize its host's immune system, and ultimately kill him, the host could spread the virus to hundreds of unknowing new hosts, whether through sexual coupling, needle sharing, or blood transfusions. And for much of that decade, the symptoms of the viral infection were so mild that the pathogen's presence remained all but unknowable. The one great defense on the side of the humans—the essential weakness of the virus's protein coat—protected humans for decades. Once the virus breached the jungle, however, and learned to travel by automobile and jet, that defense was no longer adequate.

Our story starts, then, not at the inception of the new virus, but at the moment it entered the modern world. For it was here that the virus found fertile ground to grow and spread, jumping intercontinentally in a matter of months, and growing exponentially in frequency, until it overwhelmed whole communities, towns, cities, and even nations. Our story starts in the raucous Castro and Greenwich Village neighborhoods of San Francisco and New York City in the early 1980s, where a weird amalgam of unprecedented eroticism and fierce political defiance combined to create a near perfect environ for the virus's spread.

CHAPTER 1

FIRST REPORTS

FIRST REPORTS

In June of 1981, the United States Centers for Disease Control (CDC) reported that five young men in Los Angeles had been treated in recent months for *Pneumocystis carinii* (PCP), a rare form of pneumonia. Two had later died. All were also infected with, or had been infected with, cytomegalovirus (CMV).[1] All were active homosexuals. All had had multiple sexual partners over the past several years. Several had reported using one of two sexual enhancement drugs: LSD or amyl nitrite.[2]

Two months later, the CDC reported that over 100 gay men had been diagnosed with either PCP or a rare cancer, Kaposi's sarcoma (KS), since January of 1980. Nearly half had died. Some men had been diagnosed with both maladies, others with only one. Typically, the CDC reported, KS afflicted only 1 American in 1.5 million, and the victims were predominantly elderly.[3]

The cause was unclear. Harold Jaffe, a member of the CDC group investigating the malady, queried whether this new syndrome affected only gay men, or if gay men were simply being disproportionately diagnosed. The CDC began to track the syndrome that fall, using requests for pentamidine isothionate, a drug used to treat PCP, as a means of locating the cases. Many of the diagnosed men had contracted other sexually transmitted diseases, or had been diagnosed as well with various sorts of mucosal infections and digestive parasites. The one significant factor in the cases appeared to be the number of sexual partners with which the infected men had liaised over the previous year: over 60 for the infected men versus 25 for a control group.[4]

Most troubling was the rate at which the peculiar syndrome appeared to be spreading. Case frequency seemed to grow exponentially. "If I had written this a month ago, I would have used the figure '40,' " wrote gay playwright and activist Larry Kramer that September. "If I had written this last week, I would have needed '80.' Today I must tell you that 120 gay men in the United States—most of them here in New York—are suffering from an often lethal form of cancer . . . more than 30 have died."[5] By November 1982, almost 600 cases of the strange syndrome had been reported to the CDC, with an overall mortality rate of 41 percent, and mortality rate for those diagnosed over a year previous of over 60 percent. The epidemic was doubling every six months.[6]

By that time the syndrome had a name, or rather two names—AID for acquired immunodeficiency disease, and GRID for gay-related immunodeficiency. It had been reported in nearly half the states in the United States and in several countries abroad. While the fatal part of the syndrome tended toward the two diseases initially diagnosed—KS or PCP—all of the victims were fantastically vulnerable to infection generally. GRID patients had been diagnosed with cytomegalovirus, fungal toxoplasmosis, cryptosporidiosis, eye damage, lupus, anemia, and various lymphomas and cancers. The disease did not appear to spread through airborne pathogens, and it was capable of infecting nonhomosexuals as well. In November 1982, the CDC grouped GRID victims into four major risk groups: homosexual or bisexual males (75 percent); intravenous drug users (13 percent); hemophiliacs (.3 percent); and, inexplicably, nongay or non-intravenous drug-using Haitians (6 percent). An additional 5 percent of victims fell into no known risk group.[7] GRID prevalence was 10 times higher in New York City and San Francisco than in the rest of the country.

Victims took a long time to die. The CDC physician assigned to coordinate the task force on Kaposi's reported that costs were reaching

$64,000 per patient, and that the first 300 cases produced hospital billings of $18 million.[8] During that time, their bodies weakened and wasted, as their disintegrating immune systems allowed greater and greater numbers of pathogens to invade. "I found myself bedridden with a cold that wouldn't go away, viral bronchitis, fever, diarrhea, loss of appetite, and extreme fatigue," wrote one early GRID victim. "Then I developed chronic ear infections, shingles on the backs of both legs, and a persistent sore throat."[9] Described another: "Low-grade fevers, generalized lymphadenopathy, and thrush. Weight loss—*massive* weight loss: fifty pounds! Pain, unexplained pain in my limbs, headaches, nausea, and unexplained diarrhea for seven months."[10] A New York physician described the early cases he witnessed: "It's the worst way I've ever seen anyone go. I've seen young people die of cancer. But this is total body rot. It's merciless."[11] And describing an AIDS-afflicted patient who had picked up a common parasite, the physician proceeded: "The deterioration progressed relentlessly until he couldn't carry on his job. While he was in the hospital he suffered a generalized seizure. Then another so prolonged he needed anesthesia to prevent his limbs from jerking all over. The body was still because of the drugs, but the brain never stopped seizing."[12]

The new disease left epidemiologists, infectious-disease specialists, and oncologists bewildered. What was causing this strange new illness, and how was it spreading? Researchers pondered several explanations in the early days of the epidemic, but none seemed wholly satisfactory. Gay men who contracted the disease reported using nitrite drugs at rates disproportionate to the rest of the population, but this didn't explain why nonnitrite users were also getting sick. Another theory rested on the startling number of sexual partners each of the afflicted men had coupled with—nearly 1,100 over a lifetime—and the great many infections that the men had picked up along the way, including syphilis, gonorrhea, and "gay bowel syndrome," the general term for the array of bacterial, viral, and parasitic infections that gay men tended to pick up through anal sex. This theory held that the men's bodies were suffering from "immune overload," or "sperm overload," or some other such rejection of the flood of foreign material to which they were exposed.[13] Another theory postulated that the oft seen cytomegalovirus was itself the causative agent. Still another suggested water contamination.[14] Others sought a multifactor explanation, combining in some form drugs, chemicals, viruses, and general wear and tear of the immune system.[15]

But none of these explanations accounted for the nonhomosexuals who were becoming infected, or the hemophiliacs, or the Haitians. The explanations became even less satisfying when the CDC reported in late 1982 that at least 26 infants and children had also been diagnosed. In the following months investigators began to agree that the cause was most likely a blood-borne pathogen that was frequently being transmitted sexually. Doctors began to suspect that gay men were disproportionately represented among the afflicted not because of anything unique that they were doing, but rather because of how much they were doing it. One New York doctor warned that gay men whose lifestyle consisted of "anonymous sexual encounters" would need to do some "serious rethinking," while another physician encouraged his colleagues to try to " 'rehabilitate' highly promiscuous homosexuals."[16] And a New York physician wrote in that city's gay-oriented *New York Native*: "Multiple sexual contacts with anonymous partners is especially risky now, and it should be discouraged for purely medical reasons. It's not immoral, but it is unquestionably *very unhealthy*."[17]

The blood-borne-pathogen hypothesis fit with the growing numbers of cases associated with IV drug use. These cases, making up 16 percent of all cases by early 1983, tended to be found among the poorest and lowest functioning drug users, who were more likely to administer drugs to themselves in a quasi-public "shooting gallery," where needles might be shared among dozens of users over several weeks. "You take a needle from someone else," one user explained, "rinse it off to make sure there's no blood, use it and pass it on to the next guy—like a reefer."[18]

Whatever was causing the malady, the progress of the disease was becoming clear by early 1983. The immune system in the infected patients was catastrophically and irreparably breaking down, and as it did so the numerous pathogens of the world could gain free entry to the afflicted bodies of the sick. In particular, the T cell lymphocytes, central cells in the functioning of the immune system, were dying off at unsustainable rates. As the T cells died off, and as the remaining T cells ceased to function normally, the afflicted men became sicker and sicker, and more and more vulnerable to what were now being termed "opportunistic infections."[19]

If the disease was viral in origin, what type of virus was it, and where was it coming from? Investigators were intrigued at the high rate of AIDS cases in Haitians, and speculated that a new pathogen had developed in Haiti, spread through that nation's gay community, and then been passed to gay American tourists who had visited the island on vacation. Or contrarily, the virus could have existed in Haiti for some time, but only begun to grow epidemically after entering a newly promiscuous gay community whose numerous liaisons and multiple side infections would amplify the virus's toxicity and accelerate its spread.[20]

By early 1983, researchers, particularly virologists, began to suggest that the infectious agent was some sort of derivation, or mutation, of one of several known viruses that could compromise an immune system. High on the list was the human T cell leukemia virus (HTLV)—a known retrovirus with immunosuppressive and oncogenic properties—as well as feline leukemia virus (FeLV), which caused leukemia-like symptoms in cats. A third possibility was HPV, a DNA virus (as opposed to an RNA virus) that was known to induce immune system disorders, but was not considered immunosuppressive.[21]

HTLV was the early favorite of virologists, particularly of Robert Gallo, director of the National Cancer Institute's Tumor Cell Biology Laboratory. The RNA-based virus tended to attack T cells, induced immunodeficiency and cancers, and was blood-borne. The question was whether the virus could be semen-borne as well, and thus enter its victims through tears in their rectums sustained during traumatic anal intercourse. Gallo and a team of scientists actually detected HTLV particles in cells of AIDS victims, while Harvard School of Public Health researcher Max Essex reported that nearly 25 percent of patients under observation tested positive for HTLV antibodies.[22]

But other data suggested that HTLV was not the cause. T cells taken from HTLV-infected patients did not behave the same way as T cells taken from AIDS patients. Although they grew abnormally slowly, they did not die as quickly as the AIDS-infected T cells. Furthermore, a substantial portion of AIDS patients showed no evidence of viral DNA, or of HTLV antibodies. And although Gallo hypothesized that the HTLV could not be detected in advanced AIDS patients whose T cells had largely died off, others were not convinced. Different teams hypothesized that the cause was a pathogenic variation on a thymus-infecting virus, or was some sort of autoimmune reaction, or was something new altogether.[23]

Further complicating matters was the discovery in early 1983 of an epidemic of immune deficiency in a monkey population at the University of California Primate Research Center in Davis, California. Over a third of 77 captive monkeys sharing a cage developed AIDS-like symptoms, such as swollen glands, fever, weight loss, diarrhea, and skin cancer. All of the sick monkeys died shortly thereafter, as did 60 similarly infected monkeys at Harvard's New England Regional Primate Research Center.[24]

The monkey connection led researchers to look to the region of Africa where the monkeys naturally dwelled. In fact, Kaposi's sarcoma had repeatedly broken out in an area of central Africa that also had a high incidence of CMV infection. French immunologist David Klatzmann noticed at that time that several French AIDS patients had traveled in that portion of Africa, leading University of Miami researcher Caroline MacLeod to speculate that mercenary Cuban soldiers serving in Angola may have brought AIDS back with them to the Western Hemisphere.[25]

If the AIDS pathogen was wholly new, then perhaps it was caused by a virus closely related to HTLV. French investigator Luc Montagnier isolated one that he named lymphadenopathy virus (LAV). LAV, Montagnier discovered, differed in several of its core proteins from HTLV, yet was also T cell tropic.[26] Regardless of who was right, Gallo or Montagnier, both scientists and their associated teams believed the virus to be an RNA-based retrovirus, thus narrowing the range of potential molecular structures they needed to investigate. Neither team had a model, a structure, a transmission mechanism, or even the beginnings of a cure or vaccine, yet in little over two years from first notice of the epidemic, the basic outline of the etiology had been mapped.

GAY LIFE

By 1980, San Francisco had a gay population of over 100,000, crammed into two or three heavily gay neighborhoods including the Tenderloin, Folsom Street, and Castro precincts, the last being the epicenter of gay life on the West Coast, and possibly in all of the United States. The city hosted at least 150 gay social, political, and arts organizations, 90 gay bars, and various gay churches, synagogues, clubs, newspapers, magazines, and theaters. Twenty percent of the adult population was gay, as was 25 percent of the registered electorate. Writer Frances Fitzgerald wrote at the time that the "sheer concentration of gay people in San Francisco may have had no parallel in history."[27]

Most gays were relative newcomers to San Francisco. The great migration had started shortly after the advent of the modern gay liberation era, universally dated to the famous Stonewall uprising in New York City on June 27, 1969. On that Friday night, the New York City police raided an eponymous gay Greenwich Village bar, expecting to round up the usual clientele, charge them, and then release them after fines were paid. This time, however, the crowd of men in the bar stood up to the police, emerging from the bar to protest loudly against the petty harassment, and to insist that a new era had begun for gays in America. The Stonewall protests led to the organization of the Gay Liberation Front (GLF) in New York, which soon led to brother chapters being established in Los Angeles and San Francisco. The GLF spurred the establishment of the Gay Activists Alliance, which set a new aggressive tone for gay rights activism. Gay political clubs established themselves shortly after, with San Francisco's Alice Toklas Democratic Club leading the way for Seattle's Dorian Group, and Washington, D.C.'s Gertrude Stein Democratic Club.[28]

Gay liberation resonated throughout the country, and spurred a migration of young gay men from small towns and college campuses to growing gay neighborhoods in the nation's major cities. San Francisco saw its gay population triple in the two years after Stonewall, as thousands of gays moved there to celebrate their lives within a community that welcomed and validated them. Explained one recent émigré: "I lived in Rochester. I was white, male and middle-class, and I had gone to Harvard. I thought I could do anything I wanted, so I resented having to conceal something as basic as sex. I resented being condemned to repress or ignore my homosexuality, and to live in turmoil for the rest of my life. The solution was to move here."[29] By 1975, 5,000 gay men were moving to San Francisco every year. Real estate prices in the Castro district doubled, then tripled, as businesses, services, bars, clubs, and community centers all opened to serve the growing community.[30]

Gay men organized themselves into various civic and political clubs through the 1970s, fighting to end antisodomy laws, suing to end employment discrimination, and campaigning to elect either openly gay or gay-friendly candidates who would crack down on antigay violence and fight for the interests of gays in city hall and the statehouse. In San Francisco, such organizations as the Bay Area Gay Liberation (BAGL) and the Gay Teachers Association became powerful advocacy groups, using techniques ranging from classic fund-raising and electioneering to disruption, sit-ins, and civic unrest. "I came to San Francisco to become a professional faggot," wrote gay activist John Cailleau years later.[31] The apex of their organizing came with the election of openly gay community organizer Harvey Milk to the position of city supervisor in 1977.[32]

Beyond the political organizations, however, beyond the gay synagogues and churches, gay Democratic clubs, labor unions, and gay restaurants and bars, gay men in San Francisco and New York in the 1970s began to organize themselves around sex, a "headlong gambol on the side of the human libido," in the words of one reporter, ". . . a priapic binge."[33] Although gay sex had existed as long as sex had, many residents of the nation's gay neighborhoods agreed that its essential character changed in the 1970s, becoming more central to gay existence, more defining, and simply more intense. "I can remember the euphoria of the early days," stated one community member. "We thought we were given license to be extreme."[34]

Extreme sex wasn't really so different from sex before; there was just more of it, and it was more transient, anonymous, and ephemeral. New private "bathhouse" establishments opened whose essential service was allowing gay men to couple, often with several partners per night, in a safe milieu. The number of sex partners active gay men reported having rose to hundreds per year, with lifetime partners rising into the thousands. Singer and organizer Michael Callen remembered trying to calculate his lifetime sex partners upon learning of his infected status. "I was thinking maybe a thousand, and then I was thinking, no, it can't be. Lo and behold, it was more."[35] Wrote one gay playwright: "Gay life circumvented the courtship phase. You could not pick up a boy at his house. Instead you went from sex to courtship and built the relationship backwards."[36] Wrote another: "At the beginning of this century Henry James was struck by the number of people eating candy bars when he visited New York; seventy years later, we were not eating candy bars (they were fattening), we were munching on people."[37]

For many gays, promiscuous sex was more than fun, and more than simply an effort at human bonding: it was the defining act of community building, "a force binding atoms into new polymers of affinity," Edmund White wrote.[38] Gays began to see frequent anonymous sex as the bedrock of gay liberation—an emblematic endorsement of the great liberation they had won at Stonewall, as well as a vehicle with which to solidify communal bonds. "The belief handed to me was that sex was liberating and more sex was more liberating," reflected Callen in 1983.[39] The Canadian gay magazine, *The Body Politic,* opined, "Promiscuity knits together the social fabric of the gay male community."[40] And some gays suggested that traditional views of monogamous, or at least near monogamous sex, were a vestige of heterosexist hegemony, a colonialist hangover whose time, like that of slavery and human sacrifice, has passed. "I have never looked upon 'promiscuity' as a dirty word," said Washington gay activist Frank Kameny. "It is a natural and normal style of living, while monogamy is deeply entrenched cultural overlay."[41]

Promiscuity alone did not define the new sex; it was closely coupled with anonymity. Brief, wordless exchanges had long been a component of gay sexual pickups in bars, clubs, and even parks, but the new sex reduced verbal interaction to nil. In some of the bathhouses, customers could have oral sex through a hole cut between plywood partitions, nullifying even the need for eye contact. In the booths of the bathhouses, customers could shop for young men, lying prone, waiting for someone to consume their wares. Gay activist Arnie Kantrowitz called the scene "the freedom of facelessness."[42]

Not everyone participated. Thousands of gay men had always pursued middle-class trappings and aspirations with the same steady tenacity as their straight counterparts. Gays operated businesses, practiced their professions, maintained steady relationships, attended church, dutifully looked after kin, and sought love and intimacy. Moreover, as the 1970s wore on, some who had participated, or who had at least observed, began to see the vacuousness, the basic soullessness of the wild sexual endeavor, and some dared to voice their criticisms. One older gay San Francisco resident, John Artman, mused, "I worry a lot about the young right now. They think they are free, but they are getting locked in behind their genitalia,"[43] while the protagonist Fred Lemish in Larry Kramer's play *Faggots* asked, "Why do faggots have to fuck so fucking much?! . . . it's as if we don't have anything else to do . . . all we do is live in our Ghetto and dance and drug and fuck."[44] And Kramer himself, who would later become the preeminent gadfly and ombudsman of the organized gay community, asked, "Why are we so perennially focused on our dicks? It's a very peculiar 'community' that uses sexuality as the sole yardstick of action and thought and everything."[45]

It wasn't just the quantity of sex that raised hackles; it was the increasing perversity of it. Many young gay men in San Francisco, New York, and Los Angeles in the 1970s relentlessly pursued increasingly bizarre and extreme sexual experiences, ranging from urination, to bondage, to beatings. Men had themselves tied up and bullwhipped, chained to a cross, urinated on while crouching in a bathtub, suspended in slings to be masturbated, and penetrated in every way imaginable. "Why get hung up with higher prices when all you want is a place to hang your handcuffs?" advertised one San Francisco bathhouse.[46]

Some practices seemed to invite bodily harm. Oral-anal sex or "rimming" gained popularity as the new "taste treat" in gay sex, but obviously left its partakers prone to infection with gastrointestinal parasites. The general level of promiscuity with multiple partners facilitated transmission of traditional sexually transmitted diseases such as gonorrhea and hepatitis, and the practice of "fisting," in which one partner inserted his entire hand, and even his forearm, into the other's rectum (usually abetted by heavy doses of alcohol or amyl nitrite inhalants) was a near-certain precursor to rectal tears, anal fissures, and assorted gastrointestinal ailments. By 1980, gay men in America accounted for a staggering 55 percent of all syphilis and gonorrhea cases in the country, and the San Francisco health department estimated that 70 percent of gay men in that city carried the virus for hepatitis B.[47] Callen remembered, "After a point, whenever I had sex, I got sick: syphilis, gonorrhea, hepatitis A, B, and non-A/non-B, mono, amoebas, herpes, the whole schmear."[48]

THE BATHHOUSES

As AIDS spread into the sexually active gay communities of the nation's cities, the bathhouses became a natural focus of attention. These institutions were privately run businesses that ostensibly re-created the old Roman (and more recent Russian) baths with their swimming pools, Jacuzzis, masseurs, lounges, and refreshment areas. In fact, they were unique creations designed to facilitate anonymous sex in a safe environment, away from the prying eyes of police and voyeurs. For a modest $10 entrance fee, a patron received a towel and a locker or room key, and freedom to roam the floors of cubicles and closets where he could simultaneously offer himself up to sexual liaising and also peruse the available wares. In the soft artificial light of the baths, with incessant background music shading the sounds of sex, men drifted in and out of the lounges, relaxing from coitus or scanning the crowd to seek out their next liaison. Others arrayed themselves in their rooms, doors open, inviting passersby to copulate. Writer Philip Weiss described the scene at the famous Saint Marks Baths in New York thus:

> Many occupants of the cubicles had arranged themselves on their beds with their doors open. Body language: most were on their backs, naked or decorated with the towel, eyeing the doorway; others lay on their stomachs but peered back over their shoulders at the door. The traffic in the passageways sometimes bottlenecked when a man leaned into a doorway to examine the candidate more closely. The behavior was so wordless, so pictorially reminiscent of seraglio paintings, that it seemed ancient, instinctive, acultural.[49]

The bathhouses, correctly or not, were identified by public health advocates and gay leaders as the sexual nexus of the communities, and thus attracted attention as the transmission point for AIDS.[50] Evidence supported the hypothesis. Two University of California researchers had found, in March 1983, that 1 in 233 gay men in the Castro district had AIDS; a year later the estimate was revised to 1 in 100. And by 1985, public health data suggested that more than 1 in 3 gay men in San Francisco had AIDS, a figure that later climbed to 1 in 2.[51]

Such epidemic growth called for a drastic change in the manner in which gay men had sex. Although the etiology of AIDS had not yet been comprehensively described, most people accepted that it was caused by an infectious agent, probably viral, that spread sexually. The question for many gay men became one of specifics: exactly which sexual activities needed to be modified? Most agreed that unprotected anal sex must now be considered dangerous, but what about oral sex? Was mutual masturbation safe? Or French kissing? And, if a condom was used, regularly and carefully, could these activities be undertaken with relative safety?

Over the next two years, gay men changed the manner in which they fornicated. Their average number of monthly sex partners declined from 6.3 in 1982 to 3.9 in 1984, with acts of receptive unprotected anal intercourse, the postulated most dangerous type of sex, declining from 1.9 to .7.[52] Of note, surveyed men did not reduce the number of sex acts, anal or otherwise, they participated in with a primary or monogamous partner, but only the number of partners, suggesting that the antipromiscuity message was being heard.[53]

Gay men struggled with the change. Few desisted from sex entirely, but rather most changed their sex practices, or reduced the number of partners with whom they copulated. Patronage of bathhouses declined, while use of condoms rose. Over the first half of the 1980s, nationwide condom sales rose from $182 million to $338 million. Some men began to date, in earnest, for the first time, while others abstained entirely. "Basically, I make love to my VCR a lot," divulged one gay man.[54] Others spoke of "a return to courtship and romance," and having "dropped out of the fast lane."[55] And even men who continued a promiscuous lifestyle moderated their pickup habits and venues. "It's stopped me from going to places like bathhouses, back rooms of bookstores and some of the more sleazy places," explained a New Jersey man. "People who hang out at bathhouses may have sex with 18, 19 in one night."[56]

Andrew Holleran made light of the new reality, writing of a celibate acquaintance: "I concluded he was simply more intelligent and disciplined than the rest of us. He became outwardly more calm; he left his gym, changed his friends, habits, went to school, became obsessed with a vegetarian diet, and then, three years later, tried to kill himself. Celibacy is tough."[57]

Not all men accommodated the new danger. Some men angrily condemned the antipromiscuity message as being essentially antigay, or neopuritan, or simply repressive, unrealistic, and unnecessary. "Monogamy is not for everyone, gay or heterosexual. And I challenge anyone . . . to disprove the undeniable fact that totally safe sex, practiced carefully and soberly, is just as healthy whether it is performed with dozens of partners or with a single dependable lover," wrote New York University anthropology professor Douglas Feldman.[58] Similarly, Arthur Felson declared that gays had to constantly affirm their "gayness," lest they regress to a more primitive stage. "To totally stop having sex is, for me, going back into the closet."[59] Others, however, simply admitted that frequent anonymous sex had become a sort of addiction that they were having difficulty breaking, even as they knew that continued indulgence in it jeopardized their health. One man who had tried the path of abstention and failed explained that he had found loneliness "as bad as a disease,"[60] while another responded to a question about his continuing promiscuity, "It's hard to change my sexual behavior because being gay means doing what I want sexually."[61] Overall, fewer men went to the bathhouses and participated in unsafe sex, but those who continued to go failed to alter their sex practices significantly.[62] Rationalized one forlorn man, "Men in my family tend to die very early, anyway, in their 50s—and since I'm 44 . . ."[63]

By 1983 many members of both the gay community and the public health establishment realized that continuing declines in promiscuity, and thus new infections, could only be accomplished by closing the bathhouses. Despite education campaigns and community awareness efforts, a large stubborn core of gay men continued to flock to the baths, either denying the risks entirely, or rationalizing them. A University of California research team concluded that men who were still frequenting the baths in late 1983 had changed their behavior hardly at all over the past year, although many surveyed outside the baths admitted that they no longer frequented those places.[64] The path to further public health gains, it seemed, was simply to put padlocks on the bathhouses and drive the anonymous sex back to the parks and strips where it was necessarily less efficient, or at least less pleasant.

The move, however, attracted a startling degree of antipathy from gay leaders, libertarians, civil rights activists, and even physicians. Such a move, argued opponents, stigmatized institutions without fundamentally changing people's behavior, and in doing so jeopardized communal life. "You don't get diseases from places," stated one New York psychiatrist who specialized in working with gay clientele. "You get them from activities."[65] New York Civil Liberties Union executive director Norman Siegel objected to the baths' closure because it would force gay men "underground" and make them even harder to reach.[66] And the most militant homosexuals actually labeled the effort "genocidal." San Francisco activist Konstantin Berlandt argued that "institutions that have fought against sexual repression for years are being attacked under the guise of medical strategy."[67] "I didn't become a homosexual so I could use condoms," he said elsewhere.[68]

Bathhouse owners, of course, fought to stay open, arguing that the bathhouses themselves were probably the best single venue for bringing AIDS education to the clientele at highest risk, and that by closing them they were losing the single most efficient vehicle to communicate a safe-sex message. Rather than close the bathhouses, argued the owners, it would be preferable to post signs, offer brochures, distribute condoms, and even prohibit certain types of the most dangerous activity, such as unprotected anal sex and semen swallowing. In a compromise with public health commissioners in New York and San Francisco, they offered to take off doors of cubicles to more easily monitor the activities within.

On April 9, 1984, San Francisco's health director banned sexual activity in 14 bathhouses, without actually closing them. The move drew rounds of condemnation from bathhouse owners and gay leaders, one of whom called the move "Orwellian."[69] *New York Native* publisher Charles Ortleb asked CDC AIDS director James Curran, "Now that you've succeeded in closing down the baths, are you preparing the boxcars for relocation?"[70] Various challenges over the following 16 months saw some baths reopened, some shuttered, and bizarre regulations passed in New York and California banning "dangerous sex" without actually prohibiting the existence of bathhouses. Editorial writers and pundits weighed in, with one opining that the state had no "right to interfere," regardless of how distasteful the sex acts might be.[71] One gay police sergeant in San Francisco who had supported bathhouse closure was called "homophobic pig," "morality cowboy," and "Judas Littlejohn" in letters to the local gay papers.[72] In a March 1985 civic meeting in San Francisco, 90 out of 100 gathered people voted against any bath closures, with 1 carrying a sign reading, "Today the Tubs, Tomorrow Your Bedrooms."[73] Michael Callen, commenting on the work of an inspector assigned to patrol the notorious Mine Shaft bar in Manhattan in search of unsafe sex practices, stated: "The concept of behavior inspection is anathema to me. Any state inspection of gay behavior is problematic."[74] And one letter writer suggested: "While you're at it, why not repeal the consenting adults legislation. Queer bashing and morals arrests will be making a comeback."[75]

But despite the protests, by December 1985 bathhouses in New York and San Francisco, and in most other cities, had been closed. The law was clearly on the side of public health in cases of sustained epidemic danger to the community, and statistics suggested convincingly that closing bathhouses would help slow the epidemic. "This action is being brought to save lives," stated New York City assistant city counsel Doron Gopstein.[76] Inspectors, mirrors, door removals, pamphlets, and condoms had all proved ineffective, or unworkable, in allowing the baths to remain open within limited parameters. Their raison d'être was inseparable from dangerous sex practices, and thus compromised sex was fundamentally incompatible with their continued existence. While unquestionably some gay men would continue their risky practices elsewhere, states had sent a clear rebuke to the community.

CONSPIRACY THEORIES, RIGHT AND WRONG

As the disease spread into the gay community through 1983 and 1984, gay men began to panic. First dozens, then scores, then hundreds of their friends and associates were failing in the prime of life. While many men bonded together to support each other and provide education, succor, and outreach, a growing number began to respond with anger. The free-floating ire came to rest on heterosexuals, doctors, ex-lovers, and God, but most of all it landed on the government.

Government was blamed, rightly or wrongly, for the general unfairness of the disease, for its horror, and for its spread. In a plague of seeming biblical magnitude, it seemed that only an institution as powerful as the United States government, or at least the governments of the states of New York and California, could be charged with the necessary enormity of the crime. Larry Kramer, intensely frustrated at the inability of government to cure him, or even define his illness, raged:

> For two years we've heard a different theory every few weeks. We grasped at the straws of probable cause: promiscuity, poppers, back rooms, the baths, rimming, fisting, anal intercourse, urine, semen, shit, saliva, sweat, blood, blacks, a single virus, a new virus, repeated exposure to a virus, amoebas carrying a virus, drugs, Haiti, voodoo, Glagyl, constant bouts of amebiasis, hepatitis A and B, syphilis, gonorrhea.
>
> . . . After almost two years of an epidemic, there still are no answers. After almost two years of an epidemic, the cause of AIDS remains unknown. After almost two years of an epidemic, there is no cure.[77]

Many gay men attacked the government for its seeming insensitivity to their plight, speculating that if similar numbers of nongay individuals had died from an illness, the government would have responded with greater alacrity. For these men, the spread of AIDS within the gay community hinted at broad indifference, if not active genocidal homophobia. "You can be sure that if the victims were heterosexual bankers the money would be gushing out of Washington as it did during Legionnaires' disease," wrote gay journalist Randy Shilts in 1983.[78] Another writer found homophobia at the CDC when analyzing the members of the AIDS Activity Group's personnel: "All of them are straight; one is an orthodox Jew and another a deacon in his church," he wrote.[79] And gay writer Arthur Felson grouped both government and medicine together into one conspiracy when he declared, "Mainstream medicine *is* government control."[80]

The preponderance of vitriol was aimed at the National Institutes of Health (NIH), the huge government-funded research enterprise responsible for funding nearly 80 percent of all biomedical research in the country. While the NIH's overall budget was set by Congress, the disposition of the budget was set within the NIH itself, spread in greater and lesser amounts among the 18 different institutes that comprised the agency. AIDS research had come to rest primarily in the National Institute for Allergy and Infectious Diseases (NIAID) directed by Anthony Fauci.

The NIH's budgetary priorities were shaped by multiple forces, including prevalence of various diseases, growth trends among those diseases, morbidity and mortality rates from those diseases, lines of promising research, and of course, political pressure from intrusive members of Congress. For the most part, diseases that afflicted and killed more people tended to attract greater funding; thus heart disease, cancer, and stroke attracted a substantially greater share of the budget than did rare genetic disorders. However, small diseases that appeared to be growing in prevalence were more apt to receive attention (and funding) than larger diseases that appeared stable in the population. Furthermore, "sexy" diseases with strong advocacy groups behind them—breast cancer, leukemia, diabetes—received more funding than did those without powerful constituents.

By any measure, AIDS was small. By 1984, fewer than 1,500 people had died from the disease, and little evidence existed to suggest that it was spreading into the wider population. On the other hand, within its target population, AIDS was spreading in classic epidemic fashion, growing exponentially, with no peak expected soon. It was the growth trend, and not the absolute number of AIDS cases, that drove AIDS advocates in the gay community to demand that the NIH commit more funding to basic research of the disease. In the past, small but aggressive pathogens such as Legionnaires' disease and swine flu had received disproportionate attention. AIDS, it seemed to many, deserved similar treatment.

Larry Kramer, in particular, directed his impatience at the NIH, complaining in late 1983 that the agency was planning to commit only $5 million in funding to AIDS-related projects the following year out of a budget of over $4 billion, despite having already received grant requests for $55 million. Furthermore, the NIH had committed $8 million of its budget to such research, much of which had yet to be disbursed. "During the first *two weeks* of the Tylenol scare the United States government spent $10 million to find out what was happening," wrote Kramer.[81]

Activists who were neither gay chauvinists nor gay partisans began to criticize the NIH's foot-dragging as well. In late 1983 the National AIDS Vigil Commission, which included such prominent political leaders as Senators Edward Kennedy (D-Massachusetts) and Lowell Weicker (R-Connecticut), and mayors Dianne Feinstein of San Francisco and Marion Barry of Washington, D.C., marched on Washington to focus attention on AIDS and demand greater research support.[82] Infectious-disease specialists and primary care physicians treating AIDS patients complained of lack of treatment data, and a general stalling of research. And one observer at an NIH meeting recalled the aura of homophobia that permeated the agency. "Well, I can't refer to these people as gay, that's not a good word for it. I don't find it gay or charming," she recalled hearing at a meeting.[83]

The truth was more complicated. The government did prioritize AIDS as both a research and treatment challenge within two years of the CDC identifying its existence. As early as 1983, HHS assistant secretary for health, Edward Brandt Jr., declared AIDS the "number one priority" of the PHS, while at the same time total federal AIDS funding rose to $14 million—triple that of two years previous.[84] Second, gay men refused to admit, whether through conscious posturing or honest ignorance, that their sexual mores placed them apart from mainstream America, both psychologically and physically. If AIDS was, indeed, a sexually transmitted disease, as most people in 1984 thought, then there was little reason to believe that it would spread into the heterosexual population at rates approaching its spread within the gay population. Heterosexuals had a median lifetime number of sex partners below 8—less than 2 percent of the median number of partners for sexually active gay men. Further, many infectious-disease specialists had begun to consider whether it was anal sex, specifically, that placed people most at risk for infection. If this was true, then the chance of the epidemic moving en masse into the general population was even slimmer. For all of his vitriol, Larry Kramer recognized this fact early, when he wrote in

1983: "There have been no confirmed cases of AIDS in straight, white, non-intravenous-drug-using, middle-class Americans. . . . Why isn't AIDS happening to more straights? Maybe it's because gay men don't have sex with them."[85] Even Kramer, however, couldn't quite admit that the statistical trend in the gay community would likely not be replicated in the straight one.

On the other hand, homophobia and antigay discrimination *did* exist in 1983, in all parts of the country in all sectors of the population. Many gay men lived deeply closeted lives, hiding themselves from family, friends, coworkers, even spouses. The majority of Americans, whether uneducated ruffians or highly educated and sophisticated executives, were basically uncomfortable with homosexuality and homosexuals, and preferred to avoid their company. In this milieu, gay fears about official discrimination within government were credible. Indeed, many, if not most, gay men had personally experienced antigay bias in their own lives, even from people who were charged with protecting their safety and rights. Writer Dennis Altman related how in 1984 a New York City police officer, noticing Altman holding a copy of the gay newspaper the *New York Native,* asked him, "You don't have AIDS or any of that shit, do you?"[86]

Gay men in 1984 felt frightened and abandoned, and in desperation they attacked any institution or agency that they felt could possibly help them. Ultimately, they would veer toward a more constructive course of community mobilization, self-help, sophisticated advocacy, and fundraising, but such efforts were only then in their nascent stage. Then too, many other segments of American society would soon feel the sting of AIDS, and in joining the panic would embrace the gay cause as their own. Gays would continue to be assaulted by the disease, but they would not remain alone.

[CHAPTER 2]

GROWING PANIC

While AIDS was ravaging the gay communities of San Francisco, New York, and Los Angeles, and making inroads into the populations of IV drug users and hemophiliacs, the rest of America noticed the new scourge in its midst. Across the country, people began to speak of the gay plague and to question how vulnerable they might be to its reach. Americans drew on their past experience with infectious diseases of all types—airborne, food-borne, and sexually transmitted—as they assessed the risk of their own exposure. Their reactions ranged from the sensible to the ludicrous.

The biggest confusion lay in the actual mechanism of transmission. Americans questioned whether the virus was transmittable through breast milk, or through holding hands, or by insect bites, or through touching a handgrip on a subway car.[1] Others worried over the safety of food, or food handlers, prompting at least one United States company to begin testing all food service workers on the premises.[2] In the gay vacation destination of Provincetown, Massachusetts, town officials had to reassure worried vacationers that the local restaurants were safe.[3] Priests told parishioners that they needn't eat communion wafers if they felt uncomfortable. A Canadian newsmagazine poll found that nearly half the population was either "very concerned" or "somewhat concerned" about contracting the disease,[4] while a similar U.S. poll found that 47 percent of Americans thought it possible to catch AIDS from a drinking glass, and 28 percent suspected contaminated toilet seats.[5] U.S. colleges' campus health services reported a drastic falloff in the incidence of syphilis and gonorrhea as students decreased their sexual activity. The University of California at Berkeley declared AIDS the number one health issue on campus.[6] One savvy writer described a new acronym—AFRAIDS—"Acute Fear Regarding AIDS."[7]

The public's awareness of the looming threat jumped at news of the AIDS death of movie star Rock Hudson in October 1985. Hudson, whose conventional handsomeness and humorous mien had made him a romantic lead in many films of the 1950s and 1960s, had sought experimental AIDS treatment in Paris over the summer, and collapsed there. Although he had not publicly acknowledged being infected with AIDS until a few months before his death, he had supported AIDS research and fund-raising efforts during the previous year, and his obituaries clearly attributed his death to the disease. Having been twice voted the nation's top box-office draw, his death drew the attention of many Americans to the disease for the first time.[8]

Public fear of the contagion focused particularly on the nation's schools. Parents expressed concern that their children would be placed near AIDS-infected classmates or, worse, would share their drink and food with them over lunch, or bump into them in a potentially bloody scrum during a recess soccer game. Over 50 percent of polled parents stated that they would either keep a child home from school upon learning of an AIDS-infected child present, or instruct their child to avoid the classmate.[9] Parents in different parts of the country organized rallies and protests to force school officials to remove infected children from classrooms. In Arcadia, Florida, locals rallied to protest after three HIV-infected children were allowed back into the local public school by court order. "They don't know enough about it . . . Nobody can give you no guarantees if your young-uns are going to get it or not," one father complained.[10] At one Queens, New York, elementary school, which reported an infected child among the student body, 944 of 1,100 students stayed home the first week of classes while parents protested with placards reading, "Children Want Good Grades, Not AIDS!"[11] Despite reassurances from school officials that the disease was not eas-

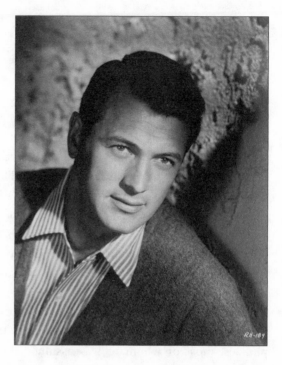

Movie star Rock Hudson in his Hollywood prime. Hudson's death from AIDS in the mid-1980s focused the nation's attention on the evolving epidemic. (Corbis)

ily contagious, one incensed parent responded: "I don't want all the medical experts telling me, 'Don't worry.' I'm worrying."[12]

Fear of AIDS percolated into professions whose members were particularly exposed to the virus: policemen, firemen, doctors, nurses, and EMTs. Many policemen began wearing rubber gloves when handling drunk or violent suspects, while others protested the requirement to administer mouth-to-mouth resuscitation in certain situations. Some undertakers in New York City refused to handle the bodies of people who had died of AIDS, and dentists and doctors who had previously simply washed hands between patients now donned rubber gloves for all interactions.[13]

Doctors and nurses lived with the added fear of a needle-stick—the all-too-common workplace mishap that had suddenly turned from a simple inconvenience to a fatal accident. One early victim recalled his reaction upon sticking himself with a tuberculin skin-test needle he had just used on an AIDS-infected patient. "I had to suppress screaming out in horror with the patient still sitting in front of me," he recounted. ". . . I recalled stories that I had heard in the Cub Scouts of mountaineers who had to amputate their own hands after snakebites to avoid having the deadly venom spread through their bodies."[14] The physician scrubbed the needle prick with scalding water and soap, had his blood tested, and donated sperm lest he be unable later to conceive an additional child.

The panic worked in reverse as well, with patients concerned about becoming infected through their doctors and dentists. Although such a scenario seemed almost impossibly unlikely, the 1987 case of Kimberly Bergalis catching the disease from infected Florida dentist David Acer drew broad attention and instigated fear. When Acer later admitted that he had infected at least nine people, six of whom had died, the public responded with near panic. Later analysis of the case revealed that Acer had been, in all likelihood, a serial murderer who had purposefully infected the patients with his own blood-soaked instruments, but the public was unassuaged.[15]

Perhaps the arena that provoked the greatest hysteria was blood transfusions. A significant minority of cases had been found in hemophiliacs, most of whom, it was assumed, had contracted the illness through infected blood products. Not understanding the mechanics of blood donation (in which a new needle was used for each donor), Americans decreased their rates of blood donations precipitating a nationwide shortage of blood products. Exacerbating the shortage, blood centers, lacking a quick and reliable method for separating contaminated from noncontaminated blood, urged donors in high-risk groups— gay men, hemophiliacs, Haitians, and IV drug users—to refrain from donating. In December 1984, the British Department of Health sent out leaflets to all regular blood donors in the U.K. asking those in high-risk categories to refrain from donating, while in the United States, National Gay Task Force leader Virginia Apuzzo suggested screening blood for hepatitis B antibodies as a proxy for AIDS detection.[16]

In fact, the chance of catching AIDS through a contaminated blood transfusion was extraordinarily low. By January 1985, only 106 AIDS cases could be traced to blood products, despite the fact that in the previous five years some 60 *million* units of blood had been transfused, leading New York physician Klaus Mayer to testify, "Statistically, you're much more likely to get run over on your way to the hospital."[17] Nonetheless, some panicked Americans began to offer "directed donations" in self-defense; storing their own blood for later use by either themselves or relatives.[18]

THE REALITY

By 1985, new AIDS cases in the gay community were actually leveling off. San Francisco, for example, was reporting 60 to 70 new cases per month: a number that had held steady for the previous six months. Efforts to curb the community's sexual practices, to make them "safer" in the new parlance, had impelled men to either reduce their sexual contacts, wear condoms while participating in sex, or refrain from anal intercourse altogether. Coupled with the bathhouse closures and a generally less sex-friendly atmosphere, the efforts had succeeded in thwarting the exponential growth of the epidemic.[19] Gay men still had much to fear, but the growth trend was encouraging.

The more urgent question was where and how the epidemic would next spread. Epidemiologists and infectious-disease specialists had recognized by that time that AIDS had a remarkably long incubation period; infected individuals could gestate the virus for up to six years while remaining symptomless.[20] Thus, reports of AIDS cases reflected not the prevalence of the virus in the population, but rather the prevalence of new outbreaks resulting from infections that had been incurred three to five years earlier. Given that efforts to thwart sexual activity in the gay community had begun only two years before, and that the virus could presumably spread into the heterosexual population, estimates for the true incidence of AIDS—recognized or not—varied widely, but were always much higher than the number of cases presently recorded. The most pessimistic modelers assumed that 90 people already carried the virus for every 1 who had reported the disease, and thus the potential number of American cases could approach 1.5 million by 1991. Even worse, Africa, where the disease had had much longer to spread uninhibited by public health education efforts, could post over 7 million cases by then.[21]

The most urgent questions for researchers attempting to model the disease lay in the efficiency of heterosexual transmission. Presumably the disease could spread through heterosexual sex; numerous reported cases attested to just that. But would it spread as quickly and efficiently among heterosexuals as it had spread among gays? Researchers were initially reluctant to assert that vaginal walls would resist the virus more effectively than rectal linings. On the other hand, heterosexuals tended to have far fewer partners than did sexually active gay men, and some researchers questioned how efficiently an infected woman could spread the virus to an uninfected man through vaginal intercourse.

Given little data, some public health advocates envisioned a worst-case scenario in which the rate of epidemic spread among gays was replicated in straights, with devastating mortality rates in young, sexually active people. Given this possibility, doomsayers urged everybody to consider the impending threat in the gravest possible way. "AIDS is a problem for everyone—gay and straight, urban and rural," warned Nobel Prize–winning biochemist David Baltimore.[22] With projections that 7 million people in Africa had already become infected, mostly through heterosexual intercourse, the warnings seemed apt.

One mechanism poorly understood in 1985, and vital to accurately projecting the growth of the epidemic, was the actual progress of the infection. Researchers understood that end-stage AIDS entailed a wholesale dissolution of the patient's immune system, creating the path for uncontrollable sepsis from multiple organisms, leading ultimately to death. Further, researchers understood that at its onset, the disease consisted of a viral attack that slowly bonded in some manner with the patient's T cell antibodies and progressively depleted their numbers. As T cell numbers and health declined, patients developed a number of minor syndromes and maladies such as swollen glands, chronic diarrhea, and weight loss, which by 1985 were known collectively as AIDS-related complex (ARC). ARC was not lethal; AIDS was. The question was, how many patients with ARC would ultimately develop AIDS? Further, how many people exposed to the AIDS virus would go on to develop ARC? Few people believed that everybody infected would ultimately die of AIDS, but nobody knew for sure.

Scientists initially speculated that 5–20 percent of people infected with the virus would develop ARC, and that perhaps only 10–20 percent of those who developed ARC would go on to develop AIDS, suggesting that AIDS cases might represent as few as 3 percent of those who had actually become infected 6–10 years earlier.[23] But by 1985, researchers were revising these estimates upward. By that time, the CDC was estimating that 5–19 percent of exposed individuals would develop AIDS within five years of infection, while 20–30 percent would develop ARC.[24]

Even more puzzling was the rate of people with AIDS who were actually reporting it. In the absence of federal reporting mandates, all reporting was voluntary except in the case of a hospital admission, and thus virtually all researchers assumed that the disease was being undercounted. Although by 1985 tests existed to detect the antibody in the blood, and thus attest to a viral presence, few people had had themselves voluntarily tested. One epidemiologist thought that only 2 percent of all viral carriers actually knew of their infection status, although other modelers were less pessimistic.[25] Describing the depth of ignorance at the time, Harvard-based investigator William Haseltine stated, "We have moved from being explorers in a canoe to explorers with a small sail on the vast sea of what we do not know."[26]

Countering the impulse to project epidemic growth onto the general population was assorted evidence that the gay community had been uniquely vulnerable to the virus. For one, anal intercourse seemed to be unusually efficient in transmitting the virus. A University of Pittsburgh research team had found that receptive participants in anal intercourse contracted the disease at least 16 times more frequently than did other sexually active gay men who did not participate as receptive partners in anal intercourse.[27] The delicate rectal wall, whose primary function was to absorb water from the feces, was simply ill-designed to receive a penis. Having the strength of wet tissue paper, and with no natural lubricants, the rectal lining almost always suffered minute tears during anal intercourse, and thus allowed the virus to easily enter the receptive partner's bloodstream. When coupled with fisting—a practice even more damaging to the lining—anal intercourse seemed almost designed to efficiently transmit the AIDS virus.

A number of researchers began to suspect by 1985 that anal intercourse, coupled with IV drug use and blood transfusions, was responsible for practically all AIDS cases in the United States. Social scientists and epidemiologists found that large numbers of professed straight men were extraordinarily reluctant to admit engagement in homosexual activities, even to a medical professional, and even when confronted with a fatal illness.[28] Wrote White House policy adviser James Warner, "It must be assumed that a large percentage of these men . . . are simply too ashamed to admit that they took drugs or had a homosexual experience."[29] Other men lied about drug use, particularly with their sex partners, male or female. Related New York health department physician Polly Thomas, "One woman said her sex partner for the past five years is straight. Then we go interview him and the most common thing is that he has used intravenous drugs, 'but not for 10 years, and please don't tell my girlfriend.' "[30]

Although anal intercourse was a particularly effective mode of transmission, all researchers agreed that heterosexual transmission was possible—the vast and growing heterosexual epidemic in Africa attested to this fact. But of great debate was how efficiently vaginal intercourse transmitted the virus. The vagina was quite different from the rectum, made of multiple layers of tough squamous epithelial cells that secreted natural lubricants. Moreover, even if a man's semen could transmit the virus into the vagina and cervix, at which time it could enter the woman's bloodstream through any tears or lesions in the vagina, how in turn could a woman then pass the virus to another man? Was the virus carried in vaginal secretions or mucus? Could it enter a man's bloodstream through microscopic wounds in the penis? Did female-to-male transmission require the presence of an existing venereal disease such as herpes, genital warts, or syphilis to open the route to transmission through chancres and sores?

Statistics were unreliable in 1985, but of some 30,000 reported cases, only about 180 involved heterosexual transmission, and of those only 28 were female to male. Moreover, at least some of these cases probably involved unreported though risky behavior such as anal intercourse or drug use.[31] Berkeley researcher Nancy Padian followed married couples engaging in unprotected sex in which one partner was known to be infected, and only 1 of 22 female partners contracted the disease after one year.[32] In America, at least, heterosexually transmitted AIDS, in the absence of drug use, was very rare, although mounting evidence pointed to a one-step transmission from an infected male drug user to his partner. If this scenario was correct, then heterosexuals really only needed to worry if their male partner was an IV drug user or had engaged in anal intercourse with a gay partner in the past five years. "Is the general population at risk?" queried the *New York Times* in the fall of 1985. "Not really. New cases overwhelmingly affect drug abusers and homosexuals. The number of cases among the rest of the public is growing, but remains at one percent of the total."[33]

If vaginal intercourse posed little risk (but for the presence of IV drugs), what other behaviors or vectors might be feared? One tropical-disease specialist proposed insect bites, but virtually no AIDS virus could be found in mosquito saliva.[34] Others suspected urine, or tears, or saliva, but again evidence of substantial viral presence in any of those substances was scant. One physician suspected that uncircumcised men could be more vulnerable, due to greater vulnerability of the foreskin to pathogens in cervical fluid.[35] This last idea drew on evidence that uncircumcised men were more vulnerable to other sexually transmitted diseases, and might explain the rising prevalence of heterosexually transmitted AIDS in Africa, but numbers in the United States simply did not support the conjecture.

But if heterosexuals in the general population were largely safe from AIDS, a few groups were highly vulnerable. IV drug users, for example, had been represented in the AIDS population nearly from the start, and their numbers had grown sharply year by year. Although the group constituted only 17 percent of the first 2,000 AIDS patients, the percentage was growing.[36] Of infected women, over half were drug users by 1986.[37] Such growth drew the attention of epidemiologists, who considered IV drug users the "gaping hole in the dike" of the general population, in the words of University of Michigan researcher June Osborne.[38]

The IV-drug-using epidemic was not uniformly spread around the country, but rather was concentrated in a few cities—particularly New York; Newark, New Jersey; Washington, D.C.; and Miami. Users in those cities clustered in "shooting galleries" where they could rent needles for a nominal fee, inject either heroin or cocaine, and then stay on until the high was complete. Needles were rented or passed around multiple times, and thus provided an almost perfect vehicle for viral transmission. Moreover, since addicts often flushed the syringe with their own blood to clear any drug remnants, and then reinjected, a clean needle on a dirty syringe was no guarantee of asepsis. Even those addicts who sought clean needles could not guarantee themselves protection, as dirty needles were often repackaged and sold as new. "IV drug users are looking for clean works, but the market forces are not really providing them," noted New York City health department physician Rand Stoneburner.[39]

The one group of heterosexuals most at risk, and which seemed capable of spreading the disease heterosexually, was prostitutes. Owing to the great amount of sexual activity they engaged in with multiple partners, prostitutes were prone to virtually all sexually transmitted diseases, including those that produced open sores on their genitals—syphilis, gonorrhea, and condoloma. Those sores, postulated researchers, were conducive to AIDS transmission, and in turn facilitated their transmitting AIDS to male partners due to the mucosal, blood, and puss secretions they produced. Diseased already, the prostitutes could both more easily get the disease as well as give it. Further, many clients preferred not to use condoms while having sex with prostitutes, and prostitutes frequently did not demand that they do so.

Early epidemiological research on heterosexual transmission pointed to the prostitute vector. Studies conducted in 1985 showed that almost all AIDS-infected men who fell outside of established risk groups had probably contracted the disease from prostitutes, and although evidence was scant, international public health experts had begun to suspect that prostitutes played a pivotal role in the heterosexually spread African epidemic as well.[40] Prostitutes did not engage in activities unique or specific to them, but they did everything in greater amounts—more sex, with more different people, with less protection. As in the gay epidemic of the early 1980s, volume, it seemed, was the necessary prerequisite to epidemic spread.

The other nongay group that was clearly vulnerable to AIDS was blood transfusion recipients. Hemophiliacs, who often required multiple transfusions, were particularly vulnerable, but virtually anybody who had received blood since 1981 was at some risk. By late 1986, the CDC estimated (using statistical modeling) that 12,000 Americans had probably been infected with AIDS through blood transfusions, although many who were infected were probably unaware of their status. Beginning in 1983 blood banks had been requesting high-risk donors to voluntarily refrain from giving, and by 1986 blood began to be tested, but the substantial nascent period in the virus's life-cycle meant that blood recipients would still be at risk for developing AIDS for at least five years more.[41]

Thus by 1986, scientific theory was inconclusive. AIDS in America could be spread through normal, heterosexual intercourse, but not very well, and more easily from male to female than from female to male. It probably could not be spread by kissing, French kissing, oral sex, hugging, sharing food or utensils, breathing, cohabitating, or casual physical contact. It could easily be spread through contaminated needles and blood products. It was efficiently spread by prostitutes, who disproportionately carried other sexually transmitted diseases which weakened their immune systems and compromised the integrity of their genitals. And, most confusing, it was efficiently spread, heterosexually, by Africans, though why and how was simply not known. James Mason, director of the CDC, summed up the confusion while testifying before Congress: "The epidemic is not spreading like 'wildfire,' but that is no reason for complacency."[42]

THE PUBLIC HEALTH RESPONSE

Although the public tended to look to laboratory research breakthroughs in combating AIDS, the more immediately available weapon was public health. Public health efforts—"sanitary engineering" in earlier parlance—had historically been the most effective approach in thwarting the numerous infectious maladies that had afflicted societies. Ranging from sewer building to food inspection and offal clearing, these efforts had drastically lowered death rates from infectious disease over the last century, to the extent that by 1985 infectious disease had practically ceased to be a threat to most residents of industrialized countries.

Public health professionals had used a variety of tactics to guard against the epidemic spread of infectious disease. In a prejet age, the sanitarians had frequently closed ports and roads, stopping European cholera epidemics repeatedly during the 19th century before they could gain a foothold on the North American continent.[43] If a disease actually managed to invade the civic arena, quarantines, evacuations, and forced relocations were frequently employed. At the same time, sanitary engineers attacked the sources of pathogens—standing pools of water, rotting animal carcasses, dung, and contaminated water—by either regulating food and drink production, mandating certain methods of disposal, or by grading streets and building aqueducts and sewers. Together, these varied efforts had increased life expectancy by over 25 years since the mid-19th century.

Underlying these many efforts was record keeping. Sanitarians had closely recorded births, deaths, morbidity and mortality rates, hospital admission rates, discharge rates, and recidivism rates since at least the 18th century.[44] Although record keeping on its own could not halt the spread of disease, in conjunction with quarantine and evacuation it was a powerful tool in tracking disease paths, and it allowed public health professionals to target their efforts where they could be most productive. Record keeping, in many ways, was the foundation of all modern public health.

AIDS clearly fell within the purview of public health. As an infectious but possibly controllable disease, it could be targeted by traditional public health techniques, whether by identifying contagious individuals, regulating their behavior, circumscribing their motions and activities, or publicizing their existence. Although nobody in the early 1980s was suggesting reopening the archaic leper colonies of old, public health professionals did consider identifying AIDS patients, warning others of their existence, regulating their behavior, and possibly limiting their freedoms. All of these techniques had proven effective in the past in controlling infectious disease, and there was little reason to suspect that they could not successfully be employed again.

By 1985, a small number of public health officials had taken actions, ranging from closing bathhouses to closing adult movie theaters, to more tightly regulating activities in adult bookstores. In San Antonio, a health official sent letters to 17 AIDS patients asking them to desist from dangerous sex practices, while in various cities politicians and civic activists lobbied for tighter restrictions on food-service workers and hospital clinicians. Other public health professionals advocated "partner notification"—the mandatory informing of past and present sexual partners about the AIDS status of a diagnosed patient.

Although all such practices were consistent with typical public health practice, virtually all were vociferously opposed by a consortium of gay community leaders, patient advocates, and civil libertarians. The opposition worried that public identification of AIDS patients would undermine their ability to enjoy basic human freedoms and rights, as AIDS was both irrationally feared by the public and also served as a proxy marker of homosexuality. These opponents argued that given the incurable nature of the disease, testing, reporting, and partner notification could not possibly benefit the patients, and were merely "meaningless political gestures."[45]

Civil libertarians were particularly adamant in their opposition to almost all traditional public health efforts at controlling the disease. In New York City, for example, the New York Civil Liberties Union counsel Arthur Eisenberg opposed the closing of pornographic theaters, despite the widespread dangerous activities taking place in them. New York City Health Commissioner Stephen Joseph described them thus:

> The movie houses showed pornographic films to an almost entirely male clientele. Inside theater seats, hallways, restrooms, and lounges were used for a wide variety of sexual acts, most between anonymous partners who cruised the theater. Mutual masturbation and oral sex was most common, but anal sex was also frequent. Often a single person would take on multiple anonymous partners. In short, the conditions were similar to those that had led to the closing of the bathhouses.[46]

Nonetheless, Eisenberg argued that closing the theaters unnecessarily violated constitutionally protected free speech, and emphasized that the theater was engaged in a "First Amendment enterprise."[47]

Gay activists were relatively silent on bathhouse and movie theater closures, but to testing and reporting they were vocally opposed. Their primary arguments rested with the simple infeasibility of such measures. Existing AIDS tests were relatively inaccurate and would produce too many false positive results if widely used. Gay men would resist testing, and ultimately eschew physician care, if forced to admit their AIDS status. Testing would force gay men back into closets where they would simply continue their unsafe behavior, without any access to modern medicine.

But unspoken was the fear of stigmatization, regardless of the public health advantages to testing and reporting. AIDS was a desperately feared and maligned disease; many Americans actually considered it a form of divine retribution for a promiscuous and morally depraved lifestyle. Gay leaders worried that AIDS reporting would mark gay men, forcing them back to the margins of society, unable to gain access to work, social networks, commerce, and succor. Gay men thus resisted even the mild reporting and notification requirements, fearful that even relatively benign legislation could be co-opted by more malignant forces and used against them. "Surely it must be possible to strike an appropriate balance between protecting the public health and protecting civil liberties," mused Joseph after the fact.[48] Yet such a balance was elusive in 1985.

The one traditional public health tool that seemed to be acceptable to the most heavily afflicted populations was safe-sex education. Safe sex initially connoted a variety of actions—abstinence, modification of sexual practices, monogamy—but it came to focus heavily on condom use. Latex condoms were capable of stopping the virus *in toto,* provided they were actually used, and used properly, and thus many public health professionals as well as gay leaders began to promote condom use and condom education through poster campaigns, brochures, leaflets, demonstrations, outreach classes, college counseling, and public posters. One pornographer produced the world's first safe-sex pornographic movie, which a critic described as "titillating as open-heart surgery."[49]

Unfortunately, condom education was most effective when presented most explicitly, and thus insulted sexual sensibilities even as it prevented the spread of disease. Condom advocates produced startlingly graphic pamphlets illustrating techniques for placing them on the penis, for taking them off, for lubricating them, for sensualizing them, and for making them an integral component of a healthy sex life. Colloquial language suffused the pamphlets, with penises becoming "cocks," vaginas becoming "cunts" and "pussies," intercourse reduced to "fucking," and oral sex translated into "sucking" and "blowing." So intent were the authors on making their literature available and accessible that condoms were frequently depicted with smiley faces, names, and personalities.

Condom advocates also subscribed to distribution as a public health effort, placing condom bowls and dispensers around singles clubs, bars, college campuses, public bathrooms, and even in high schools. This last measure raised the ire of parents nationwide, and was usually limited to nurses stations in urban schools, but condom advocates refused to back down. If over 50 percent of high-schoolers were sexually active, as statistics suggested, then ignoring condom education within this population was folly.

Comparable outreach efforts were made to IV drug users, in an effort to get them to cease sharing syringes, or at least to rinse them with bleach before use. Informational pamphlets, some produced with government funds, showed cartoon characters washing their "works" before injecting themselves with heroin, and enjoying the camaraderie of a clean, hygienic shooting gallery. Such efforts stretched public sensibilities to the breaking point when the Haight-Ashbury Free Clinic in San Francisco, using funds from various health services, published "Shooting Up and Your Health" informing patrons of the proper way to hygienically inject themselves. Although the amount of government funds used in the project was trivial, county supervisors demanded that publication and distribution of the pamphlet be halted, lest people believe the government sanctioned drug use.[50]

Public health campaigns were often ill matched with the actual risk-profile of the populations. Nascent statistics suggested that the disease was not spreading into the general population, but rather was becoming more firmly entrenched in a few high-risk pockets, such as IV drug users, prostitutes and their clients, and sexually active gay men (although it was declining in the latter group). Even so, public health and education advocates were loath to target their efforts too narrowly at one or two groups, lest they stigmatize those groups, or induce a mood of complacency in the general population. Educators seemed to see part of their duty as keeping the general population in a moderate state of anxiety for its own good, regardless of any scientific or epidemiological evidence to the contrary.

One group that was particularly attuned to the developing risk was the U.S. military. Long accustomed to viewing sexually transmitted disease as a substantial threat to the integrity of its forces, the military focused on AIDS early.[51] The military, however, faced few of the limits on civil discourse or politically correct stigmatization that undermined other public health efforts. Soldiers did not have the same rights to privacy as did civilians, and as a result were tested regularly for drug use and infectious disease, often without warning. Moreover, the Army and Navy had long taken aggressive steps to educate their forces about STDs, distribute condoms, enforce condom use, and warn personnel away from certain brothels, prostitutes, and districts, lest their fighting capability be compromised.

The Army required AIDS testing of all potential recruits starting in the fall of 1985, much to the consternation of various civil rights and gay advocacy groups. "This is hysteria," complained ACLU staffer Arthur Spitzer. "There is no evidence AIDS can be transmitted through casual contact."[52] But Army physicians disagreed. Recruitment data indicated that 1.5 of every 1,000 potential recruits were infected (most through IV drug use), and only by mass testing could the bulk of those infected be kept from active duty.[53] Moreover, the Army had a particular concern about AIDS infection, even in the absence of evidence that soldiers could spread it to each other through casual contact. Battlefield injuries, emergency transfusions, and generally hasty surgical intervention during combat all raised the potential of spreading the disease through direct blood contact. The Army's vigilance paid off. By the mid-1980s, all branches of the armed forces had posted fewer than 100 cases, cumulatively, since 1981.[54]

The other group that merited particular attention from public health educators and prevention advocates was children. Pediatric AIDS was one of the fastest-growing portions of the epidemic by 1986, with almost all cases attributable to in-utero infection (often transmitted during the birth process), and possibly through breast-feeding. Infantile AIDS was bizarre and unpredictable. Most cases resulted in extremely low birth weights, multiple neonatal and infantile hospitalizations, low white blood cell counts, and repeated infections, yet at least 40 percent of the victims lived to adolescence. AIDS babies often had malformed features—flattened nose bridges and wide-set eyes—but not always. They were usually developmentally delayed, but not always. And at least a third displayed neurological abnormalities, though the other two-thirds did not.

Pediatric AIDS cases increased as the disease moved from the gay community to IV-drug-using women. Newark, New Jersey, pediatrician James Oleske, who began studying pediatric AIDS early, admitted that the epidemiology of the disease had taken an "ominous new turn" in 1983, when growing numbers of AIDS babies began appearing for treatment in his Newark clinic.[55] Although a few experimental treatments—mostly transfusions of gamma globulin—seemed to suppress opportunistic infections in AIDS babies, the disease was as incurable in children as it was in adults. Thus, prevention and education seemed to be the best tools available to combat the insidious epidemic. Unfortunately, over three-fourths of all AIDS babies were born to IV-drug-using mothers, who often lived and functioned at the limits of mainstream society. These women usually lacked permanent addresses, jobs, partners, or spouses, and often had attenuated familial relationships. The population was difficult to identify, harder to reach, and nearly impossible to educate, and thus thwarted the efforts of most public health educators. The prognosis for progress in this population was inauspicious.[56]

By 1987, public health advocates and AIDS educators faced a frustrating set of challenges. The groups at highest risk—prostitutes, IV drug users, and infants of IV drug users—were largely unreceptive to AIDS education programs. In contrast, the educated literate public—the group most likely to take the safe-sex message to heart—was precisely that portion of the population at lowest risk. Furthermore, traditional public health tools such as testing, identification, quarantine, and isolation all seemed to be politically unacceptable to a population unaccustomed to facing the epidemic spread of an infectious disease. Only the U.S. Army had the wherewithal to ignore public sensibilities and civil-libertarian arguments and to aggressively thwart the spread of AIDS in its ranks; and thus it proved to be the single segment of the nation that was adept at preventing the spread of the disease in the first place. In the face of this tangle of conundrums, some public health professionals and physicians were forced to rethink their attitudes toward wellness and prevention. "Just a few years ago, in an excess of hubris, I predicted we were nearly finished with the problem of infection," observed famed medical writer Lewis Thomas. "I take it back."[57]

TREATMENT OPTIONS

No cure was available for AIDS in 1985, but treatments abounded. Initially, AIDS patients flocked to the municipal hospitals in the cities in which they resided—predominantly New York, San Francisco, and Los Angeles—for care of the infections that lodged in their bodies. San Francisco General Hospital and Bellevue Hospital in New York City quickly became centers of AIDS services, while smaller municipal hospitals and urban-oriented private hospitals expanded infectious-disease wards or created AIDS wards anew. In San Francisco, wards 86 and 5-B at the General Hospital provided the outpatient and inpatient services of what was reputed to be the country's "best AIDS clinic," while in New York, Saint Clare's Spellman Center for HIV-Related Disease opened in 1985 with 75 acute-care beds and a 2-bed AIDS ward for prisoners.[58] In February 1986, Johns Hopkins Hospital in Baltimore opened a 9-bed AIDS unit, and the following year 15 hospitals in New York were designated as AIDS centers and qualified for state and federal grants for research and treatment.[59]

Unfortunately, outside of general palliative care and massive doses of IV antibiotics, the hospitals could do little. The underlying causative virus was untreatable by existing therapeutics, whether they were administered in a hospital or at home. What the patients really needed, in the absence of an effective antiviral therapy, was rest, succor, and antibiotics in a hygienic environment, and hospitals were not particularly efficient venues for dispensing these services. By 1985, New York City estimated that the cost of hospital treatment over the life of an AIDS patient averaged anywhere from $80,000 to $150,000, and yet the hospitals could do little more than extend the patients' lives briefly, if at all.[60]

Hospital administrators and AIDS planners agreed that what most AIDS patients needed was not hospital care but rather palliative care—the type of care one might find in a hospice, a day care facility, or even a nursing home. Unfortunately, by the mid-1980s few long-term-care facilities were equipped to handle either the medical or social needs of AIDS patients. Other patients often insisted that AIDS patients be isolated or segregated, and untrained nurses and orderlies (and sometimes physicians) were reluctant to work with the population. New York City and San Francisco attempted to alleviate this need through the early 1980s by funding private AIDS clinics and hospices, or by creating new public institutions. As early as 1983, New York's Mayor Ed Koch proposed converting a Manhattan high school into an AIDS health center, while two years later the city worked with the local Catholic archdiocese to establish an AIDS-only shelter facility.[61]

Underlying the shortage of AIDS beds, whether inpatient or outpatient, was a crisis in health insurance for AIDS patients. Although the initial gay epidemic had affected both those who were insured and those who were uninsured, the new IV-drug-using victims were typically uninsured, and often failed to qualify for Medicaid. At the same time, most AIDS patients could not qualify for Medicare disability provisions until they had lived with AIDS for two years, by which time they were often dead. While public hospitals were committed to serving all patients, regardless of ability to pay, the rising patient load in the municipal hospitals drew heavily from municipal and county budgets.

Some of the fiscal burden was carried by newly founded charitable groups dedicated to AIDS treatment, or to gay health, or to charity health-care generally. In San Francisco the San Francisco AIDS Foundation, along with the Godfather Fund, the Bay Area Lawyers for Individual Freedom, and the Shanti Project, offered services ranging from gifts of money to legal advice to hospice care, while in New York the Gay Men's Health Crisis offered similar services as well as general social support. But the scope of the epidemic far exceeded the capacity of these community organizations to fight it, and even municipal treasuries would quickly run dry unless new funds were forthcoming. "We've allocated new monies for AIDS," noted San Francisco mayor Dianne Feinstein," "but we can't go on doing that. The times have changed. The numbers have changed."[62]

When they were not seeking help in hospitals and clinics, AIDS patients, particularly those of means, sought out experimental treatments wherever they could find them. By 1985, at least five different drugs were being touted as AIDS cures or (or at least AIDS curatives) by hucksters ranging from charlatans to well-meaning holistic health specialists. Rock Hudson, shortly before he died, had been seeking treatment in Paris with HPA-23, a tungsten-and-antimony compound used to treat Creutzfeldt-Jakob disease. Proponents of the drug theorized that it could inhibit the formation and functioning of the reverse transcriptase needed for the AIDS virus to multiply, and early results suggested that daily doses might at least reduce the growth of the virus in the body. Unfortunately, the drug seemed incapable of reducing the viral load once the disease had progressed, leading most researchers to dismiss it from the therapeutic armament. "I would be in no great rush to go to Paris," spoke UCSF physician Harry Hollander.[63] Other drugs that were considered possible antiviral contenders included Suramin (an antiparasitic), Ribavirin (used to treat Lassa fever), Alpha interferon (most promising for treating KS), and Fascarnet (used against cytomegalovirus and herpes). Coolheaded scientists, however, dismissed nearly all claims for the experimental treatments. "Drug treatment won't stop the virus," pronounced Boston oncologist William Haseltine in 1985.[64]

In the absence of reasonable drug interventions, some AIDS patients sought help from holistic, organic, and alternative healers who promised varying degrees of miracles from their concoctions and potions. Goat's milk, massive vitamin dosages, and homeopathic cures all were touted as possible cures, and all later dismissed. Failing to find pharmaceutical interventions, AIDS victims sought psychotherapy to help them cope with their depression and fear, even while the virus raged unthwarted in their systems. Support groups and specialized AIDS counseling sessions sprang up as thousands of patients sought comfort and kindness. AIDS couldn't yet be prevented, or controlled, or even treated, but perhaps it could be tolerated, both by the patients and the world around them.

BACKLASH

Fear of AIDS spreading into the general population provoked a torrent of animosity toward gays. While homosexuality had never been broadly accepted in the general population, AIDS seemed to galvanize many people's disdain for homosexual practices, and for homosexuals in general. *Time* magazine reported in 1985 that it was "open season on gays," while a *Los Angeles Times* poll found that even in the nation's most tolerant cities—New York and Los Angeles—over 60 percent of surveyed adults found homosexuality "wrong."[65] (The rate of disapproval for the country at large was 73 percent.) In the three years from 1982 to 1985, hate crimes against gays tripled nationally, while in New York City assaults on gays rose from 176 to 517 in a single year. Some of the assaults were murderous in their ferocity. In Fort Lauderdale, a pickup truck driver swerved purposefully into a patron emerging from a gay bar, while in San Francisco gay men were beaten with logging chains and cut with razors. "AIDS has provided a green light to bashers and bigots. It's a convenient excuse for those who hate us," stated Kevin Berrill of the National Gay and Lesbian Task Force.[66]

Americans, and Canadians too, grew less tolerant of general courtesy and freedoms shown toward AIDS sufferers. The *Los Angeles Times* poll found that 51 percent of surveyed adults would support criminalizing sex for AIDS sufferers, 51 percent supported quarantining AIDS patients, 45 percent supported testing all job applicants for AIDS, and 42 percent supported closing all gay bars.[67] One editorial writer wrote that although gays had in the past been a persecuted and vulnerable minority, they were "surely unjustly and needlessly protected" today. The writer reserved particular vitriol for a proposal to hide the identities of students with AIDS from school officials. "Officials! Not even parents! We are being treated as if we were wards or children and did not have the right of informed personal consent."[68]

Antigay sentiment reached a new level among conservatives who had traditionally been less willing to extend recognition to gay groups or validate a gay lifestyle. Conservative writers, columnists, and politicians called for nationwide mandatory testing, marking, tattooing, quarantining, or worse. One extremely conservative psychologist, Patrick Fagan, director of the Child and Family Protection Institute, called for deprovera* treatment of promiscuous homosexuals, and for requiring AIDS screening for all agricultural personnel and slaughterhouse workers. "AIDS positives need to be removed from jobs that bring them into body fluid contact with these animals," he wrote. He further suggested making spreading AIDS a litigable tort, and mandating AIDS testing before all weddings.[69]

*A drug known to reduce the sex drive.

AIDS raised uncomfortable questions for a number of religious institutions. The more conservative denominations—Catholicism, Mormonism, Orthodox Judaism—had long condemned homosexuality as sinful, and disallowed promiscuity or premarital sex of any kind (not to mention opiate and narcotics use). At the same time, all tended to preach messages of compassion, tolerance, and forgiveness, and emphasized visiting the sick and reaching out to the afflicted. Pastors in these denominations faced the difficult task of condemning the practices that had led to AIDS infection, while extending sympathy and kindness to those suffering from the disease. Christian authors Roy McCloughry and Carol Bebawi personified this approach in the pamphlet *AIDS: A Christian Response,* calling promiscuous sex "highly addictive," and noting that society was "fearful lest it may not be able to kick the habit." At the same time, they emphasized the Christian calling of "hope, faith, and love," and condemned those who justified homophobia by viewing AIDS as God's curse on gays. "To make AIDS the criterion of whether a person is under the judgment of God, is to use the Biblical categories to confirm personal prejudice," they wrote.[70]

The message of love and tolerance for the disease's victims rippled throughout mainstream Christianity. "You don't have to endorse the homosexual life style to agree that it's a terrible idea to turn AIDS victims into social lepers," wrote a guest columnist in the *Christian Science Monitor*.[71] One group of communal volunteers cited Christian teachings that compelled them to care for an AIDS-afflicted neighbor. "The book of Matthew says you take care of your neighbor, so we've decided to take the risk," noted one member of the group.[72] And even chaplains who had hitherto condemned homosexuality, or at least viewed it with distaste, found that the suffering of the afflicted superseded any reservations they might have about the moral caste of the sufferer. One hospital chaplain in Los Angeles admitted that homosexuals had been "abhorrent" to him, and that he had first avoided AIDS sufferers when they started to appear on the hospital's wards in large numbers. He changed his ways, however. "But as I read the Bible, I thought, 'I can't do this. I can't just avoid these men if I'm a follower of Christ.' "[73]

In quick succession, the antigay movement gave rise to a sentiment leading to an anti-anti-gay movement, composed of gay activists, civil libertarians, members of rights-oriented groups, and leftists of all types who viewed the new homophobia and AIDS phobia as despicably bigoted, if not altogether un-American. These anti-anti activists recapitulated the Christian message of separating the victim from the behavior, but then amplified the message by claiming that AIDS was a disease that afflicted all people, not just gays and IV drug users. Those who carried this message resisted the notion of "high-risk" groups, be they gay, Haitian, or hemophiliac, and instead noted that such designations belonged to the past. "There is no such thing as a high-risk population," stated one gay physician. "It is all people, period. AIDS is the greatest human threat since nuclear war."[74]

Those who rushed to protect AIDS patients from stigma and derogation sought to universalize the disease and to make it an affliction of all people, regardless of ethnicity, predilection, or behavior. Groups who had suffered so acutely in the early years, agreed the universalizers, had simply been unfortunate enough to be at the forefront of an epidemic, but that epidemic was now growing with little regard for social or demographic distinctions. "It is becoming increasingly more difficult to define those with AIDS as 'them,' wrote Harvard researcher William Haseltine. " 'Them' now includes not only Africans, not only homosexuals, not only Haitians, not only drug abusers, not only hemophiliacs, but also soldiers and Johns or Johns' wives. I am confident that we will wake to realize what problem is in our midst, but when? And how late in the day will it be?"[75]

Extending the argument to its logical extreme produced the idea that the true cause of AIDS was neither sexual activity, nor drug use, nor other high-risk behavior, but was rather "social paranoia, political prejudice, and cultural ignorance," in the words of one left-leaning editor.[76] In this alternate reality, discrimination and intolerance drove certain subpopulations to society's margins where they were cut off from information and medical care; thus, it was society at large that bore the blame for the epidemic. By the same logic, societies could cure the disease by reforming their social outlook and adhering firmly to a credo of tolerance, kindness, and social equity. "A virus does not respect the finer distinction many of us like to draw between ourselves and others," wrote NBC science correspondent Robert Bazell.[77]

But navigating the choppy shoals between these two extremes were epidemiologists, physicians, and public health professionals who could see that the data, insofar as it existed, supported neither conjecture. On the one hand, AIDS growth was leveling out in the gay population just as it was spreading into the heterosexual population. Further, the predominantly heterosexual profile of the epidemic in Africa presaged a potential mainstream outbreak in the West. On the other hand, numbers simply did not support the universalizers' model. The heterosexuals who were catching AIDS were either IV drug users, partners of IV drug users, prostitutes, or customers of prostitutes. Almost nobody more than one step removed from a clearly identifiable risk group had gotten the disease, and these numbers did not appear to be changing. A team of epidemiologists at Imperial College, London, produced a computer model that suggested that the disease could actually die out naturally, or decline to a stable low incidence within the population.[78]

In this rationalist epidemiological world, two barriers guarded the general population from a second scourge of bubonic plague dimensions. The first was the profound disparity in sexual activity between gay men who had gotten AIDS early, and the general population. "It is just essential that you recognize the great degree of sexual activity of the group at risk," noted Princeton epidemiologist Robert May.[79] Even the African epidemic seemed to be predicated on a far more promiscuous set of sexual mores than existed in the West, ranging from greater tolerance toward prostitution and extramarital girlfriends, to large numbers of migratory workers who became unusually effective disease vectors as they traveled the continent's roads and byways.

The second barrier was the developing virological understanding of the disease, which possibly foretold more effective treatment in years to come. One drug, AZT, was already proving to be mildly effective in prolonging the lives of AIDS patients, and further anti-viral therapy brought promise of breakthroughs in years, rather than in decades. Mathilde Krim, co-chair of the American Foundation for AIDS Research (AmFAR) described the future as she saw it: "We are going to be able to prevent the more serious stages of the disease and keep people alive for many years," she foretold. "They'll be healthy enough to work and function in society, although they'll require constant medical monitoring and treatment."[80]

Both the antigay activists, and the anti-anti-gay responders were guilty of misstating reality. Facts, though incomplete in 1986, did not support the extreme vision of the future propounded by either side. True, gays had gotten the disease first, but they posed little threat to the general population. The disease was not going to be a disease of "all of us," however convenient such a reality might be for the universalizers. Heterosexuals differed from homosexuals (and IV drug users) in basic comportment and behavior in exactly those areas that favored a diminishing disease presence. The idea that gays had gotten the disease first by simply randomly stumbling into it, and that the rest of the population would soon follow suit, was based on either jumbled logic or wishful thinking. The truth was, rather, that gays had gotten it, but that they were getting over it, and that the rest of the population would probably never get it in quite the same way, or in the same magnitude. Such a complicated truth was unsatisfying to most everybody, but at least a few epidemiologists were able to tease it out nonetheless.

HAITIANS AND AFRICANS

If AIDS was not going to infect the general population with the same force with which it had infected gays and IV drug users, then how could its infection of Haitians be explained? The Haitian epidemic has long been the inexplicable exception in the epidemic's growth. All evidence suggested that the disease was infectious and blood-borne, and therefore should selectively choose only those populations particularly vulnerable to blood-borne infection—and Haitians as a group could not be described as such. Did Haitians have a peculiar genetic vulnerability to the disease, or had they been engaging in hitherto unknown activities that raised their risk profile?

Cases of KS and other opportunistic infections later associated with AIDS were identified in Haiti from 1978 on, striking men far more frequently than women.[81] Early theories of the island's outbreak included general miasma, unhygienic conditions, and strange speculations of co-infection with African swine fever virus in pigs. ("There is raw sewage on the ground and rats running all around," observed tropical-medicine researcher Mark Whiteside.)[82] From 1982, Haitian nationals and Americans of recent Haitian descent were identified as being overrepresented in the epidemic, despite not admitting to IV drug use or homosexual activity at unusual rates.[83] The link between AIDS and Haitians was "baffling," in the words of one reporter, and defied initial explanation.[84]

But close investigation of the phenomenon over the following years revealed that in fact most Haitians contracting AIDS had engaged in gay or bisexual prostitution, and had failed to identify themselves as gay initially because of their desire to distance their identity from their sex work. The disease had probably originally been brought to the island by Haitians who had lived in the Belgian Congo as guest workers in the 1960s and 1970s, and who had returned to spread the disease among Haitian prostitutes. At least one investigator postulated a transmission route to the island via infected European (probably German) tourists who had infected local gay and bisexual prostitutes in the mid-1970s.[85]

Haiti's capital, Port-au-Prince, became a popular destination for gay tourists and cruise ships in the 1970s, and developed a reputation as being a sort of Caribbean gay Bangkok—a place where sex could be easily purchased in a politically stable region with compliant policemen and an accommodating hospitality industry. By 1981, the *Spartacus International Gay Guide* described Haitian men as "very beautiful and very well-endowed," and having "a great ability to satisfy, whatever it is you are looking for."[86] By 1980, wrote historian Edward Hooper, "Haiti had become very much a buyer's market, and the fairly discreet gay scene of the sixties and seventies had been transformed into something much more overt and geared toward foreign tastes."[87]

In fact, except for Haitian prostitutes and gays and bisexuals, Haitians were not a high-risk group. Data from the mid-1980s showed that Haitians had a lower incidence of AIDS than did residents of major American cities, and that the incidence was actually dropping as the widespread AIDS-information effort propounded by the Haitian government went into effect.[88] By then, however, the Haitian tourist industry had been badly damaged by the popular association of AIDS with the nation, and revenues had dropped by as much as 75 percent.

Although study of the Haitian epidemic did not reveal a virological breakthrough, it did reveal an epidemiological one. Scientists and researchers who studied the Haitian epidemic and traced its origins to Africa realized that Haiti was probably the pivot point of the epidemic—the place from which the disease had jumped into the United States. Hooper, in his exhaustive investigation of the origin of AIDS, described Port-au-Prince as the "key interchange" on the AIDS virus's "world tour," from whence it traveled north into the United States via Haitian émigrés to Florida, and south and west into the country via infected gay men in New York, Montreal, Los Angeles, and San Francisco.[89]

Regardless of how the virus arrived in Haiti, it had clearly originated in Africa, somewhere in the region of central Africa where Rwanda, Uganda, Zambia, Burundi, Congo, Kenya, and Tanzania all came together. Investigations of old blood samples from the late 1960s and early 1970s revealed the probable presence of the virus in Zaire (the Belgian Congo) as early as 1970, and in Uganda from 1972.[90] KS and cryptococcal meningitis (uncommon outside of AIDS cases) became more common in Zairian hospitals starting in 1978. Similarly, isolated cases of Europeans who had lived in central Africa in the mid-1970s and were retroactively diagnosed as having died of AIDS were cataloged. Of particular note among these cases was a 31-year-old Dane who had probably contracted AIDS in Rwanda and Burundi sometime between 1974 and 1981, and who had died of PCP pneumonia in 1983.[91] In another case of almost preternatural synchronicity, a survivor of an emergency crash landing of a transport flight over Zaire in 1976 was treated at a Kisangani hospital, where he received two units of blood. He died four years later, in Canada, from multiple infections. Years later his stored blood samples revealed that he had had AIDS.[92]

By 1986, crude incidence reporting found AIDS levels in six central African countries—Zaire, Rwanda, Uganda, Kenya, Zambia, and the Central African Republic—to range from 5 to 10 percent of the population, roughly 10 to 20 times that of the incidence in the United States. Over 51 percent of Kenyan prostitutes were infected, and nearly 20 percent of young adults in a few small towns in Rwanda were as well. In the area of densest infection, the Rakai region of southwest Uganda, 30 percent of the population was infected. While cases in the United States totaled 15,000, worst-case estimates of the African epidemic now totaled nearly a half million.[93]

The disease, frequently called "Slim" in central Africa, was devastating whole towns in the region, even as it remained ensconced in a few high-risk groups in the United States, Canada, and Europe. The population of one Ugandan town, Kasensero, dropped from 600 to 150 over four years, through death, evacuation, and attrition. Given the long incubation period of the disease, researchers estimated that as many as five *million* Africans might have been infected, resulting in as many as 1.5 million deaths over the following years. "It's difficult using these words, but we risk an apocalypse," stated a researcher of the African AIDS epidemic.[94]

Although African AIDS research was still in a nascent stage, several facets of the African epidemic were apparent in 1985. Unlike in the United States, the disease infected men and women nearly equally, with little bias toward homosexuals. Furthermore, the disease was most prevalent not among the poor and marginalized, but among the educated elite. The disease seemed to spread through a nexus of prostitutes who were most frequently patronized by employed (and therefore wealthier) African truckers and migratory workers. As in the United States, the infected were more promiscuous than the population as a whole; Zaire reported that infected individuals had an average of 32 lifetime sex partners, versus a population average of 3.[95] But unlike in the United States, infected men seemed able to easily pass the virus on through heterosexual intercourse to their wives and girlfriends. This inconsistency with transmission patterns in the United States troubled researchers, who struggled with explanations ranging from female circumcision, to ritual genital scarification, to the presence of exacerbating sexually transmitted diseases. No one explanation satisfied all the conditions.

AIDS threatened central Africa with true decimation of Black Death proportions. Moreover, the population most vulnerable was made up of exactly those individuals who were needed for continental economic development, educational and technical progress, and political leadership. Even if the epidemic could be stopped, an entire generation of leaders might already have become infected. AIDS researcher Jonathan

Mann noted: "AIDS is a threat to the social shape of Africa in a way starvation and malaria aren't. It has the potential to wipe out the urban elite. AIDS attacks the productive people society has made an investment in. It really is terrifying."[96]

By 1986, general panic in the United States and Canada had produced new outbreaks of homophobia and anti-AIDS sentiment. Whether in schools or on jobs, Americans resisted being intermingled with AIDS patients, despite virtually all evidence showing that the disease could not be transmitted through casual contact, kissing, or even most sex. In their panic, Americans looked to nationwide testing, identification, and the possibility of quarantine, despite substantial scientific and legal barriers to all of these.

They were assaulted by mixed and competing messages. On the one hand, AIDS advocates warned against a segregationist mentality, explaining that the growing epidemic would make all Americans potential victims, regardless of sexuality or status. On the other hand, new data and epidemiological modeling demonstrated that even as the disease leveled off among gays, it was becoming entrenched not in the general population, but in a marginal subpopulation of drug users and their immediate sexual partners. Heterosexual Americans who did not use drugs, did not sleep with people who used drugs, and did not frequent prostitutes were highly unlikely to get the disease.

New data on the Haitian epidemic seemed to confirm the model. Although Haitians had originally been considered high risk, they were now removed from that classification. The Haitian epidemic had really been a gay and bisexual epidemic, spreading through the nation's active sex trade to tourists and émigrés. Among heterosexual Haitians, the disease was now no more prevalent than in the general American population, and even among its sex workers the incidence of AIDS was now declining.

To everyone's consternation, however, the exploding African epidemic was markedly different. There, the disease spread easily from men to women and back, with little help from homosexuality or injection drugs. True, those who contracted the disease in Africa tended to have many more sex partners than was true of the general U.S. population, but even so the transmissibility of the virus defied early under-standing of heterosexual transmission in the United States. Something unique to Africa was lubricating the disease's progress, raising two troubling questions: would that unique something remain ensconced in Africa, and what could Africa, and the world, do for that embattled continent?

CHAPTER 3

RACE TO THE VECTOR

What was causing AIDS? At the disease's onset, speculation ranged broadly, from a strange toxic reaction to overexposure to semen, to acute response to narcotics and amyl nitrite abuse, to malnutrition, to an alien form of interferon.[1] Quickly, however, researchers coalesced around the theory of an infectious agent, most likely a virus (given the inefficacy of antibiotics in treating the disease), which was being spread through blood products, semen, and vaginal secretions. The compelling goal of AIDS research at that point became to identify the virus.

One group of researchers, personified by Joseph Sonnabend of the uniformed services medical school in Bethesda, Maryland, and Myron Essex of Harvard insisted that the virus was most likely an existing one, either the cytomegalovirus, the Epstein-Barr virus, the African swine flu virus, a mutation of the feline leukemia virus, or one of two viruses known to attack the immune system—the human t-lymphotropic virus (HTLV) I and II. Any of these seemed likely, as they were all associated with certain cancers commonly found in AIDS patients, and each had the capacity to compromise the immune system. In defense of this hypothesis, Sonnabend suggested that talk of a new viral agent had been spurred by the recently discovered infectious agent for Legionnaires' disease, but that more likely AIDS was caused by one of a number of known agents.[2]

Drawing the most attention were HTLV I and II, which belonged to a class of viruses known as retroviruses. Retroviruses were viruses that seemed to defy the laws of genetics. In most cells, in most organisms, genetic information was carried in the two-stranded DNA molecule. The DNA would periodically unfurl itself, stamp out a single-stranded RNA molecule, and this RNA in turn would synthesize new proteins for the body's use. Viruses, however, which were extremely simple organisms, could carry their genetic information in either DNA or RNA, with the RNA-based viruses simply using their RNA to create proteins and thus replicate themselves while being sheltered in a host cell. A small group of RNA-based viruses, however, worked differently. Those viruses used an enzyme called *reverse transcriptase* to create DNA from the RNA—a unique feat, somewhat akin to a tailor measuring a set of clothes to create a person, rather than the obverse. These retroviruses then inserted the newly formed DNA into their host cells' DNA, and then forced the host cell's protein production processes to create new copies of the virus for them. The whole process was analogous to an enemy agent infiltrating an automotive plant, resetting the machine codes, and then getting the enemy's machines to produce tanks and planes for his nation.

Human retroviruses had been discovered by NIH researcher Robert Gallo and his colleagues in 1976. Gallo had perfected a technique to grow lymphocytes (a central component of the body's immune system) in a lab culture, from which he was able to isolate and extract several lymphotropic viruses, including the two most closely associated with leukemia. Since AIDS always involved the dissolution of the immune system, frequently involved cancer, and appeared to have a viral etiology, a virus that was known to cause cancer and to suppress the immune system seemed a likely candidate for causing the disease. From early on, Gallo suspected that the new disease was caused by HTLV I or II, or some closely related pathogen.[3]

Gallo was known as something of an *enfant terrible* of the molecular biology world. Garnerer of multiple scientific honors, including two of the highly prestigious Lasker awards, he could take justifiable pride in

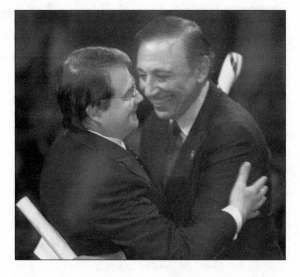

Robert Gallo and Luc Montagnier at an awards ceremony in 2000.
(Corbis)

discovering both HTLV viruses. On the other hand, he had a reputation for being fiercely—many would say excessively—competitive, and in the past several of his claims of scientific discoveries had been questioned. His results leading to the discovery of the leukemia virus (originally called HL-23) proved to be initially irreplicable, and he had repeatedly claimed primary credit for work done in his lab when much if not most of the work had been done by others. Recalled one lab associate, "With something as friendly as a lab softball game, he'd be dirty—he'd kick you in the balls if he thought he was going to lose."[4]

Gallo's great unrealized dream was to win a Nobel Prize, and discovering the genesis of a new viral disease seemed to offer the opportunity. As early as 1974, he was reputed to have tried to recruit a scientist to his lab with the line, "Don't you want to be able to say you were in a lab that won a Nobel Prize?"[5] He had aggressively lobbied members of the Nobel nominating committee, and had tried to squelch negative news stories that he felt might compromise his chance of winning the prize.

By late 1983, American researchers coalesced around Gallo's theory about HTLV viruses. Harvard biologist Myron Essex declared it the "leading candidate" for the cause of AIDS, and with coauthors trumpeted Gallo's hypothesis in the September 9 issue of *Science,* one of the most prestigious and widely read scientific journals in the world. Along with university-based researchers, both the National Cancer Institute and the Centers for Disease Control lent their imprimatur to the HTLV hypothesis, and Essex noted that only HTLV met all the criteria for an AIDS-causing virus. Further, statistics showed that the known rate of HTLV infection was 12 times as high in AIDS patients as it was in the general population.[6]

However, the Gallo hypothesis was being challenged from abroad. Working independently of the Americans, Luc Montagnier of the Pasteur Institute in Paris isolated a new virus from an AIDS patient who had maintained an unusually healthy number of T cells. This virus differed from HTLV in two significant ways: it depleted T cells (while HTLV actually facilitated their growth), and it failed to bind correctly with HTLV antibodies. These two observations led Montagnier to conclude that he had discovered a wholly new virus, albeit a member of the retrovirus family, which he would later name lymphadenopathy AIDS-associated virus (LAV). He published his findings in May 1983, in the same issue of *Science* in which the Gallo and Essex publications appeared.

Montagnier had, in fact, discovered the cause of AIDS, yet the significance of discovery was overlooked. This was partially because his prominence paled next to that of his better-known American counterparts, and thus his article was overshadowed by the two HTLV claims in the same journal issue. But more important, Gallo had engaged in a bit of chicanery. Gallo, himself, had acted as the reviewer of Montagnier's article. The article had been submitted without the necessary abstract ("in my haste I forgot to write the summary," Montagnier wrote years later) and Gallo offered to write it. In Gallo's summary, however, he described the new virus as part of the HTLV family of viruses, despite the fact that Montagnier had made no such claim. Montagnier failed to detect or halt Gallo's claim.[7]

The following year, Gallo himself claimed to have discovered a new virus, closely related to HTLV I and II, which he named HTLV III—a new and unique virus that was the true cause of AIDS. Given Gallo's prominence and renown in the virology world, his claim was quickly lauded, with Harvard Medical School professor Jerome Groopman declaring, "I think that Dr. Gallo has identified the cause of AIDS . . . and I am a very cautious, skeptical person."[8] Montagnier, however, was suspicious of the claim. Workers in his lab had found that LAV samples from different AIDS patients differed markedly, much more so than did most viral samples. Yet Gallo's HTLV III appeared to be nearly identical to Montagnier's original LAV, of which he had given a small sample to Gallo the previous summer. Had Gallo simply taken the Montagnier sample, worked with it, renamed it, and claimed it as his own?

Ignoring Montagnier's suspicions, Gallo attended a press conference in which U.S. Secretary of Health and Human Services Margaret Heckler awarded credit for discovery of the new virus to "our eminent Dr. Robert Gallo," and galled the French by declaring, "Today, we add another miracle to the long honor roll of American medicine and science."[9] Both Montagnier and the U.S. government (representing Gallo's NIH lab) now filed for patent protection for blood tests for the virus, and in May 1985 the U.S. Patent Office awarded the patent to Gallo. Montagnier sued, claiming that the two viruses were "substantially identical," and demanded access to documents from Gallo's lab. Those documents proved to be damning. One letter, addressed from one of Gallo's lab workers, alluded to the two most promising viruses in the lab as LAV, suggesting that this was how the viruses had been labeled when the worker had begun to work with them. The only viruses that could have been labeled such were the two samples given to the lab by Montagnier. Further, a series of damaging photos showed that the virus that Gallo had labeled HTLV III was clearly LAV. Although Gallo had actually published the photos in the journal *Science,* to avoid being sued, he ultimately had to recant the claim two years later in that same journal.[10]

In light of the evidence emerging that the Gallo lab's "discovery" was simply Montagnier's virus, the U.S. patent office rescinded its initial patent decision the following year, and awarded the primary patent to the Pasteur Institute. At the same time, an international group of scientists agreed that the new virus should be called human immunodeficiency virus (HIV) to distinguish it from the two existing HTLV viruses. Gallo fought to maintain the HTLV III title, but the disease primarily associated with his original two HTLV viruses was leukemia, and HIV was not associated with that particular disease. Gallo had essentially lost.

Or had he? AIDS was becoming such a prominent issue internationally that in 1986 senior officials from the French and U.S. governments began negotiations in an effort to straighten out the patent dispute and achieve a solution that would preserve the dignity and honor of all involved. In March 1987, President Ronald Reagan and Prime Minister Jacques Chirac announced that joint credit for the patent would be given to the U.S. and French teams, and that a new AIDS research foundation would be established to which 80 percent of all blood testing royalties would be paid. Further, both sides agreed not to comment on or challenge the agreement, meaning that henceforth official credit for discovering the new HIV virus would be shared equally.[11] Despite the shared credit, Montagnier wrote bitterly some years later that in fact Gallo and his colleagues had each drawn personally some $100,000 per year over several years in royalty shares, while he and his lab colleagues received nothing for several years, and then only a nominal royalty payment thereafter.[12]

THE VIRUS

What was this HIV that was proving to be so troubling to the world? It belonged to a subgroup of the retroviruses called *lentiviruses,* or slow viruses, so called because they replicated and spread slowly in the host's body, compared with some of the faster-acting cancer-causing viruses. It appeared to be closely related to the simian immunodeficiency virus, which attacked the immune systems of monkeys, and the virus singled out its attacks for the T4 lymphocyte cells of the human immune system.

HIV was comprised of a sphere with multiple protrusions on its surface, each of which contained molecules of a protein called gp120. This gp120 protein was particularly well adapted to bonding with CD4 proteins in the surface membrane of the T4 lymphocytes—the target cells of the immune system. Once bonded, the virus breached the T4 cell wall and injected its contents into the lymphocyte, including the two strands of RNA that carried the genetic program for making more viruses. Inside the T4 cell, the RNA quickly began the process of reverse transcription

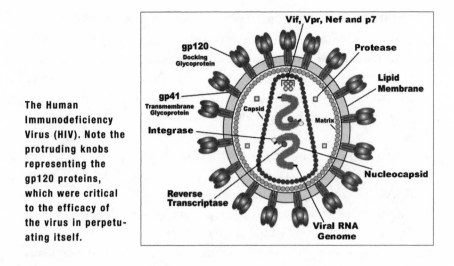

The Human Immunodeficiency Virus (HIV). Note the protruding knobs representing the gp120 proteins, which were critical to the efficacy of the virus in perpetuating itself.

using a reverse transcriptase enzyme. The newly created DNA, which now carried the genetic code for the virus, was then incorporated into the host cell's own DNA, where it could begin the job of creating new viruses.

HIV was a particularly formidable viral foe in two ways. First, unlike most retroviruses, it seemed more robust in its ability to incorporate its DNA into the host cell's DNA. While most retroviruses could perform this incorporation trick only when the host cell was in the process of replicating its own DNA in order to divide (*mitosis*), HIV was able to incorporate its DNA into the host cell's DNA at other phases of the cell's life. This meant that HIV was more infectious, and more virulent for a greater portion of the C4 cell's life than another retrovirus would be.

But from a treatment standpoint, it was another component of the virus's biology that proved so troubling. All cells periodically make mistakes in the course of replicating their own DNA, usually at the rate of 1 error per each 1 billion base molecules in the DNA. Such mistakes, called *mutations,* are periodically advantageous to the cell, and thus are selected for survival and transmission to future generations. Such is the process of evolution.

But HIV appeared to mutate nearly 100,000 times faster than did most cells—at a rate of 1 error per each 10,000 base molecules. The reason for such a high error rate was weirdly simple—the virus replicated in the host cell so quickly that it quite literally ran out of basic molecular material from which to create new DNA, and thus was forced to use incorrect substitutes. At such a ferocious rate of mutation, the virus was able to adapt to potential vaccines and antiviral treatments much more quickly than could other viruses, and thus was far more difficult to annihilate. This was, incidentally, also the reason that, when Gallo's original HTLV III virus proved so nearly identical to Montagnier's LAV, the discovery aroused such suspicion.

Consistent with this discovery of mutation rates was Montagnier's discovery in 1986 that a related but clearly unique virus existed in west Africa (as opposed to central Africa) that was causing AIDS-like symptoms. The virus, which did not show up on AIDS antibody tests, was eventually isolated in Montagnier's lab from patients from Guinea-Bissau, and proved to be so closely related to HIV that Montagnier dubbed it HIV-2. HIV-2 was possibly the original AIDS virus, as it shared at least 50 percent of its genetic material with the prototypical immunosuppressant virus, SIV, a virus that exclusively infected macaque monkeys and that had possibly given rise to HIV sometime in the last century. The problem with HIV-2, from an epidemiological standpoint, was that two unique viruses (and there could be more) might not necessarily respond to the same vaccine or viral treatment, if one was ever developed.[13]

Last, the virus had a number of proteins within it that enabled it to more effectively commandeer the host cell's replication machinery to its own end. The most important of those proteins was called *nef*, which was capable of the important trick of suppressing production of the host cell's CD4 proteins. With few CD4 proteins being produced, the host cell was unable to recapture some of the newly produced HIV, and thus virtually all of the new HIV was available for release to spread to new T4 cells, and further propagate the infection. Further, nef seemed capable of activating a T cell, and thus making it available for HIV DNA replication. Without this capability, HIV would still infect T cells, but at a much slower rate.[14]

In short, the new virus fit neatly into a known group of viruses, but appeared to have certain adaptations that would make it a formidable foe for both treatment and inoculation. Evasive and protean, the virus was capable of evolving out of danger from almost any antiviral agent that an infected person could either ingest or inject. Moreover, it seemed superbly able to commandeer the host cell's protein production machinery for its own end, and thus spread relentlessly throughout the human body.

The virus had several serious weaknesses, however. It could not survive in air, it was largely untransmissible through saliva and tears, and it could not penetrate healthy skin or intact epithelial membranes. Thus, the virus could really only spread itself through certain types of sexual contact and blood exchanges: a mechanism far less effective than the airborne droplets that carry the common cold. AIDS was lethal, but relative to other viruses, quite slow to spread.

RAMIFICATIONS

One of the remarkable aspects of the AIDS story is the degree of complacency with which the general population received the discovery of HIV. Whereas the discovery of the pathogenic origins of other infectious diseases throughout the ages—anthrax, smallpox, polio, and influenza, to name a few—had been treated as near miracles, the discovery of HIV seemed almost pedestrian to many people. Not so among microbiologists. To those who understood the complex challenges facing a would-be discoverer of a new pathogen, the discovery and description of the new virus was a modern-day miracle. The *New England Journal of Medicine* termed it a "triumph of biologic science," and predicted that the discovery presaged a workable vaccine or treatment.[15] Lewis Thomas proclaimed: "In a long lifetime of looking at biomedical research, I have never seen anything to touch the progress that has already been made in laboratories working on the AIDS virus. Considering that the disease was recognized only seven years ago and that its agent, HIV, is one of the most complex and baffling organisms on earth, the achievement is an astonishment."[16]

Vaccine development faced enormous challenges from the beginning, however. Vaccines can be of several types—live-attenuated, killed, or subunit. In killed vaccines, the virus is killed, then injected, and there-after prompts the immune system to create antibodies to proteins specific to the virus that will ward off future viral infections. Killed vaccines are safe, but not always effective; a large number of viruses are incapable of stimulating the immune system while dead.

In live-attenuated vaccines, the virus is cleaved or distorted in such a manner that while incapable of causing infection, it can still stimulate the immune system to create virus-specific antibodies. Unfortunately, for most viruses live-attenuated vaccines are capable of causing illness in a small minority of patients, and for some viruses, in a majority of cases.

Subunit vaccines were still quite experimental in 1984, consisting of a cleaved portion of the virus that was just enough to stimulate the immune system. It appeared safe, and in fact one drug company had been recently approved to market a subunit vaccine for hepatitis B. Unfortunately, not all viruses were susceptible to subunit vaccine technology, for the subunit needed to be capable of stimulating the immune system to create antibodies against a whole virus, while incapable of causing disease.

HIV appeared to resist vaccine development for a number of reasons. First, as a retrovirus, it was a member of a family of viruses that in the past had proven difficult to vaccinate against. Because retroviruses inserted their DNA into the cell's DNA, they could remain dormant in cells until by some unknown mechanism they could turn on the host cell's replication machinery and begin perpetuating themselves. The viruses could presumably hide out in the nuclear material of cells throughout the body, safe from antiviral treatments and vaccines, until a later date, perhaps years in the future.

Second, as already mentioned, the virus mutated extraordinarily rapidly, meaning that even if an effective vaccine could be developed, HIV could almost certainly mutate itself into an adaptive strain that could overcome the newly produced antibodies in the host's body. Antibodies tend to be highly specific, comporting themselves to the unique shape of a particular protein or proteins in the virus's coating. A few new amino acids could change the shape of the protein enough to make it unrecognizable to an antibody, while still allowing it to go about its grisly business of infecting and creating disease. With 1 mutation for each 10,000 base pairs of DNA nucleotides, the chance of HIV creating an adaptive strain was very high.

Third, specific to HIV, the virus infected exactly those cells—the macrophages—that were critical to the functioning of the immune system. One horrible possibility of fighting HIV was that new antibodies whose production a vaccine would induce would become attached to the macrophages while also being attached to the HIV, allowing the HIV to infect the macrophages more aggressively and effectively than they could without the antibodies being present. Further, because the virus infected T4 cells also—a central component of the immune system—even a small amount of infectious virus could compromise the system whose functioning was necessary to ward off the targeted virus. It was a little like using machine guns to fight an enemy whose prime weapon was its ability to render gunpowder useless.

Last, HIV had a tremendously powerful affinity for certain proteins in the T4 cell coat called CD4 proteins. To prevent the spread of a virus, an antibody would have to interrupt the virus's ability to bind to these CD4 proteins, and thus would have to block the active site on the viral protein coat. Unfortunately, the antibody would itself have to resemble the CD4 proteins, and could thus stimulate the production of a second round of antibodies that could attack the CD4 proteins itself. This kickback reaction could threaten the integrity of the vital T4 cells as ominously as could the original HIV.[17]

Rather than seek a vaccine, one possibility was to look for pharmaceutical intervention. Gallo, himself, suspected that one possible treatment route was attacking the reverse transcriptase with some sort of inhibitor. The transcriptase was vital to the functioning of any retrovirus, as it allowed the RNA to produce the DNA that would be inserted into the host's genetic material. The transcriptase was a complex protein which could conceivably be adulterated or inhibited, and thus negate the action of the virus. Because the transcriptase had a unique shape and structure, and was potentially more susceptible to pharmaceutical inhibition than were other proteins that could mimic the body's own proteins, it was an alluring treatment target.[18]

Treatments and vaccines were far in the future in 1984, however. Molecules were neither in testing phases nor "in the pipeline," to use a phrase common in the pharmaceutical industry. HIV had been described, but much of its mechanism at the molecular level was still unknown. The little "knobs" affixed to the viral coat, made of protein gp120, seemed like a promising target, as did the reverse transcriptase, but how to specifically disable the virus's ability to attach to C4 proteins, infect macrophages, or disable T4 cells was still unknown.

THE INSECT VECTOR

About the time that HIV was definitively identified as the cause of AIDS, a number of researchers began to speculate on the possibility of an insect vector. HIV was clearly blood-borne, had originated in the African tropics, and, in Africa at least, appeared able to spread to people not participating in high-risk activities. These facts together suggested that HIV might possibly be carried by insects. When Rockville-based Bionetics Research found that mosquitoes that ingested AIDS-contaminated blood harbored live virus in their stomachs two days later, the possibility seemed a likelihood.[19]

Evidence for this conjecture was found in the 3–6 percent of all American and Western European AIDS victims who fell into no known risk group, as well as the much larger portion of Africans who were similarly uncategorizable. One zealous malpractice lawyer writing on AIDS invoked the rule of Occam's razor to argue that when considering various explanations for an unknown phenomenon, "the most likely is the simplest," in this case insects.[20]

But arguing against the insect hypothesis was the simple fact that AIDS cases did not mirror the usual demography of insect-borne disease. Pathogens spread by insects, such as malaria and dengue, infected all sectors of the population equally, regardless of age or gender. But AIDS infected the very old and the very young hardly at all, seeming to wholly ignore the nonsexually active component of any population. This fact was inconsistent with insect spread, and was hard to reconcile with the zealousness and creativity of the insect theory. One theorist hypothesized that head lice spread the disease differentially to blacks and whites depending on the shape of their hair follicles, while another suspected bedbugs. Responded a skeptic in frank frustration, "If a science-fiction writer had invented AIDS and the scientists in the book were behaving as these scientists are, the writer wouldn't find a publisher, because no one would find the behavior credible. Nobody in science fiction would get away with this crap."[21]

This much was known by 1987. AIDS was caused by a virus. The virus was called HIV. HIV was a retrovirus. It mutated rapidly. It attacked the body's T4 cells (specifically rooting to the CD4 proteins) and macrophages. It was spread through sexual activity, through contaminated blood products, and through either the uterus or vagina to a growing fetus. All else was still speculation. Even this limited information, however, brought the possibility of treatment, inoculation, or vaccination substantially closer than it had been only four years before.

CHAPTER 4

CONSERVATIVE BACKLASH

SOUNDING OFF

In the early years, despite isolated incidents of homophobia and antigay violence, AIDS and AIDS victims attracted more support than opprobrium. Certain agencies and individuals, such as the Centers for Disease Control (CDC) and many members of the infectious-disease research community, had rushed in at the onset to try to understand the disease, prevent its spread, and diminish its effect. Other bodies, such as Congress, the National Institutes of Health (NIH), various state legislatures, and health-care officers in the Reagan administration, had dutifully raised budget allocations for research and prevention, albeit after initial reluctance and with some distaste. But overall, the nation had refrained from exploiting AIDS to attack homosexuals.

By 1987, however, this reluctance had faded. Religious and political conservatives, leading a larger block of conservative moderates, began to attack homosexuality and homosexual behavior in a concerted effort to demonize gay lifestyles and portray gays as self-indulgent, irresponsible, and morally depraved. This conservative backlash had been simmering for a half-dozen years, and now it exploded in vitriolic and self-righteous attacks on the branded culprits. At Dartmouth College, for example, conservative students celebrated Rock Hudson's death with a sorority party, while at the University of Kansas "Fagbusters" T-shirts were proving popular.[1] With more discretion, editors at the *National Review* deemed AIDS a "prominent skeleton at the feast of sexual liberation."[2]

The first step for conservatives was to reeducate the public into understanding that AIDS still, in 1987, infected predominantly homosexuals and drug addicts, and to remind the public that homosexuality violated basic laws of nature and transgressed God's intention. Homosexuality was, in short, perverted, and needed to be identified and understood as such if AIDS was to be alleviated and banished. Catholic theologian Eugene Clark reminded his readers in May 1987 of the "unmentionable fact" that "promiscuous sodomy is the root cause" of turning a viral attack into a modern plague, and that sodomy (not "anal intercourse" as was the preferred term among public health officials) was simply at odds with Christian teachings—"an essentially unsanitary act."[3] "There *is* a body of Judeo-Christian thought regarding homosexuality," Clark implored. "Sodomy is not a birthright. Like adultery and running a red light, it is a voluntary act. And like them, it has consequences."[4] Other religious leaders went further, and actually accused the gay community of actively denying their culpability in a deliberate campaign of disinformation. "Homosexuals and the pro-homosexual politicians have joined together with the liberal, gay influenced media to cover up the facts concerning AIDS," wrote Moral Majority founder Jerry Falwell in a mass mailing in 1987.[5]

AIDS became fertile ground for political conservatives, an issue that allowed them to prove their credentials and score hits against an unpopular minority. Never shy about denigrating homosexuality, many conservatives took the existence of AIDS as proof of the rectitude of their political philosophy, and as vindication of their personal biases. Ex–White House staff member Pat Buchanan had decreed as early as 1983, "The poor homosexuals. They have declared war on nature and now nature is exacting an awful retribution,"[6] and *Commentary* magazine editor Norman Podhoretz described the AIDS research funding efforts as "giving social sanction to what can only be described as a brutish degradation."[7] And in England, Manchester's chief constable James Anderton declared in December 1986 that AIDS was spread by the "obnoxious practices" of homosexuals. "Everywhere I go," related Anderton, "I see increasing evidence of people swirling about in a human cesspit of their own making."[8]

Some conservative critics were a bit milder in their attacks, condemning not so much homosexuality per se, as gay flamboyance, indulgence, and general fecklessness. "A generation ago homosexuals lived mostly in the closet. Nowadays they take over cities and parade on Halloween and demand equal rights for themselves," wrote *National Review* editor William F. Buckley in the summer of 1986.[9] Other prominent conservatives, such as Phyllis Schlafly, questioned the strategy of the gay lobby in pressuring governmental agencies to create AIDS-friendly regulations and programs, rather than fighting the disease in the most direct and effective (albeit possibly painful) manner. "Why are young boys and men not warned that all who engage in homosexual activities can expect to become infected with AIDS," demanded Schlafly, and "Why is AIDS presented by the media as a homosexuals' civil-rights problem instead of as a public health problem which the government can isolate and treat?"[10] Buckley continued in the same vituperative vein when he wrote in March 1986, "Everyone detected with AIDS should be tattooed in the upper forearm, to protect common-needle users, and on the buttocks, to prevent the victimization of other homosexuals."[11]

In a certain sense, gays had left themselves open to such vitriol, at first through sexual excesses, and later through impolitic protestations. Many people who harbored vague homophobic feelings might have expressed some sympathy for the beleaguered community, had they not discovered the extremes of some gay sexual activity. As the statistics became more widely published—means of over 100 sex partners per year, lifetime partners of 1,000 or more, strange and bizarre sex practices—even the most libertarian and tolerant straights began to question or condemn the moral acceptability of America's gays. Gay Liberation Front founder Jim Fouratt acknowledged the community's political insensitivity when he commented, "The problem the gay AIDS leadership refused to confront until recently—the sex issue, the life-style issue—created a vacuum for the homophobic moralists."[12]

The moderate backlashers focused on two components of the epidemic that they found offensive: the effort to universalize it as a disease of all, and the gay community's general insensitivity to community mores. By 1987, AIDS was most certainly spreading out of the gay community, but the spread was largely toward prostitutes and their clients, and IV drug users. Little evidence suggested a broad spread into the non-drug using heterosexual community, and some straights took offense at the insinuation that they and their ilk would be the disease's next victims. Further, statistics on current AIDS cases indicated that by 1987 almost three-quarters of all AIDS victims were still sexually active homosexual men, even if the profile of the coming epidemic was far more skewed toward IV drug users. Savvy conservatives who took the time to understand the epidemiology harped on this fact, and blamed gay leaders for spreading misinformation on the disease's threat to heterosexuals. "AIDS is not the pandemic its publicists would like us to believe," wrote physician and columnist Charles Krauthammer. Rather, it was a "relatively small public health problem" that had been exaggerated for political ends by the gay community.[13]

More moderate conservatives resented the special treatment they believed gays had received, including extensive efforts to protect the confidentiality of AIDS victims, and the passage of local ordinances to protect gays and AIDS victims from discrimination. Los Angeles, for example, had passed an ordinance in 1985 making it illegal to discriminate against any AIDS sufferer. Similarly, the Reagan Justice Department argued in court that federal antidiscrimination law could not protect AIDS-infected workers from dismissal as their infection constituted a true threat to the integrity and safety of the workplace. The Supreme Court ultimately ruled against the government.[14]

But it was in the area of sexual mores that the more balanced conservatives took the most offense. Even if they accepted gays' demands to be left alone to conduct their sexual relations as they saw fit, they rejected the idea that these practices were normal and that they reflected larger social mores, and they outright resented the suggestion that society as a whole ought to accept and even endorse the lifestyle. In this sense, the gay leadership had sorely overestimated society's general sympathy toward their plight, or toward their lifestyle choices, and had exacerbated this hostility with abrasive rhetoric and publicity. For example, Los Angeles's Gay and Lesbian Community Services Center had distributed a safe-sex pamphlet entitled *Mother's Handy Sex Guide* in 1985, which raised the ire of the county supervisor's office. The material "goes beyond all boundaries of good taste and decency," wrote the supervisor. "The material is not educational; it's hard core pornographic material."[15] And the conservative *National Review* reported with disbelief (or possibly prurient glee) of the self-proclaimed monogamous gay man who had been infected with AIDS—monogamous except for the one evening a week that he and his partner agreed that each could sleep with whomever he wished. "Once a week every week is half a hundred partners," pointed out the *Review* writer. "Ten years of that takes you halfway to Don Giovanni's *mil e tre*. In a heterosexual, that is promiscuous."[16] Even the staid *New England Journal of Medicine* published a letter quoting the eminent 19th century physician William Osler, who had advised: "Idleness is the mother of lechery; and a young man will find that absorption in any pursuit will do much to cool passions which, though natural and proper, cannot in the exigencies of our civilization always obtain natural and proper gratification."[17]

Conservative legislators joined the backlash by introducing restrictive legislation to various state and federal bodies governing the manner in which AIDS patients should be identified, quarantined, prohibited from donating blood, marked for identification, and generally tagged as responsible for their own plight. The most visible examples of this were perennial presidential candidate Lyndon Larouche's proposed California ballot initiative to quarantine AIDS victims and Florida state legislator Tom Woodruff's proposal to jail all AIDS patients who knowingly donated blood, but more mainstream politicians proposed bills as well.[18]

The most persistent legislative efforts against gays came from California congressmen William Dannemeyer and Robert Dornan, who actively fought to defeat federal budget outlays for AIDS research and prevention in late 1985. Dannemeyer exemplified many of the most conservative critics of AIDS victims in claiming to be concerned not with gay sex, per se, but rather with the public's health. "There are those in the homosexual community, in the public health establishment, and at the [Los Angeles] *Times,* who put greater emphasis on the perceived civil rights of AIDS victims and high-risk groups than on either the civil rights of potential victims or the health of the general public," he wrote in early 1986.[19]

Although Dannemeyer's argument sounded relatively value neutral, his bills masked a history of blatant homophobic remarks and assertions. He had repeatedly claimed to speak for "traditional family values," and on the floor of Congress had asserted, "God's plan for man was Adam and Eve, not Adam and Steve."[20] And the previous year he had hired outspoken antigay psychologist Paul Cameron to conduct AIDS research. Cameron, who had advocated quarantining AIDS victims, had been expelled from the American Psychological Association, and been reprimanded by his local psychological association. "The hiring [of Cameron] is akin to relying on the Ku Klux Klan or the American Nazi Party for advice," stated Orange County gay community leader Werner Kuhn.[21]

A significant weakness in Dannemeyer's and Dornan's arguments, and in those of other prominent conservative politicians, was that although some of their proposed policies for containing the AIDS epidemic fell within the accepted range of accepted public health techniques, their motives were suspect. Technically, they were simply proposing restrictions on the movements and behaviors of AIDS victims that had been used repeatedly and successfully to control infectious diseases for hundreds of years. But many conservative politicians had a history of embracing antigay positions, which incited the suspicions of gay leaders and AIDS-patient advocates. Conservative Washington lobbyist Paul Weyrich exemplified this position in stating: "I'm not for gay-bashing. I have compassion for those people who've gotten themselves into a reprobate mind-set."[22]

Some anti-AIDS legislators were simply exploiting a perceived "AIDS-fatigue" among their constituencies for their own political ends. Even the most tolerant and open-minded of Americans had begun to question by 1986 whether the supreme consideration in the face of the epidemic ought to be protecting the privacy of those who already had contracted the disease, or aggressively *ensuring* their employment, civil rights, and general freedom to move about and participate in society. During previous epidemics, the welfare of the general community had taken precedence over the comfort and welfare of the ill, yet in this one few public health proponents seemed willing to actively advocate for the welfare of the broader community. Such reluctance created a vacuum in public health leadership, which was easily exploited by opportunistic politicians, homophobic or not. "We have a sick public health community that has been frankly intimidated by the homosexual lobby," stated conservative fund-raiser Richard Viguerie.[23] And in a wholly sensible platform, Christian columnist Kerby Anderson proclaimed that in the absence of definitive knowledge about the etiology and epidemiology of the disease, "the benefit of the doubt should be given to society, not the AIDS victim. This is a medical issue, not a civil rights issue."[24]

By 1987, Republicans as a group began to view AIDS—previously a politically untouchable issue—as possibly fertile ground for their 1988 platform, due almost entirely to the excessive zeal of the "patients' rights" defenders who had so long dominated debate about the disease. Americans might not care what sort of sexual practices their neighbors engaged in, or even whether or not they injected drugs, but many deeply resented being told, implicitly or explicitly, that the civil rights of others took precedence over their claims to good health. Such priorities defied common sense, and Americans with middling sensibilities resented being accused of bias, prejudice, or homophobia for simply looking after the well-being of their children and friends. A full year before the 1988 presidential election, the republican political consulting firm Charlton Research produced a policy memo describing the political opportunities that AIDS had created for candidates in swing states. "If we are low-key, sound logical, and stress the importance of 'protecting' families from the disease," wrote the memo's author, Chuck Rund, "then we could find ourselves in excellent shape in '88."[25]

AIDS IN THE REAGAN WHITE HOUSE

To the surprise of many observers, the Reagan White House had mobilized substantial resources to fight the disease by 1987. Although their political base demanded generally downplaying the issue, administration officials and congressional allies had managed to substantially increase funding for research, education, and drug treatment every year since the disease was first identified by the CDC, to the point where it was drawing the most federal money per patient of all contagious diseases. And although Reagan himself publicly eschewed association with the disease, in private he endorsed efforts within his administration to expand research and prevention programs, and generally increase funding to levels deemed appropriate by public health experts.

Critics of the Reagan White House were loath to give any credit to the administration for these efforts. From the onset of the disease, liberals and moderates alike perceived administration officials to be extremely uncomfortable with a disease that disproportionately affected marginalized groups (particularly gays) and that was closely associated with unseemly habits and practices. The centrist *New York Times* excoriated the administration for its "inappropriate apathy," and for having "yawned through the first two years of the crisis," while more radical critics implied that the administration was practically guilty of mass murder.[26] "They tend to see health in the same way that John Calvin saw wealth; it's your own responsibility, and you should damn well take care of yourself," observed American Public Health Association former President Stanley Matek.[27] On a less philosophical note, one liberal Senate health staff member decried the pathetic AIDS alleviation efforts of HEW secretary Margaret Heckler. "The idea of Heckler sitting down to brief Reagan on AIDS is like the stupid leading the senile," he said.[28]

The truth was more ambiguous. On one hand, Reagan himself was not concerned with the issue and devoted almost none of his personal time to educating himself about it or to engaging in AIDS policy debates with his staff, members of Congress, or the public. He did not publicly say the word "AIDS" until 1987, and devoted only one speech in his entire presidency to the topic. Although he never articulated a personal homophobia, his profound lack of personal concern for victims of the worst infectious disease to emerge in nearly a century bespoke indifference to the welfare of America's gay citizens.

On the other hand, various agencies under Reagan's purview clearly articulated the importance of AIDS treatment, research, and prevention from an early point in the epidemic's development. By 1983, the Public Health Service had defined AIDS as its "number 1 priority,"[29] and Secretary Heckler herself deemed the disease her "top priority."[30] In August of that year, when the disease was afflicting almost exclusively sexually active homosexual men, Heckler appeared at the bedside of a 40-year-old AIDS victim in New York's Cabrini Hospital and stated: "The person with AIDS is bearing a very heavy burden. We ought to be comforting the sick rather than afflicting them and making them a class of outcasts."[31] William Roper, chairman of the Reagan administration's Domestic Policy Council's health policy group, reported that Reagan had "acknowledged that AIDS is a major public health problem," and had pledged appropriate resources.[32]

Federal funding for AIDS grew astronomically from 1982 to 1987, despite the president's reluctance to publicly identify himself with the disease. Public Health Service AIDS resources grew from $5.5 million in 1982 to $204 million in 1986, with an additional $133 million pledged that year to the NIH, $55 million to the CDC, $10 million to the FDA, and $7 million to the Alcohol, Drug Abuse, and Mental Health Administration. All of these sums were slated to rise substantially over the following two years, with the General Accounting Office estimating that the 1988 Public Health Service AIDS budget would top $900 million.[33]

Despite critics' complaints about the administration's foot dragging, the coffers had opened up nearly at the onset of the epidemic. As early as 1983, the NIH devoted nearly $15 million to AIDS research: a sum, noted Assistant Secretary of Health Edward Brandt, nearly equal to the total sum spent on Legionnaires' disease since its discovery seven years earlier.[34] The prestigious *Science* magazine reported in 1983 that the federal government was "pouring money into AIDS research."[35] And NIH grants to AIDS laboratories in that early year ranged from $300,000 to $500,000. The following year, Brandt's recommendations prompted Congress to add $14.6 million to previously calculated budget recommendations, despite challenges from other institutes within the NIH.[36]

From whence did the administration's reputation for niggardly disbursals of AIDS monies arise? In part, Reagan's base among Goldwater Republicans and family-value advocates had roused the suspicions of the gay community from the start. Then too, the general unwillingness of either Heckler, Brandt, or CDC director James Mason to closely align themselves with the gay community exacerbated the administration's reputation for callousness. But part of the reason for this reputation was simply ordinary bureaucratic malaise and political infighting. True, the NIH was devoting substantial funds to fighting AIDS, but the demand for such funds was nearly infinite, and underfunded researchers loudly assigned blame for their inability to win even larger grants to the administration's homophobia. Budget analyst David Kleinberg noted: "The worst offenders are the medical bureaucracy. The guys who want the brand new labs and 12 new research assistants."[37]

The administration's purported passiveness on the issue was belied by the actions of White House staffers and cabinet members in fomenting federal AIDS policy after 1985. While Reagan, himself, demurred from publicly commenting on the issue until nearly the end of his second term, the administration's Domestic Policy Council addressed AIDS policymaking repeatedly after 1985, with consensus developing around a well-coordinated federal strategy consisting of education, research, treatment, public health funding, and prevention. In those closed meetings, virtually no member of the cabinet or White House staff suggested that the White House might be excused from confronting the challenge owing to its predominantly afflicting gays and drug users.[38] And in a 1986 Public Health Service AIDS meeting and retreat in Coolfont, West Virginia, 85 experts developed a series of recommendations for federal AIDS programs that comported almost precisely with recommendations from the most progressive public health specialists: education, voluntary testing, research, drug treatment, blood screening, and vaccine development.[39]

On the other hand, critics of Reagan's efforts were correct in accusing the administration of drawing morality lessons from the epidemic. If the public health community insisted on depriving the epidemic and its victims of any moral taint, Reagan staffers insisted, to the contrary, on imposing moral judgment on the disease and its victims, and on applying such moral judgment to efforts to thwart the disease. Various White House planners insisted on developing AIDS prevention programs that stressed "values,"[40] and the president himself ultimately endorsed an AIDS prevention program that encouraged "responsible sexual behavior"—"fidelity, commitment, and maturity, placing sexuality within the context of marriage."[41] (At an earlier DPC meeting, he had referred to a public health specialist who had emphasized to him the importance of "individual responsibility" in combating the disease.")[42]

In a sense, criticism of Reagan administration AIDS policy did not hinge so much on actual actions taken as on whether or not traditional family values had a role in health policy formation. Many in the public health community had spent their careers improving the lives of people whose behavior and proclivities defied accepted social norms: alcoholics, drug users, victims of and perpetrators of domestic violence, unwed mothers, and the like. Underlying their work was a credo of moral neutrality, in which all victims of disease, social pathology, and violence merited equal levels of compassion and treatment. The conservative revolution, spearheaded by Reagan, in contrast, demanded that discussion of morals be returned to public discourse. In his one public speech on AIDS, the president stated: "Values are how we guide ourselves through the decisions of life. How we behave sexually is one of those decisions . . . if children are taught their own worth, we can expect them to treat themselves and others with greater respect. And wherever you have self-respect and mutual respect, you don't have drug abuse and sexual promiscuity—which, of course, are the two major causes of AIDS."[43]

In April 1987, the Domestic Policy Council recommended the establishment of an AIDS commission to advise the president on AIDS policy as well as to mediate between the public and the administration on actions involving the disease. From the start, many administration critics worried that the council would be little more than a foil to deflect accusations that the administration was resisting taking action on the epidemic, and noted that as the commission's report would be released shortly before the 1988 presidential elections, it could hardly have a substantial impact on administration policy. On the other hand, the council would be immune to political reprimand, and thus would have the freedom to make recommendations that could exceed proposals emanating from the Public Health Service and other federal agencies.[44]

An uproar ensued when the names of the 13 AIDS commission members were released. None had academic expertise in HIV; none had been drawn from a list of proposed members created by Assistant HEW

Secretary Robert Windom, many were outspoken conservatives, and only one, Frank Lilly of the Albert Einstein School of Medicine, was an admitted homosexual. Several of the commission members possessed such conservative and homophobic bona fides as to wholly discredit the committee in the eyes of the gay community: among them New York City's Archbishop John Cardinal O'Connor, State Representative Penny Pullen of Illinois; California sex therapist Theresa Crenshaw, and *Saturday Evening Post* publisher Cory Servaas. O'Connor had been an outspoken critic of condom distribution as a method to prevent AIDS transmission and had been generally critical of gay sexual practices; Pullen had sponsored legislation in Illinois calling for mandatory AIDS testing; Servaas had reported in her magazine that an AIDS-infected doctor had successfully treated himself with amino acids and drugs; and Crenshaw had publicly discussed quarantining AIDS-infected individuals and expelling AIDS-infected children from school, and derided condom use as "putting a mere balloon between ourselves and a deadly virus."[45] The appointed chairman was Eugene Mayberry, CEO of the Mayo Clinic in Rochester, Minnesota, and an acquaintance of White House Chief of Staff Howard Baker. The *New York Times* dismissed the panel as a "motley group" incapable of devising a comprehensive AIDS policy.[46]

KOOP

Into the sluggish malaise of the Reagan AIDS policy team stepped Surgeon General C. Everett Koop. A figure seemingly drawn from central casting, the former chief of surgery at Philadelphia Children's Hospital vitalized the usually moribund and marginal office of surgeon general, and used the office to speak candidly and frequently about the need to confront the epidemic with education, condom distribution, and frank talk. He steadfastly refused to overlay the epidemic with a moral taint, citing his primary role as a public health officer as opposed to moralistic sentry. And responding to his many critics concerning his advocacy for greater sex education, he noted, "You can't teach young people about AIDS until you've taught them something about their own sexuality."[47] In doing so, he drew the ire of conservatives both within the administra-

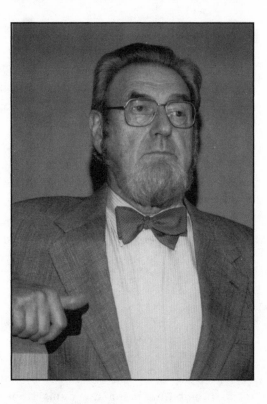

**Surgeon General
C. Everett Koop.**
*(National Library of
Medicine)*

tion and in the general public, while winning plaudits from public health professionals, gay activists, and proponents of sex education.

Koop's role in combating the AIDS epidemic was all the more surprising in that part of his appeal to Reagan had been his staunch and outspoken opposition to abortion, and his generally socially conservative outlook. The post of surgeon general had historically been more honorary than substantive, and few modern surgeon generals had used the position for anything more than a pulpit from which to articulate vague and uncontentious warnings about smoking, nutrition, fitness, and disease prevention.

In February 1986, President Reagan requested that Koop prepare a comprehensive AIDS report on the state of the disease. Nearly a year later, the report startled government observers with its candor, frankness, and progressive recommendations. Centering on education in fighting AIDS, the report emphasized comprehensive sex education in elementary and secondary schools, condom usage, home-based family discussions on sexuality, and monogamy. Ignorance regarding sexuality in general, and the spread of sexually transmitted diseases in particular, were deemed the most substantial barrier to controlling the disease. "This silence must end," emphasized Koop in a follow-up article.[48]

Koop's report offended constituencies across the political spectrum. He pointedly explained that blacks and Hispanics had contracted AIDS in numbers disproportionate to their presence in the population, and recommended education programs designed to target these groups exclusively. He also recommended sex education programs aimed at all primary and secondary school students in the country, constituting 95 percent of all of the nation's children, in an effort to banish sexual ignorance. And although he stated that abstinence and monogamy were the preferred patterns of sexual activity, he emphasized that condom use could significantly limit the spread of AIDS. Further, he argued that AIDS could not be spread through kissing, touching, or other casual contact.

Not surprisingly, the surgeon general's report raised the ire of conservatives. Congressman Dannemeyer recommended copious emendations, including recognizing the importance of "conscience, morality, and ethics in sexual liaisons."[49] He demanded that the report recommend prohibiting blood donations from all members of high-risk groups, and argued that the report's conclusions regarding the difficulty of contracting the disease through casual interactions be removed. Moreover, he wanted any sex education program in the public schools to contain "moral and ethical arguments for avoiding homosexuality," and argued that the report's recommendations vis-à-vis condom use were pernicious. "[The report] does not note the failure rate of condoms in preventing conception (10% failure rate); nor does it point out that the AIDS virus is a tiny fraction of the size of a sperm."[50]

Individuals within the administration also voiced their differences with Koop's seemingly "value-neutral" approach to AIDS and sex education. Within the Domestic Policy Council, White House counselor Gary Bauer stated that he did not want the government preparing educational materials that could be "offensive" to people who were "concerned about their children's education."[51] White House counselor Robert Sweet wrote to Koop, "It is a fact that sex education, as it is currently being taught in public schools, downgrades the true nature of sexuality and is destructive to the spiritual and moral values most Americans believe in," and that there was growing evidence that sex education was "responsible for the increase in teenage pregnancies, psychological problems, and venereal diseases."[52] One White House domestic policy adviser stated, "I don't see why a third grader needs to know anything about condoms or sexual practices—and I'm not about to give the go-ahead to the local school to talk to my 9-year-old daughter about sodomy."[53]

Outside the administration, the most scathing critique of the Koop doctrine of broad sexual and AIDS education came from noted conservative writer Phyllis Schlafly, whose monthly *Phyllis Schlafly Report* was distributed across the United States. Schlafly had long argued against sex education, claiming that the courses "shred the girls of their natural modesty . . . by forcing them to discuss sexual acts, techniques, devices, and parts of the body, with explicit vocabulary in a coed classroom."[54] In a 1986 column, Schlafly had targeted school-based sex education courses as misrepresenting the entire concept of "responsible" sexual activity claiming, " 'responsible sexuality' means enjoying promiscuity without guilt and without having a baby."[55]

Although nothing in the Koop report stipulated that children and teenagers be taught that premarital or promiscuous sex was permissible or even laudable, Schlafly preemptively attacked the report for even leaving open the possibility that AIDS-related sex education might disseminate a message of permissible premarital sex. Rather, Schlafly stated, the Koop report should explicitly state that all sex education programs eschew mention of sex outside of marriage, and of condoms or other contraceptives preventing pregnancy or AIDS, lest it "offend the first amendment rights of those who believe that all sex outside of marriage is morally wrong." Schlafly further promoted modesty as a constitutional right, demanding that the right to modesty be given treatment under the law equal to that accorded church-state separation and free speech. "The moral child has the constitutional right to be protected against the embarrassment of being in a public school classroom when others are discussing sex activities, contraceptives, abortion, or other sex practices which he believes are morally wrong," Schlafly wrote. She also argued that children needed to be protected against embarrassing topics and exhibits, such as those using explicit language and photographs, and "psychologically disturbing films such as the birth of a baby."[56]

Amid the shrill protests of ideological stalwarts, however, emerged the voices of moderates, who also opposed the type of compulsory and comprehensive sex education that Koop advocated, but on firmer grounds. These voices of reason questioned the need to educate children as young as 8 or 9 who rarely engaged in sexual activity in the explicit details of sex acts, contraception, and AIDS transmission, and questioned why it was necessary to strip sex education of all moral weight. Personifying this more thoughtful approach was Secretary of Education William Bennett, who argued that all education, emanating from both schools and parents, bear some sort of moral message urging self-control, discipline, self-abnegation, and emotional restraint. In Bennett's philosophy, children needed to be given clear divisions between right and wrong, and be taught that engaging in wrongful behavior carried with it consequences for both the child and for those around him. Insofar as children were capable of comprehending their own actions, they needed to be held accountable for them from a young age. "Teach restraint as a virtue," urged Bennett repeatedly in speeches and articles. "Demonstrate moral standards through personal example . . . Demonstrate responsibility for others in personal relationships."[57]

Army viral disease researcher Robert Redfield urged a similar toned-down message of restraint and morality when presenting sexually explicit information. In his pamphlet *AIDS and Young People,* the physician counseled teaching teenagers to avoid sexual contact beyond hand-holding and kissing, and to eschew a message of "safe sex," which he felt to be misleading. "Don't engage in intimate contact at all," he wrote. "If you have had that kind of contact in the past, stop now. That is truly the only 'safe sex.' "[58] And reinforcing Bennett's message of responsibility for one's actions, Redfield wrote: "You make choices, and you are expected to make the right choice. And your sexual drives are no different. You can control them, and you should control them."[59]

Both Bennett and Redfield spoke for a silent majority in their mild opposition to explicit references to homosexuality and condom use in the nation's public schools. Despite the national hysteria surrounding AIDS that had emerged a few years previously, most American parents simply did not view an aggressive and comprehensive sex education curriculum as a desirable or reasonable approach. Parents around the country voiced their dissent alone and in groups, and principals found themselves facing irate parent groups when the topic came up at PTA meetings and parent-teacher conferences. Reported National School Boards Association president Nellie Weil: "I've talked to school superintendents in the Southern states, in the Midwest and in the Far West, and, with rare exceptions, they do not want AIDS education to broach homosexuality or safe sex practices. As far as they are concerned, that's unconscionable."[60] Shrill though Schlafly may be, she spoke for a large constituency who viewed an assault on public mores as more threatening to their children's well-being than the AIDS virus.

Buttressing the protestations of these more moderate critics of the Koop report was a growing body of literature that cast doubt on the efficacy of sex education generally. By 1987, sex education had been taught in public schools across America in value-free curricula for some 25 years: long enough for dependable data to be collected regarding its effect on sexual behavior. Initial conclusions undermined arguments for expanding sex education. A 7-year study conducted by Mathtech found that sex education appeared to have minimal effect on "contraceptive use, views on premarital sex, or such social skills as assertiveness and self-understanding," while a study of high schools in Indiana, Texas, and Mississippi conducted by the Center for Population Options found that such courses had no consistent effect on teenage participation in sexual intercourse.[61]

Education efforts aimed at the gay community seemed similarly futile, with studies showing that condom use among gay men engaging in anal intercourse was correlated hardly at all with sex education efforts.[62] In fact, although 90 percent of gay men who had engaged in anal intercourse in the previous six months knew that condom use could diminish their exposure to AIDS, over 65 percent had engaged in unprotected sex during that period.[63] Such results correlated with experiences of servicemen during both World Wars I and II, when education efforts surrounding syphilis and gonorrhea proved ineffective in dissuading servicemen from engaging in unprotected sex with infected prostitutes.[64] In the end, both the U.S. Army and the U.S. Navy had resorted to aggressive use of preventive oral sulfathiazole and follow-up antibiotics, rather than rely on educational efforts, to retain the fighting integrity of their ranks. Concluded one physician in a White House memo: "The answer is obvious—public education in the use of condoms is not going to increase their use to the extent that it will stop an HIV epidemic."[65]

Offsetting these pessimistic studies was conclusive evidence that condoms, when used properly, worked extraordinarily well to stop HIV. Despite the ominous warnings of "Russian roulette" fatalities in condom use delivered by conservatives, almost all data showed that common latex condoms used before their expiration dates were impermeable to HIV, and that heterosexual couples with one infected partner who regularly used condoms vastly reduced the chances of infecting the noninfected partner.[66] Unfortunately, most of the studies examined condom usage in vaginal intercourse exclusively, leaving researchers unsure of the efficacy of condoms in retarding the spread of HIV during anal intercourse. And although several condom manufacturers were working to develop tougher condoms, none of the companies was willing to guarantee its products when used in anal intercourse. Potential risk exposure was too great, and fears of damaging "product image" haunted them as well.[67]

THE PAMPHLET

Despite general opprobrium from administration conservatives, Koop cleaved to almost all of his initial conclusions in preparing a pamphlet, *What You Should Know About AIDS: America Responds to AIDS,* to be distributed to every household in America. The pamphlet emphasized that AIDS was difficult to catch, was not spread through casual contact, and could be stopped through abstinence, consistent monogamous behavior, condom use, and refraining from sharing needles. The pamphlet explained that AIDS, per se, did not kill, but rather destroyed the body's ability to fight off other infections that could kill. Further, the pamphlet suggested that people refrain from deep "French" kissing, whose risk was not precisely known. The pamphlet recommended that young people abstain from drug use, always, and abstain from sex until ready to enter into a "mutually faithful, single-partner relationship."

The pamphlet also suggested that people concerned that they might be infected should have themselves tested.[68]

Despite the socially conservative tone of the pamphlet, administration conservatives, particularly AIDS Commission member Theresa Crenshaw and White House counselor Gary Bauer, strongly objected to the pamphlet. Crenshaw protested the lines "AIDS by itself doesn't kill," and "Fortunately AIDS is hard to catch . . . ," preferring language less reassuring lest the public develop a false sense of security.[69] Similarly, Bauer protested to Koop, "Parts of your current report fail to bluntly disabuse people of the false confidence that condoms will protect them."[70] And the White House Health-Policy Working Group (of which Bauer was a member) recommended changing the text as follows: "Replace the last sentence with 'If you or your sexual partner are concerned, using a condom is less dangerous, but it isn't safe. Since the AIDS virus can kill you, you need to ask, is it really worth the risk.' "[71]

The combined weight of the objections led the White House to veto the pamphlet in fall of 1987, and recommend redrafting it by the following spring to comply with a congressional mandate that AIDS education pamphlets be sent to all American households.[72] A revised brochure, *Understanding AIDS,* was mailed out the following spring with compromise language. Although *Understanding AIDS* emphasized abstinence more than had the previous pamphlet, it devoted an entire section to condom use, and asserted that condoms were the best prevention "besides not having sex." It also suggested using lubricants with condoms, avoiding lambskin condoms, and choosing condoms with spermicidal coatings for added protection. It asserted that AIDS could not be contracted through casual contact, kissing, or mosquito bites. And it continued to insist that Americans most at risk were those who engaged in risky behavior: needle sharing, anal sex (with and without a condom), vaginal sex with a drug shooter or participant in anal sex, sex with prostitutes, and any unprotected sex.[73]

In writing the final pamphlet, Koop favored neither gay and AIDS-patient community groups, who preferred language stating that AIDS posed an equal threat to all Americans, nor conservative groups, who cleaved to the idea that AIDS really posed a threat only to gay men and IV drug users (and their partners). The pamphlet asserted that "who you are has nothing to do with whether you are in danger of being infected," but rather "what matters is what you do." While technically correct, the assertion belied the statistical reality that "who you are" was highly correlated with "what you do." Certain groups practiced high-risk activities at rates disproportionate to the general population, and thus membership in those groups served as a dependable proxy for behavior. The surgeon general was making a specious distinction in separating the activity from the person—a distinction designed more to placate constituent groups than to assist in improving the public's safety.

QUARANTINE AND REPORTING

The conservative backlash extended to local governments and authorities as well. From 1986 on, state legislatures, city councils, and private citizens through public referendums introduced a variety of bills calling for quarantines, testing measures, and mandatory reporting procedures in an effort to identify and isolate AIDS patients, and putatively "protect" the public from the threat they posed. Conservative coalitions of lawmakers and constituent groups fought gay lobbies and liberal public health administrators, claiming the concern over the rights of the afflicted had become excessive. "People don't have a license to kill," stated New Jersey assemblyman Walter Kern, who called for five-year prison terms for those who knowingly transmitted AIDS. "If need be, these people will have to be incarcerated to save others."[74] California citizen activist Paul Gann stated more succinctly, "Who in the hell has the right to give you a virus that is going to kill you?"[75]

More extreme was a proposal by Lynwood, California, councilman Robert Henning calling for mandatory quarantine of all AIDS patients. Quarantine had been a popular tool for containing contagious diseases through the 19th century, but generally the quarantined patients had remained infectious for only a few days or weeks, meaning that the quarantine could be imposed on an individual's house, and then only temporarily. When faced with the challenge of quarantining individuals for the remainder of their lives, Henning refused to acknowledge either the logistical or the ethical challenge. Who would submit to such quarantine, and where should the municipality or state put the quarantined individuals? "Where we put them is not my concern. They'll find places," snapped Henning.[76] "It is not fair to the public to be subjected to such silliness. I don't want them cooking my food or have them bumping into me."[77]

More popular were a variety of proposals calling for mandatory reporting by physicians of any patient who had tested positive for the virus. Colorado ratified such a bill in June 1987, and other states (notably California) considered similar proposals. Proponents of those proposals stood on firm historical ground, for reporting of disease cases had been one of the primary responsibilities of public health agencies since their founding in the last century. If AIDS reporting was made mandatory, public health officials could track when and where individuals had contracted the virus, and identify other infected individuals. Education efforts could be aimed at high-risk areas, and individuals and groups could be given condoms or warned against high-risk behavior. Moreover, health departments could better plan for future service demands, hospitals could invest in appropriate infrastructure and staffing, and legislatures could better understand possible future budget demands. On many levels, the reporting requirements were consistent with successful public health practices of the past, and promised to provide useful and constructive data.

Others insisted that requiring reporting would simply force AIDS patients to resist being tested. The stigma of AIDS was still so great in 1987, they argued, that individuals would go to great lengths to protect their anonymity. "Enforced contact-tracing will make people afraid to be tested," concluded Harvard researcher Jerome Groopman. "That would be a much greater disaster than the occasional, rare case of some infected prostitute who's still working the street."[78] Gay advocates worried that not only would the measures fail to produce useful data, they would actually dissuade infected individuals from seeking treatment, thus exacerbating the epidemic. "Ultimately this bill is going to kill people," stated Denver lawyer Dennis Brinn about the Colorado reporting measure.[79]

In fact, nobody really knew. AIDS was unique in the annals of infectious disease for the length of its latency period, for its extraordinary fatality rate, and for its targeting of some of the most despised and oppressed members of society. Fear of stigma for gay men was very real—almost all had experienced discrimination firsthand for simply being gay, and AIDS-infected gay men had experienced added hostility. Given that in 1988 effective treatment for the disease was nonexistent, the men had little incentive to comply with the new rulings, and great incentive to avoid formal contact with either public health authorities or private physicians. Early data appeared to confirm that in the presence of mandatory reporting laws, gay men became notably less visible.

An isolated incident from the U.S. Navy confirmed the worst fears of gay men when hospital corpsman Bernard Broyhill was found, in a routine Navy physical, to carry the AIDS virus. Assured that confidentiality would be maintained, he admitted his homosexuality to a Navy physician, and reported the names of individuals with whom he had had sex. Within days Broyhill was charged with practicing homosexual acts, a criminal offense in the military punishable by dishonorable discharge. "As a general rule," noted Pentagon health affairs specialist Robert Gilliat, "there is no doctor-patient privilege in the military."[80] Yet even in civilian life, gays worried that state reporting measures would undermine *traditional* doctor-patient privilege, and make them as vulnerable as their military counterparts.

TESTING

The most hotly contested component of AIDS policy in the late 1980s surrounded mandatory testing. Two antibody tests had been developed in 1985 that, used in conjunction, were capable of screening out nearly all individuals infected with HIV. Unfortunately, the *specificity* of the tests, though high, was inadequate to claim with certainty that all persons found to be infected actually were, and testing was expensive.

The first of the two tests was known as the "enzyme-linked immunosorbent assay" (ELISA), which used beads or micro titer wells coated with antigens to produce a colored precipitate when exposed to HIV-infected serum. The coloration was then read by a spectrograph, which determined which of the samples were HIV-positive. The test had a false-positive rate of .18 percent, meaning that of every 10,000 HIV-negative specimens read, 18 would result in an HIV-positive reading.

All positive test samples from the ELISA were thereupon tested through the second test, the "Western Blot," in which viral antigens were "blotted" to nitrocellulose paper. The test serum was then applied, and specific antigens could be identified by band. This test, while more *specific* than the ELISA (fewer false positives) was less *sensitive* (more false negatives). The two together promised nearly 100 percent specificity, and nearly 100 percent sensitivity. That is, when the two tests were used in conjunction, nearly all people who were in fact HIV-positive were detected, and almost nobody who was confirmed HIV-positive was in fact HIV-negative.[81]

Initially, the ELISA test promised to be more useful. Fast and cheap (planners thought they could obtain the kits for as little as 75 cents each in bulk orders), the test's sensitivity promised to be very effective in screening out tainted blood in blood donation centers, while the relatively low specificity seemed fairly benign in such a situation—about .5 percent of all samples that were HIV-negative would be discarded owing to improper specificity.[82] The FDA approved the test for blood screening in summer 1985, confident that the early hysteria over tainted blood products could be alleviated.[83]

Blood donation administrators were not so sure, however. Even with anonymity guaranteed, they worried that potential donors, knowing that their blood would be tested for AIDS antibodies, would be dissuaded from donating, fearful of being labeled HIV-positive, or perhaps fearful of even finding out their seropositivity status themselves. Early polls among potential blood donors in New York City indicated that 23 percent would cease to donate if mandatory blood testing was applied during donations.[84] The poll may have been misleading, however. Blood products were already routinely tested for hepatitis and syphilis, with little effect on donor intentions.

Using ELISA widely to ferret out HIV-positive Americans was far more problematic. It's initial lack of specificity meant that if 1 in 1,000 Americans was actually HIV-positive (as was estimated in 1987), then each 10,000 people tested would result in 28 positive "hits," of which 10 would truly be HIV-positive and the remaining 18 would be false positives. Thus, the accuracy of the testing was only 35 percent—an abysmally low rate. The Western Blot follow-up on these 28 could be expected to remove nearly all of the 18 false positives, but at much greater cost; the test would cost nearly $35 per trial. Thus universal testing, which would entail the lab and serum costs of each test, plus an estimated $75 in counseling fees for each person double-testing positive, would run to nearly $18,000 per each infected person detected. By contrast, if only high-risk people were tested (with a true prevalence of approximately 20 percent), the cost of detecting each infected individual dropped to $128. On a cost basis alone, universal testing appeared to be prohibitively expensive and intrusive.[85]

Despite the costs and privacy issues involved, large numbers of Americans advocated universal (or at least widespread) testing. "This is not a civil rights question," wrote cancer physician Burton Lee. "This issue . . . is clearly one of the most serious public health crises this country has ever faced. This infection is contagious, and it is *fatal!*"[86] Other physicians concurred, with the American Medical Association breaking precedent and recommending that physicians notify sex partners of HIV-positive patients of their patients' status.[87] Regardless of cost in both monetary and legal terms, stopping AIDS required the most aggressive efforts known to public health and medicine. Education could have only a negligible effect, argued some, with statistics showing that nearly one in two gay men continued to engage in unprotected anal sex, *despite understanding the risks involved.*[88] Moreover, testing might help AIDS-infected patients too, as AZT therapy could be initiated earlier in the disease's course, and opportunistic infections (particularly tuberculosis) could be treated more aggressively.[89] One physician even suggested that lack of universal testing would frighten people from engaging in sex, thus leading to declining marriage and birth rates.

Perhaps the most prominent advocate for universal testing was Vice President George H. W. Bush, who articulated his support for the measure in a televised speech in June 1987. The vice president was perceived, generally, as more socially tolerant than President Reagan, and would later speak frequently on the need for greater government support for AIDS research and treatment. But his fundamental pragmatism in policymaking drove him to support broad, if not universal, testing for AIDS, if such a measure could possibly save lives and inhibit the disease's spread.[90]

Bush's stance drew substantial derision; he was openly heckled, and gay advocacy groups tried to portray him as homophobic and possibly fundamentalist. His speeches drew support too, however, and many viewers wrote in to articulate their pleasure. "I do believe the average American is not as stupid as the audience you were unfortunate enough to be faced with—who must believe in magic," wrote one Florida voter.[91] Wrote another: "You were booed by the audience, and I simply could not believe my ears. It should be obvious . . . that the first step toward the control of any infectious, epidemic-like process is to identify *all* the carriers."[92]

Policymakers in the Reagan White House strongly supported testing, arguing that eschewing it was an abnegation of the government's obligation to protect the public. Various White House advisers argued that most of the objections to testing were specious, and all could either be negated or were worth the cost in order to control the epidemic. White House adviser Gary Bauer suggested, for example, that AIDS testing needn't carry a stigma if it were truly applied universally, while the Domestic Policy Council suggested that a testing regime that could protect confidentiality and identify false positives could be designed if the will existed.[93] Overall, the counsel argued, precise knowledge of the disease must supersede virtually all other considerations if an immense catastrophe was to be thwarted. Advised a White House staffer to the council, "It is not hyperbole to suggest that this is the most important question before government today and must remain so until it can be shown, with certainty, that the security of the nation and the life of the human species is not at risk."[94]

Ultimately, Reagan deferred to the states on the issue. While strongly urging states to develop testing requirements for admitted hospital patients, STD and substance abuse clinic patrons, and marriage applicants, he refrained from issuing a binding federal injunction. He did stiffen Immigration and Naturalization Service (INS) testing protocols and demanded that AIDS be added to the list of contagious diseases for which an alien or immigration applicant could be denied entry to the United States, and he demanded testing of all federal prison inmates. (The armed services were already testing all inductees.) But he stopped short of demanding nationwide testing for state and local inmates, and eschewed universal testing requirements altogether.[95]

Testing advocates drew added ammunition from foreign examples: particularly the Soviet Union and Cuba. By 1987, the best statistics available (which were admittedly questionable) indicated that AIDS had made almost no inroads into the Soviet Union.[96] While differing social mores and diplomatic isolationism explained some of the phenomenon, the country's aggressive efforts at testing and identification were partially responsible as well. In September 1987, the country began requiring involuntary testing on demand for both citizens and foreign residents: resisters could be forcibly detained in a clinic, or expelled from the country. Moreover, infected persons who knowingly spread the virus could be imprisoned for up to eight years. The country had already deported numerous students (mostly from Africa) who had tested positive, and was warning its citizens to avoid having sex with Americans and resident diplomats.

More compelling for testing advocates was the case of Cuba. Unlike the Soviet Union, Cuba maintained relatively open borders, lay proximate to the United States, and nearly touched one of the epicenters of the early stages of the AIDS epidemic—Haiti. Yet Cuba had been extraordinarily successful in limiting the epidemic, despite being poor by Western standards, with limited access to the most modern medical techniques and resources.

Although Cuba did not mandate universal testing, its physicians had the latitude to test anybody they chose, without permission, and to initiate aggressive contact tracing (as they could do with all STDs). Cuban doctors actively inquired into risk factors in their patients (inmates, pregnant women, known drug users, carriers of other STDs) and ordered testing when the patients' profiles indicated it. When HIV was detected, its carriers were forcibly incarcerated in the nation's well-developed sanitarium system, in which they were reported to be treated humanely. The whole system was designed to protect the public's health, while also according as much dignity as possible to the diseased patients. "I as a doctor don't have to have someone's permission to test them," stated infectious disease doctor Jorge Perez. "I don't ask. Testing isn't mandatory, but I simply prescribe a test when I have good reason."[97]

Although skeptics questioned the "humanity" with which Cuba treated its patients, and doubted the efficacy of the program, disease prevalence records ultimately vindicated its policies. The nation would never have the funds to purchase the expensive antiviral treatments that became available in the United States and other industrialized nations over the next decade, but it maintained one of the lowest incidences of AIDS in the world. By 1997, fewer than 1,700 Cubans (out of a population of 11 million) had been infected, and only 442 had died. By that time, 362,000 Americans had died of AIDS. Cuba's per capita death rate was an astounding 1/24 as large as America's. Stated one American epidemiologist: "Cuban figures are absolutely reliable and dependable. Surveillance is quite good because they have essentially universal testing and an excellent tracking system. We trust the Cuban figures more than any other country's."[98]

Opponents of mandatory testing argued their case just as vociferously. Testing would benefit AIDS victims hardly at all, given the limited efficacy of AZT, while little evidence supported the conjecture that patients tested under duress would voluntarily desist from activities that could spread the disease. The high cost and persistent problem with false positives also argued against universal testing, as did the questionable practice of testing without counseling and follow-up behavioral-modification programs. Instead, almost all opponents argued for broadly available voluntary testing accompanied by support services for those found to be seropositive. "Scarce public funds could be better spent providing anonymous voluntary test sites," wrote Surgeon General Koop in April 1987,[99] and elsewhere he stated, "I would think anybody who is getting married today would want to be tested and would want to know."[100]

Besides the civil rights argument, which appealed more to libertarian zealots than to the general populace, the most persuasive argument against testing lay in the experience of the gay community. Through community-based initiatives, self-policing, and expansive educational efforts, the gay community had practically stopped AIDS in its tracks. Although the incidence of AIDS followed by some years actual HIV infection (owing to the long incubation period), all statistics indicated that the spread of AIDS had begun to slow among gays by 1985, and that new cases of HIV infection were declining by 1987. More available STD proxy markers showed extraordinary declines, with the incidence of rectal gonorrhea (to choose one) declining by 83 percent in the mid-1980s.[101]

In fact, proponents on both sides of the issue were getting their facts wrong. True, many gays continued to have unprotected anal intercourse in the aftermath of condom education, but they were sharply reducing the numbers of partners with whom they had sex, thus limiting their risk. And yes, the gay community had been highly successful in changing its ways and practices, but only after health and medical authorities had applied pressure repeatedly. Yes, the ELISA test did result in high numbers of false positives, but nearly all of these could be eliminated by following up with the Western Blot test. On the other hand, many people testing falsely positive would be traumatized by the experience, even if ultimately "cleared," and targeted (as opposed to universal) testing could prevent many of these unfortunate happenstances in the first place. Misunderstanding and misinformation about costs, techniques, results, and the efficacy of various programs all complicated the discussion considerably.[102]

Perhaps most forgotten in the debate was whether the information gleaned from a universal testing program, even if accurate and reliable, could actually prove useful. Testing (or other forms of disease identification) historically had been used as a precursor to intervention—usually in the form of a quarantine, isolation, or port closure. Such actions made sense when the threat posed by the disease was short-lived, as in the case of smallpox or cholera. AIDS, however, was a permanent condition. Patients would need to be quarantined for life: an action that defied all precedents in modern industrialized societies. Almost nobody in the United Stated considered widespread and permanent quarantine a reasonable option in intervening in the AIDS epidemic—editors of the *New England Journal of Medicine* deemed it "atrocious" and feared that its very mention "fuels public fear."[103] In the absence of such will, universal testing seemed senseless. Better to test those who wished to be tested, in the hope that they would voluntarily refrain from high-risk activities, inform previous partners, and generally bear the mantle of responsibility that an HIV diagnosis brought.

TROUBLE WITH HEALTH INSURANCE

Conservatives and liberals also locked horns over health insurance. Although most Americans who had health insurance in 1986 received their insurance through a group (usually their employer) or the government (in the form of either Medicaid or Medicare), a significant minority continued to purchase their policies individually. Those individuals, usually self-employed professionals and small business owners and employees, ran through a gamut of questions and probes constructed by health insurers to make sure that they did not pose an excessive risk to the company. If a high-risk factor was discovered, such as prior history of cancer, stroke, or heart disease, either the insurance premiums were adjusted accordingly, the condition was excluded under a "preexisting condition" clause, or insurance was denied altogether.

Not only was this type of risk-profiling allowable, it was the essence of the insurance industry. Insurers made their money by assessing and assigning risk in such a way that subscribers were able to pay the lowest premium possible for their particular risk profiles. The exception to this was a form of insurance pricing known as "community rating," in which insurers derived a risk profile of an entire community (a town, a state, or some other division) and required all beneficiaries to pay equal premiums, regardless of individual risk profiles. (Group insurance purchased through an employer was essentially community rated, with the community defined as the employees of that particular firm.) Historically, Blue Cross/Blue Shield plans had used community rating pricing in exchange for receiving certain types of tax preference by the states. For-profit firms had always priced based on individual risk profiles.

To say that AIDS was correlated with higher risk is almost a tautology—it practically *defined* high risk. For example, a random group of 1,000 American males in their mid-30s selected in 1986 would be expected to produce 7.5 deaths per year. By contrast, a group of 1,000 AIDS patients in their mid-30s would produce 200 deaths per year. The AIDS group carried with it 26 times the risk of death of the non-AIDS group. Moreover, even those who did not die would draw disproportionate payments from the insurers in the form of hospital, physician, and medication bills.

Recognizing the extraordinary risk posed by AIDS patients, health insurers, starting in 1983, began to aggressively screen out such patients by asking them directly whether or not they were infected with HIV, by having them tested, or by demanding to see their prior medical records. When AIDS victims resisted providing answers, insurers began to seek proxy markers for AIDS, such as intravenous drug use and homosexual activity. And when those proxy markers became unavailable to insurance companies, they resorted to secondary proxy markers, such as residence in specific (heavily gay) neighborhoods, or involvement in certain professions disproportionately populated by gay men such as hairdressing or floral arranging. The Great Republic Insurance Company, which lacked the foresight to keep such policies unwritten, had required its salesmen to be wary of "single males without dependents . . . in occupations that do not require physical exertion."[104] Other insurers did not aggressively select out gays, but rather capped benefits for AIDS treatment at extremely low levels—for example, $5,000 per year, with a lifetime maximum of $15,000 in the case of one insurance company.

These types of discriminatory practices raised the ire of gay advocacy groups, but also of liberals in general. Many Americans who had long propounded some sort of national health plan viewed health insurance as a vehicle for redistributive justice. In the decades when Blue Cross plans had dominated the market, the tax exempt status of the plans and their highly regulated operations and pricing had accomplished just that.[105] But for-profit insurers, whose market share had increased during the 1980s, operated for the benefit of their shareholders and their individual subscribers: not for the general welfare. For these companies, not only was competitive pricing necessary to ensure profits, it was necessary to remain viable. "If we charged the premiums necessary to cover AIDS claims," noted Provident Indemnity president James Hellauer, "our premiums would be beyond the affordability of most small businesses."[106] And in response to accusations of homophobic bias, company executives responded that their whole business was based on bias, albeit against diseases rather than people. Explained Metropolitan Life vice chairman Philip Briggs: "We see this as just a disease problem. . . . So it is not a question of discriminating against gays, it's a question of underwriting a risk which can affect really any number of people."[107] Rob Bier of the American Council of Life Insurance stated the insurers' credo more succinctly: "It's bad business to write off entire groups—we want to sell insurance."[108]

In an effort to protect the more socially expansive characteristics of health insurance, several states began regulating against AIDS testing or anti–AIDS discrimination in any form by insurance companies starting in 1986. Heavily Democratic Washington, D.C., was first to pass such a law, with California, Massachusetts, and New York following closely. In each of these states (or districts), insurers were prohibited from testing, inquiring, or in any other way adjusting insurance premiums based on HIV status. Further, in Washington, insurers were prohibited from adjusting rates based on zip code, occupation, or marital status.

Such actions quickly backfired. In Washington, for example, many insurers simply stopped offering individual policies entirely, or else excluded all AIDS benefits.[109] Members of Congress exerted enormous pressure on the D.C. City Council to rescind the testing ban, with Senator Jesse Helms (R-North Carolina) threatening to freeze the entire municipal budget unless the ban was removed.[110] In Massachusetts, Governor Michael Dukakis came to the aid of insurers by reversing the ban on testing, although his insurance commissioner resigned in protest over the policy.[111] And although the nation's insurance commissioners had issued recommendations for states to bar AIDS testing as early as 1986, few states proved willing to impose the guidelines lest they jeopardize local insurers.

The posturing surrounding the legislation was largely political. Although testing bans could be issued, insurers could either deny AIDS benefits outright, reduce them to inadequate levels, or find proxy markers for AIDS. Insurers were exquisitely sensitive to statistical risk profiles, and maintained reams of data allowing them (through sophisticated statistical testing) to determine the likelihood that a potential applicant posed a high risk for AIDS. Furthermore, the high cost associated with treating AIDS created strong inducements for insurance companies to exclude any high-risk individual from their rolls. The real burden of the antitesting bans fell on those individuals who displayed a high-risk profile, but were in fact HIV-negative. Those individuals would have been able to purchase insurance had testing been allowed, but were now effectively excluded.

THE COMMISSION'S REPORT

Early in 1988, President Reagan's AIDS commission, whose leadership early on had passed to retired Navy admiral James Watkins, issued its final report. The gargantuan document, replete with 597 recommendations, was far more liberal than many government watchers had expected, with emphasis on new antidiscrimination laws, confidentiality, and assurances of civil rights. The commission firmly argued against mandatory testing and reporting, and suggested that partner notification was an inappropriate activity for health-care providers. And, it argued for new federal protections to maintain the anonymity of people who tested positive for AIDS. In short, the report advocated against nearly all measures promoted by conservative AIDS watchers.

The commission emphasized that AIDS was rapidly moving from gays to IV drug users and their partners, and strongly recommended that drug treatment programs be expanded. It also recommended fast-tracking new pharmaceuticals (through the FDA clinical testing process) and strengthening the nation's long-term care infrastructure. And (to the relief of conservatives) it recommended criminalizing the act of knowingly passing on the AIDS virus.

Reagan administration officials responded with lukewarm enthusiasm, thanking Watkins and other commission members for their "excellent" work, while suggesting that many of the recommendations needed to be considered, pondered, and perhaps implemented slowly, if at all. "We need to prepare ourselves for the long haul," noted White House adviser Ian McDonald. Many of the commission's recommendations were perhaps "best left to the next Administration."[112] The acerbic *Economist* newsmagazine described the report as "another rebuke" to the administration.[113] By contrast, AIDS advocates and civil rights organizations were generally, and unexpectedly, pleased with the commission's recommendation for better protections against discrimination, with Lori Behrman of the Gay Men's Health Crisis calling it "excellent, very compassionate, fair and aggressive."[114]

Over the following six months, Reagan officials fomented a response to the report, trying to abide by the spirit of the recommendations while taking little concrete action. They planned a series of "consensus conferences," took steps to inform recipients of blood transfusions that they were at risk, increased allocations to drug treatment programs, and devised a plan to facilitate FDA testing for "fast-track" drugs. Moreover, they issued plans for a large new building on the NIH's Bethesda campus as well as several new buildings at the CDC's headquarters in Atlanta. Further, they increased allocations to the various government agencies conducting AIDS research and relief, with total federal AIDS funding slated to double between 1987 and 1989.[115] On the other hand, the administration eschewed almost entirely the commission's central recommendations concerning antidiscrimination legislation and protections of anonymity.

Astute AIDS watchers noted that many of the commission's recommendations had been presaged by the Institute of Medicine's (IOM) 1986 document, *Confronting AIDS*. The IOM, a subsidiary of the National Academy of Sciences, had similarly recommended expanded drug treatment and needle exchanges, and protections against testing, quarantines, discrimination, and screenings.[116] Both organizations had advocated more funding for research, pharmaceutical development, and the ubiquitous educational efforts.

That the IOM had so vindicated liberals was to be expected. Its base in the academic and public health communities suggested it would cleave to the traditional path. But the Watkins commission surprised almost everybody. Watkins, himself, was known as a traditional and conservative Catholic, whose personal mores and military conduct seemed to presage a more moralistic approach to the epidemic. Furthermore, most government watchers agreed that Watkins had almost single-handedly molded the commission and forced it to consensus. Like Koop, Watkins had investigated the facts of the epidemic, and concluded that the most effective interventions and actions (among a panoply of mostly ineffective options) involved education, treatment, social networks, and a hope that the future would bring more effective medical interventions. Disciplining AIDS victims or forcing them to the margins of society would, in the conclusions of both men, be counterproductive and inhumane.

Americans, it seemed, more or less agreed with the commission's recommendations, despite vocal opposition from ardent conservatives. A radical ballot proposition in California (No. 102) calling for mandatory disclosure of AIDS victims and requiring contact tracing failed badly at the polls in late 1988. Congressman Bill Dannemeyer's repeated efforts to pass legislation requiring reporting and testing for prisoners, patients, and marriage applicants were repeatedly defeated as well. And although many Americans privately agreed with Dannemeyer's vociferous pronouncements about "embracing the heterosexual ethic," most did not wish to grant either federal or state governments broad powers to test and demonize AIDS victims.

In the end, Reagan's record on AIDS was middling to poor. Although he eschewed the vitriolic gay-baiting rhetoric of the Far Right, his reluctance to fully embrace the disaster in all of its magnitude exposed his latent homophobia, or disengagement, or both. In his one public speech on AIDS (to the College of Physicians in Philadelphia in April 1987), he noted how U.S. scientists were making rapid progress in identifying and fighting the virus, suggesting that a viable vaccine would soon be available, and then quickly moved on to extol the miracles that American medicine was producing.[117] Although he greatly increased government spending on all aspects of AIDS between 1983 and 1988, he consistently failed to spend the entire budget allotted to him by Congress. People who were well informed on the epidemic recognized Reagan's basic decency, but also his incompetence in this area. "The White House record on AIDS . . . is one of confusion and neglect, complicated by an almost willful refusal to face the facts," noted Congressman Henry Waxman (D-California).[118] Seagram and Company senior executive Stephen Herbits, a committed Republican and veteran of the Nixon and Ford administrations, wrote critically: "The simple truth is that the President has a moral and probably constitutional imperative to trigger America's best defense from this plague. He has yet to exercise it."[119] And when Vice President George Bush won the White House in November 1988, much to the chagrin of gay and AIDS advocates, even the liberal (and ardently Dukakis-biased) *Boston Globe* projected an improvement in federal AIDS policy. "He cannot possibly do less than President Reagan, and there is reason to expect that Bush will do far more."[120]

CHAPTER 5

ORGANIZING AND SELLING

As the epidemic took hold in the early 1980s, gay men coalesced informally to commiserate and share information. In the major AIDS centers of the nation, before the disease even had a name, small groups began to organize themselves into information clearinghouses, educational resource centers, and political lobbying teams. San Franciscans organized the KS/AIDS Foundation and People with AIDS in late 1981 and early 1982, while in New York City gay activists Michael Callen and Richard Berkowitz organized Gay Men with AIDS. Representatives of these groups, along with other nascent organizations, attended a conference of other People with AIDS (PWA) organizations in Denver in 1983 to define lobbying goals and discuss political tactics.[1]

At the same time, a small group of men organized a fund-raising dance in New York in April 1982 to support AIDS-related research. The men, who had all attended a lecture by local physician Alvin Friedman-Kien in writer Larry Kramer's apartment the previous summer, organized themselves as the Gay Men's Health Crisis (GMHC) with the intention of supporting research, providing health-related information, and facilitating patient care for AIDS patients. Distinct from the PWA groups, GMHC did not view itself as a lobbying organization, and generally eschewed advocacy activities beyond a narrow clinical mandate.

Within the year, the Whitman-Walker Clinic, a Washington-based venereal disease clinic that had been serving the gay community since the early 1970s, reoriented itself to serving the needs of AIDS patients. And in Chicago, Boston, and Los Angeles, local gays organized the Fenway Clinic, the Howard Brown Memorial Clinic, and the Gay and Lesbian Community Services Center, respectively. All of these grew rapidly over the following decade. Under the leadership of local attorney Jim Graham, for example, Whitman-Walker ballooned from 5 staffers in 1984 to 115 a decade later, providing dental and medical services, housing, street outreach programs, educational literature, and pharmaceutical support.[2]

Perhaps the most comprehensive service foundations could be found in San Francisco. In that city, the AIDS Foundation grew from a nearly identical ferment as GMHC, with gay men raising money beginning in April 1982 to fund informational flyers and a KS help line. Within a year, it had received a contract with the San Francisco Health Department to provide AIDS education and information, and within five years it had several dozen staffers drawing from a multimillion-dollar budget to operate a clinic, a hot line, a crisis intervention service, and assorted educational programs. At the same time, the Shanti Project, a San Francisco community organization founded in 1974 to help people contend with issues surrounding death and dying, focused its resources on AIDS and also contracted with the San Francisco Health Department. Besides providing mental health counseling, volunteers for Shanti provided emergency food and transportation services, and generally strengthened the porous social safety net into which AIDS victims often fell.[3] By the late 1980s, the AIDS Foundation was operating satellite centers in northern California, and had also begun to provide food, housing, pharmaceuticals, and family services. Like the GMHC and Whitman-Walker, both Shanti and the AIDS Foundation had transformed themselves from informal community groups to sophisticated bureaucracies in the space of half a decade.[4]

All of the community AIDS organizations relied heavily on volunteer labor, ranging from low-level sick visits and shopping assistance to sophisticated pro bono legal and medical services. Volunteers initially came almost exclusively from the gay community, but as the epidemic progressed they came from the outside community as well. People were drawn to serve for many reasons, but many volunteers had seen friends and relatives touched by the disease, and felt compelled to intervene in whatever way they could. Reflected one GMHC volunteer: "I deeply identified with these men. I wanted to offer the support I hope that I would get if I were to come down with it. There is a sense of taking care of one's own."[5] In a similar vein, one of the directors of the GMHC referred to the organization as "a family of healers."[6]

As the disease progressed, these service organizations began to sort themselves into one of three types, oriented toward either social or clinical services, or research.[7] While most of the organizations began with a mission of education and outreach as well as providing psychosocial support, several, such as the GMHC and the Whitman-Walker Clinic, began to allocate large portions of their resources to clinical services. The move resulted in part from the simple fact that a surprising number of AIDS patients appeared to be living beyond the predicted one- to two-year life span of an HIV-infected individual. By 1987, CDC researchers realized that while half of all AIDS victims were dying within a year of diagnosis, at least 15 percent appeared to be living five years or more. And a very few, perhaps 1 to 2 percent, appeared to show no signs of deterioration at all.[8]

INPATIENT RESOURCES

Although AIDS per se could not be treated except with the largely ineffective AZT, the opportunistic infections that afflicted AIDS patients could be treated, as could the AIDS-related dementia that afflicted nearly 1 in 10 AIDS patients.[9] As the infections attacked the bodies of AIDS patients, the patients sought help from their physicians in the form of powerful antibiotics, fungicides, chemotherapeutic agents, and even ultraviolet radiation. Initially all treatments were dispensed on an outpatient basis, but ultimately the patients almost always resorted to inpatient treatment in the infectious disease ward of a general hospital. Patients might spend their final weeks or months in an ICU, or be transferred to a long-term-care facility or hospice. Regardless, the treatment tended to be extraordinarily expensive (averaging $40,000 per patient by 1987) and difficult to tolerate.

AIDS patients sought treatment from a variety of sources, primarily their own private physicians and local hospitals. Large numbers of doctors, however, were unfamiliar with the disease and its symptoms (sometimes purposefully so) and thus referred patients aggressively to infectious-disease specialists or to internists with established practices in gay-related ailments. But by 1987, many of these physicians were overwhelmed with the surge in cases, and many had capped their practices.

Exacerbating the shortage, a number of doctors actively resisted treating all AIDS patients for fear of their own safety. In dealing with AIDS, a common needlestick could be fatal, and even contact with the usual fluids and bloody rags that suffused general hospital wards posed unknown risks. One particularly alarmist physician at San Francisco General Hospital required her surgical team to wear a panoply of protective coverings, ranging from double-thickness plastic shoe guards to reinforced disposable hospital gowns, sleeve guards, and helmets with their own internal air supply when operating on AIDS patients. Some physicians began taking AZT prophylactically, while others walked off the job altogether.[10] Surgeon General Koop derided this latter group as a "fearful and irrational minority" who engaged in "unprofessional conduct."[11]

A large number of patients were ultimately treated in the local public hospital, either because no other hospital would accept them, no other hospital had the expertise or the staff to treat AIDS, or because the patient had exhausted his or her insurance benefits and savings. Starting in the mid-1980s, indigent AIDS patients flooded the wards and emergency rooms of the nation's municipal and county hospitals, which had no choice but to admit them. Some had been transferred ("dumped") from private hospitals, some had been admitted directly from private physicians, and many had admitted themselves through the emergency rooms. These patients tended to be more advanced in their symptoms, less robust in their underlying health, and frequently afflicted with a host of exacerbating problems such as drug abuse, homelessness, poverty, or other chronic diseases.

For public hospitals, the rising caseload threatened to exhaust their bed space and their financial resources. In some urban areas, 40–50 percent of medical (as opposed to surgical) beds in public hospitals were occupied by AIDS patients by 1987, leaving fewer beds for remaining patients whose private insurance policies could help the hospital defer the costs.[12] A few hospitals with large infectious-disease practices declared bankruptcy, or quietly closed, while others pleaded with city councils or state legislators for additional emergency funds.[13] Even when funds were forthcoming, they were often inadequate. In heavily hit Newark, New Jersey, for example, the public University Hospital found that it was losing between $300 and $400 per day on each drug-addicted AIDS patient, even when the patients were covered by the state Medicaid program. Total losses per patient approached $9,000, and with nearly 20 percent of all beds in the hospital devoted to AIDS care by 1987, the losses threatened to undermine the hospital's solvency.[14] As AIDS cases mounted, the hospital's residency programs were threatened as well, as young medical graduates began to shun the program. In a survey that year of 24 fourth-year medical students interested in internal medicine who were rotating through University Hospital, 22 admitted that they would not apply for an internal medicine residency there. "It's begun to hurt the program," admitted the president of the affiliated medical school.[15]

In this environment, Whitman-Walker and GMHC began to consider expanding their clinical services. For Whitman-Walker, which had evolved from a preexisting VD clinic, the decision was natural; for GMHC, it required a realignment. Yet by 1988, both organizations were providing high levels of clinical services to the AIDS-stricken community, often drawing on unparalleled treatment expertise. In that year, Whitman-Walker (to cite one example) treated 811 inpatients, 329 dental patients, tested nearly 4,500 people for HIV antibodies, and provided direct social services such as case management, housing, legal assistance, home companions, and financial assistance to over 1,000.[16] To produce those services, the clinic employed a staff of 60 full-time employees, and over 1,000 volunteers.

Money for these patient services came from a variety of sources, including Medicaid reimbursement, private insurance, fund-raising, and philanthropy. Medicaid was most important, for although gay men did not lack private health insurance significantly more than did the nation at large (with a 15-percent uninsured rate), they did more frequently exhaust their insurance coverage, and thus were forced to "spend down" to Medicaid eligibility. By the time many patients arrived at Whitman-Walker or GMHC, they had exhausted their private insurance benefits as well as their personal savings, and had fallen onto the medium-soft landing of their state's Medicaid benefits.

Medicaid benefits could be generous or stingy, depending on the state, as states set their own eligibility levels and reimbursement schedules. Fortunately for AIDS victims, the majority lived in three of the states with the most generous Medicaid reimbursement levels in the nation: California, New York, and New Jersey, with the District of Columbia close behind. Thus, although the prerequisite poverty necessary to qualify for Medicaid was quite harsh, the reality was that purchasing care with Medicaid money in those states was reasonably easy. So long as the professional expertise and bed space existed (and this was by no means assured), Medicaid benefits could cover a substantial portion of the costs.

Medicaid did not cover all of the program costs these organizations incurred however, and to fund the balance they turned to fund-raising and philanthropy. Fund-raising efforts were frequent and imaginative in the early 1980s, with the organizations drawing on the sympathies of the gay community. GMHC, in particular, became known for its successful fund-raising events in those years, such as renting out all of Madison Square Garden for a performance of the Ringling Brothers Circus in 1983, or the $1,000-per-seat "Best of the Best" event at the Metropolitan Opera House two years later. GMHC also started its annual "AIDS Walk" in 1987, bringing substantial publicity as well as funding to the organization. By 1990, the event was grossing nearly $4 million annually and attracting 25,000 walkers who garnered donations from nearly 200,000 sponsors. Other events included all-night dance-a-thons, and the "Music for Life" concert (featuring Leonard Bernstein and James Levine).[17]

ACT UP AND THE LAVENDER HILL MOB

Underlying the rich ferment of community activity, however, lay rifts. Gay community leaders, newly energized and politicized, quickly began to disagree about priorities, missions, and styles. Even as patient-service organizations posted impressive gains in their capacity to treat, nourish, and provide succor, some gay activists and community leaders suggested that the organizations had either lost their way or had drifted from their initial purpose, or perhaps had misdefined their purpose to begin with. Reflected Arthur Felson: "I can't pick up a local gay paper without getting supremely depressed—not about AIDS statistics but because gay men have been reduced to horrid little infighting sessions, blaming each other for screwing up the AIDS Foundation or selling somebody-or-other down the river."[18]

No one so angered his peers and comrades as activist and playwright Larry Kramer. The driving force behind the establishment of GMHC, by 1984 Kramer was regularly protesting that organization's emphasis on direct patient services, and lambasting its board and director for their unwillingness to turn to lobbying and political activism. Calling GMHC board members "equal to murderers" at one point, he was ejected from that body and failed to regain membership despite repeated efforts.[19] "THERE IS NOTHING IN THIS WHOLE AIDS MESS THAT IS NOT POLITICAL!" he wrote in an open letter to GMHC executive director Richard Dunne in 1987. "How can you deny this fact and assert that your role must remain unpolitical?"[20]

Demonstrating a similar rift in Washington, Whitman-Walker director Jim Graham drew widespread criticism for inviting First Lady Barbara Bush to visit the clinic. Hoping to win support from Congress and enrich his fund-raising network from the visit, Graham drew harsh invectives from activists. "Her candles are not enough to solve the torment of people with AIDS grinding their teeth in writhing pain," wrote gay columnist Stephen Smith. "Jim Graham, j'accuse. I charge you with treason! Your treachery offends people with AIDS. You have made a pact with the evil one, signed with our tainted blood."[21]

Kramer's response was to found the AIDS Coalition to Unleash Power (ACT UP) in 1987, a quasi-guerrilla organization dedicated to public disruption, attention-getting antics, and extreme protests. The group's activities ranged from humorous to offensive, with members necking in the office of Republican senator Jesse Helms, creating traffic jams, and disrupting trading on the New York Stock Exchange. The group gained notoriety when it disrupted communion during mass at New York's Saint Patrick's Cathedral and crumbled communion wafers on the floor. In response to criticism from more genteel gay organizations, an ACT UP member claimed, "It is ACT UP's job to be disruptive and it is the job of the other AIDS groups to pick up the pieces."[22]

Paralleling the activities of ACT UP, the Lavender Hill Mob, a similar radical gay activist organization, carried out its own protests and media stunts in the mid and late 1980s. Led by several older veterans of some of the original gay liberation groups from the 1970s such as Marty Robinson and Henry Yaeger, the Lavender Hill Mob carried out "zaps" at the Alfred E. Smith Dinner (the annual gathering of New York's Catholic Democratic Party leaders) in 1986, at Saint Patrick's Cathedral, at the offices of Senator Alphonse D'Amato (R-New York), and at the headquarters of the CDC in Atlanta. Their antics included dressing as priests to gain access to the pulpit at Saint Patrick's, buying a table at the Alfred E. Smith Dinner to gain entrance for the purpose of protesting the speakers, and placing mock arrest warrants in Senator D'Amato's office for the murder of the thousands who had died from AIDS. At a conference at CDC headquarters, two "mobsters" entered the hall dressed as concentration camp inmates, including pink triangle patches.[23]

Some of the protest activities merited applause, regardless of the tactics. The groups attracted high levels of media coverage to the AIDS epidemic, garnered the attention of the FDA and of Congress, and generally raised public awareness of the ongoing tragedy. In its most tangible victory, ACT UP persuaded the Burroughs-Wellcome pharmaceutical company to lower the price of AZT from $8,000 to $6,400 for a year's supply of the drug. And it forced the Pentagon and various companies to at least reconsider their policies regarding homosexuality, partners' health-care benefits, and discriminatory practices in hiring.

On the other hand, ACT UP and the Lavender Hill Mob alienated

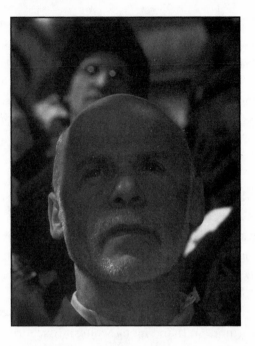

Activist and author
Larry Kramer.
(Stockphoto)

the preponderance of people who witnessed their actions, possibly damaging the cause of AIDS more than it helped. "Larry Kramer is about as rotten a person as I've ever encountered," stated Dunne. "He's shrill, tiresome, and a bully."[24] And others worried that ACT UP's focus on AIDS, to the exclusion of all other challenges facing homosexuals, would ultimately prove destructive to the community. Even as gays were dying of AIDS, they continued to face limits on their civil rights, discrimination in hiring, lack of access to marital protections, and not-infrequent outbursts of violence. "The increase in anti-gay violence, the perpetuation of sodomy laws and civil-rights abuses are going to destroy more lives than AIDS will ever destroy," predicted gay activist Darrell Yates Rist.[25]

To his credit, Kramer admitted his own irascibility, even if he unapologetically insisted on his rectitude. On his split with GMHC president Paul Popham, Kramer noted: "He knew he was right and I knew I was right. He was a much better team player than I'll ever be."[26] At the same time, Kramer felt that given the magnitude of the disaster, aggressive action was the only reasonable response for gays. "I was out to attack every perceived enemy in sight," he explained.

"Reagan, doctors, the NIH, the AMA—you name it, I was after it."[27] But Popham and others differed, feeling that cooperation and subtle persuasion would prove to be the more constructive tools. Kramer felt that Popham was wrong. Ironically, the playwright had pleaded to fellow gays at the onset of the epidemic, "There is one thing we must not allow AIDS to become, and that is a *political* issue among ourselves."[28]

MINORITIES AND LESBIANS

Blacks faced different challenges in combating AIDS, and began developing their own communal response in the mid-1980s. Disproportionately afflicted with poverty and drug use problems, they quickly began to contract AIDS in numbers disproportionate to their presence in the population. In addition, a general cultural discomfort with homosexuality (more so than among whites) dissuaded gay black men from disclosing their sexuality, while at the same time deterring traditional black communal institutions from confronting the crisis. Although by 1987 AIDS was proving to be the worst health crisis ever to hit black America, neither the NAACP, the Southern Christian Leadership Conference, nor the Urban League was devoting anything beyond trivial sums to combat it.

The community responded by establishing new organizations, such as the Minority Task Force on AIDS (New York), the San Francisco Black Coalition on AIDS, the Minority AIDS Project (Los Angeles), and Blacks Educating Blacks about Sexual Health Issues (BEBASHI) in Philadelphia. These organizations, underfunded and manned nearly entirely by volunteers, were incapable of replicating the type of clinical and case management services provided by the major AIDS organizations. Rather, they focused on educating black youths and adolescents on sexuality and safe-sex techniques, and on drug use. In 1988, the CDC provided $7 million to agencies and organizations specifically addressing minority AIDS concerns.[29]

Black AIDS community groups faced particular challenges in confronting high degrees of homophobia, or simple denial, within the black community. Gay blacks, more so than gay whites, kept their homosexuality hidden, and were more likely to lead unreconciled and inconsistent sexual lives, hiding their preferences from those around them. At the same time, black community leaders (particularly ministers) were reluctant to discuss black homosexuality, or even admit its existence. Homosexuality ran counter to the basically conservative morality code of the black church, and to the image of the community. Moreover, in a community grappling with substantial social pathologies, AIDS seemed less compelling, or perhaps simply too much to contend with. "We've got enough stigma," stated one leader. "We don't need to add AIDS to it."[30] Similarly, the Reverend Carl Bean of Los Angeles's Minority AIDS Project related: "People walk in with AIDS, but they also walk in with poverty. We're dealing with mothers who have to grease the crib legs and place them in cans of oil to keep the rats off the crib, kids who still hunt down soda bottles to buy potato chips for a meal."[31] But such sentiments did not win over all adherents. After years of this sort of quasi-institutional denial, Ronald Johnson, director of the Minority Task Force on AIDS exploded: "There's not one black or Hispanic legislator who has done a goddamned thing about AIDS in this city, state, or country. And that's disgusting."[32]

But most paradoxical was the lesbian response to the epidemic. From the beginning, AIDS was exclusively a problem for male, rather than female, homosexuals. Differences in sexuality, promiscuity, and simple biology dictated that HIV would spread quickly among sexually active gay men, but hardly at all among lesbian women. Nonetheless, lesbians had long aligned themselves politically with gay men in their fight for equal rights, partner benefits, and general antidefamation legislation, and thus many felt compelled to partner with their male compatriots in fighting for AIDS funding, services, and research.

AIDS exposed the underlying enigma of lesbian identity: the pull between forging alliances with feminists on the one hand or with gay rights activists on the other. In many ways, lesbian women followed the politics of the broader feminist movement, albeit in a more "rejectionist" mold. They played an active role in mainstream feminist organizations and coalitions (NOW director Patricia Ireland was a known bisexual), and many saw their sexuality as an extension of their politics.

On the other hand, women who led exclusively lesbian lives faced many of the same prejudices as did gay men, ranging from job discrimination to inability to get marital benefits for their partners. Thus, lesbians had long allied themselves in certain areas with gay activist groups in a partnership born more of political necessity than of great collegialism and empathy. Consistent with this history, several lesbian women worked for AIDS organizations with the understanding that the type of discrimination shown toward AIDS victims could quickly bleed over to general chauvinism for heterosexuals. "A good deal of AIDS phobia is simply disguised homophobia. When thinking about the AIDS crisis, I often see images from Bergman's movie about the black plague in the Middle Ages, 'The Seventh Seal'—images of witch-burnings, flagellation, and the superstition that abounded at that time," stated Margaret Nichols, the director of the Hyacinth AIDS Foundation in New Jersey.[33] ACT UP member Mary Lucey opined more succinctly, "AIDS is a political disease."[34]

Most lesbians were unimpressed with this argument, however, and in general lesbians did not take active leadership roles in AIDS community organizations. Many lesbians had long disapproved of the promiscuity in the gay community, and felt alienated from the cult of physicality that abounded there. Some simply didn't like gay men, feeling that the culture was in some ways more "male" then general heterosexual culture. "Straight men at least have an incentive to pretend they respect women," joked one prominent lesbian.[35] But more generally, lesbians simply didn't view the epidemic as a threat to their well-being. Women who were not prostitutes or IV drug users simply did not frequently contract AIDS: lesbian women, all the less. The handful of lesbian women who had caught the disease were seen as aberrant, and even suspect. One lesbian who had tested positive for HIV felt the need to defend her sexuality to her skeptical lesbian associations, who had confronted her with the evidence of a heterosexual relationship. "Does that make me less of a lesbian if I did [have sex with a man]?" she demanded.[36] And one HIV-infected lesbian described being verbally attacked after discussing the need for safe sex among lesbians at a gay pride rally. "Where do you get your information about female to female transmissions? This is not a fact. Where is that written?" demanded the angry spectator.[37] Many lesbians agreed.[38]

THE SELLING OF AIDS

With the establishment of community-based AIDS organizations came a flowering of fund-raising. Once the afflicted (mostly gay) community realized that it had both the opportunity, and probably the obligation, to take action, it turned its attention to raising money to support its new programs. And in doing so, it managed to publicize the cause of AIDS to both potential donors and the public at large.

Perhaps the least controversial and most compelling form of AIDS fund-raising in the early years was for basic research. The cause of research fit neatly into a form of long-established charity that was at once linked to prestigious organizations (such as research universities and medical schools) without being hampered by images of actual AIDS patients. Research was apolitical, for whatever one felt about the people who actually contracted AIDS, nobody could dispute the validity of furthering scientific understanding. Moreover, the people actually being supported by the research funds were scientists, rather than AIDS patients, allowing donors to associate their philanthropy with brilliant individuals rather than men (and women) of questionable character.

One of the first and most successful research organizations to garner AIDS charity was the American Foundation for AIDS Research (Am-FAR), which began life in 1983 as the AIDS Medical Foundation. Founded by Memorial Sloan-Kettering researcher Mathilde Krim, along with her husband United Artists chairman Arthur Krim, the organization managed to raise over a half-million dollars within three months to support basic AIDS research. Hurrying about from congressional hearing to Hollywood fund-raising party to New York policy meeting, Krim quickly became one of the most visible advocates for AIDS research outside of the gay community, and managed nearly single-handedly to legitimize the disease as a charity for more establishment-minded philanthropists. "I personally didn't believe for a minute that being gay could cause it," Krim recalled in an interview. "It was a scientific and medical puzzle that attracted my attention."[39]

In a similar mold, Elizabeth Glaser, wife of television star Paul Michael Glaser, started the Pediatric AIDS Foundation with friends Susan DeLaurentis and Susan Zeegen in 1988 after discovering that she and

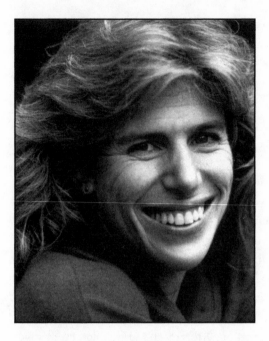

Pediatric AIDS activist
Elizabeth Glaser, who
galvanized Hollywood's
interest in the disease.
(Pediatric AIDS Foundation)

her two children were all HIV-positive. Glaser had contracted the virus in a 1981 blood transfusion, and then unknowingly passed it to both her daughter and son while breastfeeding. Blessed with high visibility in Hollywood, great public sympathy, and a tenacious commitment to fund-raising for her cause, Glaser managed to raise $3 million within two years of establishing her foundation, while lobbying Congress, appearing on national television, and generally winning over the public's sympathy. "Who is going to vote against Elizabeth Glaser?" asked AIDS Action Council head Tom Sheridan. "She has the public image that members of Congress respond to."[40]

Fund-raising for AIDS research soon became one of the most visible activities of New York and Los Angeles socialites, as movie celebrities began wearing red bows on their lapels and AIDS balls emerged on the fashion charity circuit. In New York, AIDS events were held at Lincoln Center, Carnegie Hall, and Christie's auction house. "People who wouldn't be caught dead at an AIDS benefit a few years ago are now begging to be invited," remarked AmFAR director Elizabeth Kummerfeld.[41] Fund-raising events included walks, runs, parties, dance marathons, performances, skate-a-thons, swim-a-thons, art auctions, and all-night raves. Reflected playwright Paul Rudnick a decade later, "It was soon possible to attend the Ringling Brothers circus, a Jessye Norman recital and the Mr. Leather New York contest, all with checkbook in hand."[42] David Seidner, a New York–based writer, observed wryly, "Never in history has so much schmalz been generated around an illness."[43]

Of course, the splendor of Hollywood parties meshed awkwardly with the reality of AIDS. While the creative professions, particularly the performing arts, had long been disproportionately gay, the reality was that by 1987, when fund-raising was accelerating rapidly, AIDS was already moving from gays to IV drug users and their partners. Even as speakers at fund-raisers spoke of the universality of the epidemic, and of how AIDS was a threat to all, the virus was becoming more and more firmly embedded in a small group of economically insignificant and largely invisible people. By 1987, by which point AmFAR had disbursed more than $8 million in research funds, the rate of HIV infection among Americans who belonged to no known risk group was 1 in 2,500, and actually diminishing. Wrote conservative writer Michael Fumento, "One would never know from all this that the profile of the typical victim of heterosexually transmitted AIDS is a lower-class black woman who is the regular sex partner of an IV drug user."[44]

A spectacular success in the effort to "sell" the epidemic was the AIDS quilt, which developed as a cause célèbre through the late 1980s. Conceived by San Franciscan Cleve Jones in 1986 upon the death of his longtime partner, the quilt was composed of a series of 3-by-6-foot panels, produced individually by many thousands of bereaved partners and family members, each memorializing an AIDS victim. The panels were sewn together into 12-by-12 foot parquet squares, which could be unfurled on a flat surface, individually or by the thousands, for a quilt display. Jones recalled his vision of the quilt as "bulldozing the Castro leaving only corpses lying in the sun." Each square was roughly the size of a grave, and when laid out by the thousands for a full display, portrayed the immensity of the tragedy.[45]

By October 1987, when the quilt was unfurled on the National Mall in Washington, it already memorialized 1,920 victims and measured 150 by 470 feet.[46] Within a decade, the quilt weighed 43 tons, covered

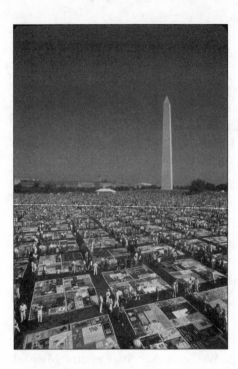

The AIDS quilt being displayed on the National Mall in 1993.
(Stockphoto)

24 football fields when fully displayed, required 12,000 volunteers to load and unload, and included 21 miles of walkway between the panels. Writer Andrew Sullivan described viewing the quilt thus:

> The quilt has to be entered in order to be understood; a piece of interactive architecture of both public and private space . . . The quilt is a buoyantly colorful, even witty monument. . . . [It is] a kind of chaotic living room, in which the unkempt [loose fragments] of human beings—their jeans, photographs, glasses, sneakers, letters—are strewn on the ground, as if expecting the people to whom they belonged to return. People walk over this cluttered landscape, looking like tourists, caught between grief and curiosity, saying little, peering intently down at the ground. . . . The point of it all . . . is not merely to release grief, but to affirm the dignity of those who have died so young and in the face of unique public disdain.[47]

But even as Hollywood and the arts communities embraced AIDS, much of the public was unwilling to accept the tragedy as their own.

AIDS in art and culture percolated up through small poetry reviews and fringe photographers, but major purveyors of art and entertainment eschewed the epidemic as subject matter through the 1980s. Despite a few noted exceptions (particularly Larry Kramer's AIDS-based play *The Normal Heart,* which opened to good reviews in Los Angeles in 1985), major movie studios and television networks avoided confronting or presenting AIDS, despite many leaders in the industry being themselves gay, and having been personally touched by the disease.[48]

Attitudes changed over time, however. As the decade drew to a close, several AIDS-oriented novels and plays, among them Robert Ferro's *Second Son,* William Hoffman's *As Is,* and Robert Chesley's *Jerker* all achieved some success, with *Jerker* airing in part on a California radio station. Television allowed AIDS to seep onto the air in a few episodes of *Midnight Caller* and the TV movies *The Littlest Victim* and *Intimate Contact.*

AIDS-in-art achieved some popular success with the release of the movie *Longtime Companion* in 1990, which chronicled the early AIDS epidemic. Although lacking big stars, and released to only limited numbers of theaters, the film's modest success convinced movie executives that the industry would not be irreparably tainted by presenting the AIDS epidemic, and might in fact even earn money and plaudits. Three years later, TriStar Pictures released the starkly realistic *Philadelphia* about a corporate lawyer fired by his firm after he had contracted AIDS. The movie, starring the highly recognizable actors Tom Hanks and Denzel Washington, earned substantial profits and garnered the best actor Oscar for Hanks. Even so, some gays complained that the homosexuality of the movie had been sanitized, and that scenes between Hanks's character and his on-screen lover (played by Antonio Banderas) were wholly omitted from ads and trailers, or else "poeticized" into a sort of ethereal dance sequence. The movie was in many ways a deft Hollywood compromise—alluding to difficult material while masking it in melodrama and plot.[49]

Thus by the early 1990s, America had learned about AIDS, and to some extent accepted it as part of the cultural fabric. AIDS could be mentioned in polite company, and millions of Americans understood the necessity of monitoring their sexual activities and asking frank questions. Nonetheless, America continued to hold AIDS, and homo-sexuality, at arm's length. The majority of AIDS art—be it performed or exhibited—remained nestled in art theaters, avant-garde galleries, and intellectual salons. Efforts to move it into the mainstream, the success of *Philadelphia* notwithstanding, drew modest protest, or indifference. As late as 1989, the National Endowment for the Arts withdrew a $10,000 grant from a New York City art gallery that was being used to subsidize an AIDS exhibit called "Witnesses: Against Our Vanishing," while that same year patrons protested Southwest Missouri State University's production of *The Normal Heart,* and arsonists set fire to the home of a vocal supporter of the production. "I think that what went wrong in Springfield," mused the play's author Larry Kramer, "is another example of the kind of bigotry Hollywood studios practice when they won't make movies about AIDS, or when our government refuses to put anyone in charge of the epidemic. It's all part of the same homophobia."[50]

THE CHURCH

One source from which community-based organizations did not originate was the Catholic Church. Long the champion of poor and oppressed people everywhere, the Catholic Church in America rejected AIDS and its victims from the beginning as almost wholly unworthy of its attention. Linking the disease with immoral acts, individual archbishops dictated that the only reasonable response was to urge monogamous heterosexual intercourse, within the confines of marriage, without a condom. "Good morality is good medicine," preached New York City archbishop John Cardinal O'Connor, and dictated that a Catholic approach to AIDS should "confront the moral dimensions of sexual aberrations or drug abuse."[51] In a similar vein, Cardinal Bernard Law in Boston suggested that Catholic parents pull their children from AIDS-awareness classes in the city's schools, deeming explicit discussion of condoms "amoral."[52]

AIDS challenged Catholic doctrine on both condom use (soundly rejected by the Vatican) as well as on homosexuality. Even as the epidemic grew in the mid-1980s, the Vatican reasserted its rejection of homosexuality, and in 1986 ordered local bishops to cease any support they may have been giving to homosexual groups or to homosexual activity among their congregants. Accusing homosexual groups of "deceitful propaganda," the Vatican's missive declared: "Departure from the church's teaching, or silence about it, in an effort to provide pastoral care is neither caring nor pastoral. Only what is true can ultimately be pastoral."[53] In succeeding months, the Los Angeles archdiocese withdrew support from the AIDS Project in Los Angeles for advocating condom use, and the following year the United States Catholic Conference explicitly condemned the practice of safe sex. "Human sexuality, as we understand this gift from God, is to be genitally expressed only in monogamous, heterosexual relationship of lasting fidelity in marriage," the conference resolution stated.[54] And although the conference's guidelines allowed for the possibility of teaching that condoms could possibly prevent AIDS, bishops in Boston, Detroit, and New York City, among other dioceses, quickly condemned the loophole.

Although individual priests, bishops, and even archbishops preached compassion for AIDS sufferers, the church's general discomfort with homosexuality prevented it from taking active measures to serve the afflicted. In March 1987, for example, the New York archdiocese forbade granting of communion to members of Dignity, a group of open Catholic homosexuals. And even when Pope John Paul II condemned discrimination against AIDS sufferers in a 1989 address, he reiterated his previous stand that promoting condom use to prevent AIDS was "morally illicit" and a violation of "the authentically human sense of sexuality."[55]

At least part of the discomfort with which the church faced AIDS was born of tensions within its own ranks. Homosexuality among the clergy, often discussed and alluded to but rarely actually recorded, was becoming more difficult to ignore. By 1987, at least two dozen Catholic priests and "brothers" (who had also taken vows of chastity) had contracted AIDS, and the most likely source was homosexual relations.[56] At the same time, Maryland psychologist Richard Sipe released figures from a study demonstrating that 20 percent of Catholic priests had been homosexual (of whom half had been sexually active) through the 1970s: a figure that had possibly climbed to 40 percent since, or even 50 percent in urban dioceses.[57] Given the extraordinary hypocrisy of a wholly heterosexist belief system being preached by a near majority gay clergy, the church proved incapable of meeting the crisis directly. Confronted with direct evidence of homosexual activity, the church turned to a policy of total denial, even within the realm of the sick and afflicted. Commented Dignity president James Bussen: "The church hierarchy cannot admit that its priests are dying of AIDS. It would be hard for them to argue that all the victims had blood transfusions or that they were shoving dirty needles into their arms. They are left with only one alternative: homosexual activity."[58]

Moreover, the church often seemed oblivious to the ravages of the disease, even when it was not actively condemning the life habits of the afflicted. Writer Andrew Sullivan vividly recalled a Mass he attended at a parish church in a relatively gay part of Washington, D.C.—a neighborhood that had lost dozens of young men to AIDS over the previous half-dozen years. The priest, addressing the incident of Jesus' healing the lepers, began his sermon, "Today, few of us know the meaning of a plague like leprosy." When confronted by Sullivan at the end of the service about the relevance of AIDS to the day's homily, the priest responded, "Well, I didn't think it would affect anyone here."[59]

The Catholic church was not alone in its disavowal or continued condemnation of homosexuality, and by extension AIDS patients. The Southern Baptists proved equally intolerant, condemning homosexuality in their 1988 convention as "a manifestation of a depraved nature," and "a perversion of divine standards."[60] And while they admitted that homosexuals could "receive forgiveness and victory" along with other sinners, the Baptists also took pains to designate homosexuality as "a chosen lifestyle," meaning that gay men and women had freely chosen to follow their own course, despite alternative options.[61] Similarly, fundamentalist Protestants took actions in 1989 to stop passage of California's Proposition S, which would allow gay couples (and other unmarried duos) to record their partnerships with municipal record offices, and give them bereavement leaves and hospital visiting privileges accorded to married couples.[62]

But more progressive Protestant denominations did begin to provide programs and pastoral comfort to AIDS victims and their families. Both laics and their ministers expanded meals-on-wheels programs to include AIDS patients, welcomed AIDS patients into their congregations, and paid calls to comfort the sick. In San Francisco, the Golden Gate Church of the Nazarene began a Saturday morning prayer group specifically focusing on supplications for AIDS victims, and then established the group as a social service agency for the purpose of providing child care to families afflicted by AIDS.[63] A nearby church established Family Link to house visiting parents of young gay men suffering from AIDS.[64] And in Washington, D.C., Episcopal bishop John Walker called for leadership and compassion from the church in reaching out to AIDS victims. "Our God is a God of forgiveness and reconciliation," he said. "If He visited all of those who sin with fatal diseases or natural disasters, the human race would have been wiped out long ago."[65]

Overall, the role of organized religious organizations in providing AIDS care fell neatly into established political divisions. The most progressive congregations, both Jewish and Christian, tended to extend existing social action programs to the disease's victims. Home care, hospital visitation, pastoral counseling, emergency funds, homeless shelters, and emergency meals—already provided to the sick and needy among them—were now simply offered to the community's newest victims. Among more conservative congregations, such as Orthodox synagogues, Catholic dioceses, fundamentalist Christian churches, as well as the more conservative of the established Protestant sects such as the Mormons and Southern Baptists, AIDS posed problems because of its close links with homosexuality. Few members in these congregations were themselves active homosexuals, and those who were tended to carefully hide their activities. Thus, AIDS could be safely ignored, or viewed generally as an affliction of those external to the community. Sympathy might be offered, but usually at arm's length.

GROWING DESPAIR

By 1990, community-based AIDS organizations had established a record of accomplishments and success in diverse spheres. Many of the oldest had grown rapidly, with GMHC boasting a new six-story headquarters housing 100 full-time staff members and 1,600 volunteers, and AmFAR making research grants at the rate of over $10 million per year.[66] At the same time, a plethora of new, more localized organizations had been established supporting a broad network of constituencies, ranging from minority and ethnic groups to specific professions, and providing a range of specialized services such as legal counseling, arts support, cultural support, access to experimental drugs, emergency housing, and child care. In heavily gay Provincetown, Massachusetts, for example, the Provincetown AIDS Support Group provided weekly support groups, transportation, meals, counseling, home care, and liaisons with Boston-area hospitals.[67] Across the social and temperate divide, Dallas, Texas, now hosted the Dallas AIDS ARMS Network promoting a similar mix of services, while New York claimed within its parameters Lawyers Against AIDS which provided pro bono help to AIDS sufferers who had been victims of discrimination.[68] The rich panoply of organizations prompted New York City health commissioner Stephen Joseph to comment, "When the story of New York's AIDS epidemic is written, that self-help effort will be the bright part of it."[69] The same could be said for many other cities around the country.

But the success of these organizations masked the underlying tragedy, which was that the institutions were growing precisely because the epidemic was growing. Although new infections among gay men had declined dramatically by 1990, new infections among other high-risk groups had increased even faster. And although physicians were getting slightly better at treating AIDS and the opportunistic infections accompanying it more aggressively with AZT and newer antibiotics, the sheer volume of patients threatened to overwhelm the organizations that had pledged themselves to help. In San Francisco, for example, exhausted volunteers and program administrators pleaded for more state and city funding, even as the city's AIDS Emergency Fund cut cash disbursements from $1,000 to $100 per patient, while the Shanti Project turned away patients seeking housing. "It feels like a tidal wave," admitted Shanti Project executive director Eric Rofes.[70]

For all of their hard work and fund-raising, the organizations had been unable to either contain the epidemic's spread, find a cure or vaccine, or even discover a particularly effective treatment. While AZT, used early and often, could possibly extend the life of an AIDS victim for up to a year, little else could be done. Organizations, instead, concentrated on nursing the sick, caring for the kin, comforting the survivors, and subsidizing the scientists, in hopes that somebody soon could provide a breakthrough.

Even in these activities, however, the organizations faced growing challenges. "AIDS fatigue" had afflicted both the gay community and its straight benefactors. Either through indifference, emotional self-protection, or pure boredom, donors became less generous as the decade came to a close, and board members were forced to pursue funds more aggressively from their established donor bases, or look to new sources of funding such as government and foundation grants, cash reimbursement for services, or fees and associated charges for certain types of charity previously offered for free. A former chairman of Los Angeles's AIDS Project admitted that there was simply a limit to his grief and empathy. "Five years ago, if a friend had died it would have been a major event in my life. Now, it almost has to be my best friend."[71]

In the meantime, the victims of AIDS could do little but fight off despair and hope to squeeze what life they could out of their remaining days, but in these activities the organizations could help. It was no wonder that AIDS victim Christopher Sherman advised his fellow afflictees in 1988: "My best piece of advice is to make contact with an AIDS service organization as quickly as possible. They will provide you with services and support that you may otherwise not be able to get."[72] And for all of his anger at the internecine fighting that had torn asunder the founders of GMHC, Larry Kramer reflected back in later years, "It was one of those rare moments in life when one felt completely utilized, useful, with a true reason to be alive."[73]

CHAPTER 6

DRUGS

DESPERATE MEASURES

From the onset of the epidemic, patients looked for cures. Desperate to take action against the inexorable progress of the disease, AIDS victims leaped from rumor to rumor, clinging to even the most tenuous and bizarre tales of alleviation and remedy. And while in most cases the drugs and regimens they found were worthless, the mere act of seeking seemed to assuage the need for action.

Charlatans, quacks, and naive do-gooders responded with brews and potions from around the world. A Munich-based physician was reported to be "hyperoxygenating" patients' blood with ozone, which could kill the virus by "inactivating" molecules in the organism's outer membrane.[1] Naturalist healers promulgated chest thumping (to stimulate the thymus gland), bleach bathing, hydrogen peroxide injections, and cow fetus cell treatments. A Bahamian physician advertised his "immunoaugmentative therapy" in which he injected a protein mix that he claimed could stimulate the immune system.[2]

Some of the claims seemed more reasonable than others. One U.S. physician claimed to have cured his own AIDS using a regimen of the amino acid lysine, along with the known antiviral agent acyclovir (used to treat herpes viruses) and the stomach medication Tagamet. The claim seemed plausible, given past evidence that lysine was effective in treating the herpes virus.[3] Several Japanese scientists claimed that the common anticholesterol medication Dextran appeared to prevent the spread of HIV between cells in a test tube.[4] And a number of patients claimed to have found a cure with "Compound Q," an extract of Chinese cucumber root that was reputed to deactivate the virus.[5] Upon FDA investigation, none of these claims was found tenable.

More reasonable were those who claimed to have found ways to bolster the body's underlying resilience, either by strengthening the immune system or by using medicines to target specific opportunistic infections. In New York, for example, reputable pediatric AIDS physician Arye Rubenstein recommended gamma-globulin injections for his young patients in the hope that the regimen could buttress their bodies' efforts to fight opportunistic infections.[6] In London, doctors at Saint Mary's Hospital reported on efforts with imunovir to treat both ARC and herpes.[7] And many gay men claimed to have found improvement with egg lipids or egg lecithin (sold under the name AL721), which several Israeli studies indicated could be effective in retarding the virus's spread.[8]

All of these interventions lacked sound bases in molecular biology, and all were eventually proven to be ineffective. But several putative cures that appeared in the mid-1980s grew from a solid understanding of viral physiology and whatever specific knowledge existed about the AIDS virus. Most AIDS researchers agreed from an early point in the epidemic that an eventual cure would probably be based on one of several known groups of antiviral medications, most likely one that could deactivate the virus's reverse transcriptase enzyme. Several large pharmaceutical concerns began experimenting with drugs in this class by 1986, with the French company Rhone-Poulenc working with HPA-23 (antimonotungstate) and Institut Merieux experimenting with immuthiol (sodium diethyldithiocarbamate).[9] In Switzerland, Hoffman-La Roche began experimenting with interferon alpha, a known antiviral agent that could possibly be used to treat Kaposi's sarcoma directly in addition to attacking the AIDS virus.[10] Other drugs in the experimental pipeline by 1986 included Newport's Isoprinosine, ICN's Virazole, and Imreg's Imreg-1.[11]

Besides being generally ineffective, many of these early drugs and interventions were actually harmful. One claimant's pills were found by the FDA to contain toxic doses of lead, while the Bahamian doctor's cell infusion was found to harbor both herpes and HIV![12] Some of the regimens produced painful and damaging side effects such as nausea, dizziness, chills, and general lethargy. A patient who was placed on an experimental course of Alpha Interferon reported of the experience: "Within two hours of the first injection, I had severe chills, followed by high fever, and reversion back to chills. . . . Over the 30-day course of treatment, I noticed myself becoming profoundly more fatigued and depressed. Where just before the course of Interferon I was still running four miles a day, there were days now that I barely wanted to get out of bed."[13]

The most promising of the early interventions was the well-known antiviral drug Ribavirin. Already in use for over a decade when the AIDS crisis broke, Ribavirin was licensed for use in over 30 countries, and was actually legal for use in American hospitals for treatment of viral respiratory diseases. Initial informal trials of the drug on patients with AIDS-related complex (ARC) indicated that it seemed to slow ARC's progression to full-blown AIDS, and might in fact partially reverse the course of the disease. In 1985, the FDA approved clinical trials of the drug for use in early stages of HIV infection, and the following year approved designation of the drug as a "treatment IND [investigational new drug]," which would allow the drug to progress to the next level of clinical testing while at the same time allowing it to be administered to certain AIDS patients on a "compassionate basis."[14] The designation did not come quickly enough for many AIDS patients, however. For at least two years, AIDS patients had been buying the drug in Mexico and illegally importing it to the United States. [15]

AZT

The first drug to prove truly effective in fighting AIDS was Burroughs-Wellcome's AZT (azidothymidine, sold under the brand name Retrovir), an analogue of the 24-year-old molecule ziduvodine first synthesized in 1964. Originally developed as an antiretroviral drug for use in fighting leukemia, the molecule was not found to be clinically useful, and was ultimately shelved. In 1985, National Cancer Institute scientists observed its properties in fighting HIV, and the following year Burroughs-Wellcome filed for patent protection on the AZT form, and began both producing the drug and preparing it for clinical trials.[16]

AZT was a far from perfect drug. Although both in laboratory tests and in clinical trials the drug reduced viral loads, it proved to be highly toxic to bone marrow and often induced the need for blood transfusions over time. Worse, the AIDS virus appeared highly adaptive to AZT presence, and usually began developing resistance after six months of AZT therapy. For these reasons, AZT seemed to be effective only if administered early on in the course of the disease, at which point it generally delayed the onset of symptoms (and eventual death) by no more than a year. Nevertheless, this limited victory against the virus was the first evidence of progress, and prompted a small degree of optimism among AIDS victims and their advocates. "After five years of basically no hope, we now have a ray of hope," noted GMHC deputy director Tim Sweeney. He cautioned, however, that the ray of hope was "extremely volatile."[17] The following spring, the FDA, working with unusual alacrity, approved the drug for general prescription sales.

AZT was initially marketed by Burroughs-Wellcome at $3.00 per pill, producing annual costs (at typical dosages) of between $8,000 and $10,000.[18] While much of this cost was initially shouldered by the private health plans insuring the preponderance of AIDS victims, most IV drug users and many longtime AIDS sufferers were insured through Medicaid programs, which could use discretion over which drugs they would or would not pay for. AIDS activists strongly protested the high cost, charging Burroughs-Wellcome with profiteering off of the deadly disease. Burroughs-Wellcome defended itself by citing its high costs of production (the process required seven months and 23 separate chemical reactions), and its need to recover its research costs.

The research cost argument, however, was specious. The ziduvodine molecule had been in the public domain for over a decade, and had only been repatented when Burroughs-Wellcome filed for protection under the Orphan Drug Act in 1985. This act, which had been passed by the FDA a decade before, was intended to encourage pharmaceutical companies to develop drugs for "orphan" diseases—rare disorders with too few patients to induce drug companies to develop targeted remedies—by awarding them special patent and tax protections. But AIDS, with its burgeoning patient rolls, was a poor fit for orphan drug protection. Within two years of its filing for AZT patent protection, Burroughs-Wellcome stock had quadrupled in price, and its sales of AZT were increasing by 50 percent or more per year.[19] "With an envisioned doubling of AZT's user pool, there is a lot of money to be made," noted one Wall Street analyst in 1987.[20]

The excessive price of the drug drew widespread condemnation from AIDS groups, and Burroughs-Wellcome ultimately lowered it. Even in the midst of the controversy, however, the pharmaceutical breakthrough drew accolades and inspired hope. At the National Cancer Institute, pediatric oncologist Philip Pizzo began administering the drug to children as young as 16 months in hopes of forestalling the onset of symptoms, and within a year had discovered that the treatment appeared to actually reverse AIDS-induced dementia in children.[21] Dr. Samuel Broder, also of the National Cancer Institute, reflected: "It shatters the doubt that pervaded this entire field. There was general belief that it would be impossible to stop the AIDS retrovirus from replication without damaging the patient. That *has* been shattered."[22] And Vice President George Bush, always more comfortable with AIDS than was his boss, visited a Burroughs-Wellcome laboratory to laud the workers. "When Marty St. Clair observed in a petri dish that the AIDS-type virus did not grow in the presence of Retrovir, you were on your way to scoring the world's first significant victory against AIDS," Bush said.[23]

BARRIERS AT THE FDA

The limited success of AZT, coupled with its toxic side-effects, raised questions as to what role the federal government should play in the regulation or encouragement of new drug development. Then and now, all prescription pharmaceuticals sold in the United States were required to pass through a rigorous multistage testing process, administered by the Food and Drug Administration (FDA), which generally took 8–10 years to complete. The process was geared toward preventing any substance from reaching markets that could prove toxic or fatal in even a small percentage of prospective patients. Past horrors such as the thalidomide and sulfanilamide debacles of previous decades had ensured that the FDA considered patient safety first, and other goals such as the development of new drugs or shortened trial periods second.

This set of priorities had seemed sound when it was developed in the post–World War II decades. The FDA, established in 1906 with the Pure Food and Drug Act, had initially done little more than ensure that the ingredients listed in patent medicine formulations were accurate and honest. It acted, essentially, as a sort of Better Business Bureau of the medical world, checking ingredients and policing manufacturers for false advertising claims. One general counsel of the agency noted of its early work, "A drug manufacturer under the 1906 act did not even have to inform the Food and Drug Administration that it was in business."[24] This changed in 1937, when enterprising chemists at the Massengill drug company dissolved antibiotic sulfa drugs in antifreeze in an effort to make a liquid formulation that was palatable to children. The formulation, sold as Elixir Sulfanilamide, killed more than 100 patients before it was pulled from the shelves. In response the following year, the federal government passed the Food, Drug and Cosmetic Act, which required that new drugs be certified safe and effective by the FDA before being offered for sale to the public.

The Food, Drug and Cosmetic Act established the general principal of government oversight over drug development, but placed relatively lenient guidelines on the process. As late as 1960, the agency employed only one staff physician to approve new drug applications, and maintained only six full-time and four part-time physicians to analyze collected data provided by drug companies in support of their new formulations. The whole process from application to approval took a little more than half a year, and was managed by an agency with an annual budget of only $11 million.

The tenor of drug regulation changed drastically with thalidomide. The sedative drug, marketed broadly in Europe and Canada, was prescribed to over 20,000 Americans between 1958 and 1961, including 624 pregnant women. Over the following two years, women on the drug gave birth to hundreds of severely deformed babies, causing public outcry and demand for stricter drug regulations. In 1962, under the leadership of Tennessee senator Estes Kefauver, Congress passed amendments to the 1938 legislation requiring not only that drugs demonstrate their immediate safeness, but also their effectiveness and long-term safeness. The FDA expanded rapidly, and the new-drug testing period increased from months to years.

By 1985, FDA testing standards were so strict that fewer than 1 in 5,000 new molecules developed in industrial pharmaceutical labs actually made it to market. The full panoply of required clinical trials could take up to a decade, and generally cost $60–$80 million. At each stage of the trials, I (for general safety), II (for dosing and effectiveness), and III (for long-term safety and effectiveness in comparison with a placebo), only one-third of the drugs under observation were retained, and this was after the majority had been discarded during prestage animal trials.[25] The program had prevented more thalidomide-like disasters, but it had also created a highly conservative pharmaceutical industry, unwilling to bring products to the FDA unless they carried with them the potential for enormous profits. Moreover, the system ignored the needs of desperate and terminally ill patients who might be willing to try nonapproved formulations but for the vigilance of the FDA. "It is as if I am in a disabled airplane, speeding downward out of control," related one frustrated patient. "I see a parachute hanging on the cabin wall, one small moment of hope. I try to strap it on when a government employee reaches out and tears it off my back, admonishing, 'You can't use that. It doesn't have a Federal Aviation Administration inspection sticker on it. We don't know if it will work.' "[26]

From 1984 on, AIDS advocates questioned the relevance of such strict standards in the face of an untreatable and fatal disease. The phase III trials, which could last for years, were designed to determine effective doses and long-term toxicity of drugs and thus were irrelevant to the needs of the target group. AIDS patients struggled to get accepted into experimental trials, or sought advice from doctors who might have personal connections with FDA officials or with investigators overseeing the clinical testing. Pressure increased when AZT trials quickly demonstrated that those on the drug were dying at much lower rates than patients on placebo. In response, the FDA began to cautiously make the drug, still in the phase III trial stage, available on a "compassionate" basis to nearly 4,000 AIDS patients, and in 1987 formalized a system of accelerated trials in those situations where drugs could potentially remedy a life-threatening disease.[27] And although AIDS activists argued that the changes had not come fast enough, in fact AZT had come through the testing process faster than any drug in history. It had been granted Investigational New Drug (IND) status (initial approval for testing) within five days of application, and phase III trials had lasted only six months before approval was given for general sale.[28]

ACT UP

Within the AIDS community, the paradoxes of the FDA-approval process became apparent in the mid-1980s, in all of their absurdity. Patients who were certain they would die begged access to experimental drugs, or drugs not yet for sale in the United States, or even substances not considered drugs at all, yet were routinely thwarted by the FDA. Women victims, still a minority within the epidemic, found themselves unable to qualify for "compassionate use" trials because certain experimental drugs were as yet unproven to be safe and effective in women, while children were often excluded from tests based on similar circular reasoning. One father of a two-year-old AIDS patient testified before Congress that his daughter was in a controlled study of pediatric use of gamma globulin, 50 percent of the children in which study were being given placebos. "Who has time for a placebo?" the man demanded, as his child exhibited signs of AIDS-induced brain damage. And when the family applied for access to AZT on a compassionate use basis for their daughter, the request was denied.[29]

The bureaucratic barriers provoked ACT UP into action. Members staged "die-ins" in front of FDA regional offices and scrawled chalk outlines of bodies on the pavement. They set up intravenous feeding equipment in front of the home of Massachusetts governor Michael Dukakis, and sponsored a condom day at New York's Shea Stadium. In a highly effective poster campaign, ACT UP members plastered billboards around New York City with side-by-side pictures of Cardinal O'Connor and a used, semen-filled condom with the caption "Know Your Scumbags" emblazoned in large block letters.

Leading the charge was Larry Kramer, the founder of ACT UP, who launched invectives at New York City mayor Ed Koch, National Institute of Allergies and Infectious Diseases director Anthony Fauci, CDC director James Mason, and FDA director Frank Young. Kramer used anger "the way Jackson Pollock worked with paint; he'll fling it, drip it, or pour it on any canvas he can find," wrote one profiler.[30] In an open letter to Fauci, Kramer wrote:

> After three years, you have established only a system of waste, chaos, and uselessness. Now you come bawling to Congress that you don't have enough staff, office space, lab space, secretaries, computer operators, lab technicians, file clerks, janitors, toilet paper; and that's why the drugs aren't being tested and the network of treatment centers isn't working and the drug protocols aren't in place. You expect us to buy this bullshit and feel sorry for you? YOU FUCKING SON OF A BITCH OF A DUMB IDIOT, YOU HAVE HAD $374 MILLION AND YOU EXPECT US TO BUY THIS GARBAGE BAG OF EXCUSES![31]

The histrionics, while obviously offensive, brought enormous publicity to the plight of the dying. "In American medicine, there are two eras," admitted Fauci. "Before Larry and after Larry . . . There is no question in my mind that Larry helped change medicine in this country . . . When all the screaming and the histrionics are forgotten, that will remain."[32] In a similar vein, New York City health commissioner Stephen Joseph praised ACT UP in 1990: "There's no doubt that they've had an enormous effect. We've basically changed the way we make drugs available in the last year."[33]

As time passed, ACT UP shifted from exclusive focus on the FDA approval process to a general lobbying stance for AIDS-related research. In 1990, for example, the organization fought against the government's use of a specific contractor to conduct clinical trials on alternative (nontraditional) cancer interventions for AIDS. The contractor, a private research firm called Emprise, employed several principal members known to be biased against alternative therapies. Its president, Grace Monaco, a lawyer, had been involved in several lawsuits against alternative therapy providers, and remained a partner in her law firm during the clinical investigations in question, which, in turn, represented several insurance agencies predisposed against paying for alternative therapies. Similarly, the firm's scientific director, Saul

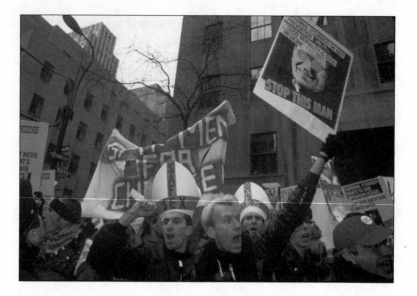

ACT UP demonstrating at St. Patrick's Cathedral, New York City. (Stockphoto)

Green, had consulted with insurance companies interested in disallowing claims for alternative therapies.[34] ACT UP staffer Bob Lederer wrote to Fauci in January 1990, "Emprise, which claims to be interested in 'objective evaluation' of alternative treatments, has both a strong predetermined bias against them and a built-in conflict of interest in assessing them."[35]

Members of ACT UP testified at hearings conducted by the National AIDS Commission, suggesting that the FDA remained overly focused on AZT—a problematic and toxic drug—even as other potential interventions lay untested. As the organization matured, it coupled more staid policy analysis and lobbying work with its "zap" tactics, becoming more effective in the process. "Some of you will tell me that, in the world of drug research and approval, it's never gone so quickly as it has with AIDS," Jim Eigo testified to the AIDS commission. "I will tell you that in some neighborhoods of this country people have never died so often so young of diseases so ugly as cryptosporidiosis, in which people can actually defecate themselves to death."[36] The tactic wasn't quite as publicity-getting as the Saint Patrick's sit-ins, but ultimately proved equally important to the organization's work.

THE FDA RESPONDS

The FDA responded to the pressure placed on it by activists, scientists, and members of Congress in fits and starts. In one of its first concessions to the unique demands of the AIDS epidemic, the agency acceded to the demands of National Cancer Institute director Samuel Broder and the research scientists at Burroughs-Wellcome to speed AZT through its approval process in a scant 108 days—lightning fast compared with the usual 760 days that new drugs required.[37] The FDA assured observers that additional drugs would soon follow.

Even as wartime freneticism worked to accelerate the process, however, numerous facts and episodes argued against caprice and carelessness. AZT, for example, soon showed itself to be so highly toxic—inducing extreme anemia and horrific fevers—that it promised to be intolerable to certain patients. Soon thereafter Interleukin-2, a promising experimental cancer drug initially shown to be effective in certain difficult-to-treat cancer cases, was found to be highly toxic as well. And another promising AIDS treatment, the antirejection drug Cyclosporine, which had shown promise in early trials, proved intolerable to many patients.[38] Warned NIH researcher Fauci, "If you want to get the drug earlier to people, they've got to understand that the risk of toxic side effects is going to increase proportionately to the time that you give it earlier."[39]

Fear of liability, too, worked to thwart the efficacy of the fast track. A year after the FDA officially inaugurated its new "treatment IND" process (essentially a formalization of its existing "compassionate use" policy), it found that few drug companies were applying to make use of the new pathway, for fear of liability lest its fast-track-approved drugs prove harmful. Further, the FDA found that the treatment INDs destabilized the symbiotic relationship between the agency and the large pharmaceutical companies. For all their complaints about overly restrictive FDA policies, large drug companies had enjoyed a sort of quasi-oligopoly created by the extremely expensive clinical trial process. With treatment INDs now in place, smaller drug companies could more easily afford to enter the market with experimental drugs, undermining a historically comfortable business relationship. With such a threat apparent, drug companies did their best to understate the significance of the new policy.[40]

But even scientists with a professional interest in seeing their breakthroughs produce tangible benefits offered reservations. The FDA clinical trial protocols had been developed over decades, in response to real experiences with dangerous and fraudulent drugs, in an effort to protect the public, maintain ethical standards within the drug development industry, and better serve all patients. While the growing calamity demanded a new response, more conservative scientists were reluctant to discard a generation's worth of gleaned wisdom regarding the best way to develop, test, and ultimately deliver new drugs to the public. For every patient whose life was saved, or at least prolonged, by the new treatment IND process, another might die for lack of detailed information regarding drug interactions, long-term toxicity, and harmful side-effects. The new process "would only create false hopes and delay accumulation of accurate knowledge that would save lives," remarked Massachusetts General Hospital physician Martin Hirsch. Too many early releases could make it "impossible to conduct properly controlled trials of drug safety," warned Hirsch, "only delaying licensure of effective therapeutic agents."[41]

The new treatment IND track was announced in March 1987, and the following year the FDA agreed to make available trimetrexate, an experimental drug used to treat PCP pneumonia. But the new guidelines were somewhat illusory. Despite celebrating the new availability of the pneumonia drug, AIDS activists soon realized that the drug would be made available only to patients who had tried two existing pneumonia treatments and displayed adverse reactions to both. Patients for whom the two existing drugs proved ineffective, but who did not actually suffer deleterious side effects, would fail to qualify for trimetrexate. "This not only defies common sense, it is contrary to the aim of the regulations," protested Lambda Legal Defense lawyer David Barr.[42] When protesters approached FDA regulator Ellen Cooper about the Byzantine regulation, she held firm. "If this community thinks that it's going to get much earlier access to drugs under these regulations, it's fooling itself," said Cooper to AIDS activist Martin Delaney in a contentious meeting.[43]

The agency seemed at war with itself, or else to be purposely deluding the public. Even as Cooper remained adamantly obstructionist, Commissioner Young testified to the White House AIDS commission that its new treatment IND would "allow broader use during the second phase of clinical testing of drugs for immediately life-threatening diseases," and listed the 178 potential AIDS drugs currently in the FDA testing pipeline.[44] Despite the ongoing debate over trimetrexate, Young specifically singled out the drug as representative of exactly the type of drugs that the FDA wished to make quickly available through the program. And when Cooper was confronted with the fact that her regulator pronouncements lay in direct conflict with her boss's intentions, she stood her ground. "I think he has raised some false hopes there," she said of Young.[45]

The problem seemed to be one of culture. Over decades the FDA had developed a highly risk-averse approach to new developments, drugs, breakthroughs, and scientific claims. Acting from a vantage of extreme skepticism, appropriate to an agency whose genesis lay in fighting patent medicine fraud, the FDA had nurtured a generation of regulators who instinctively understood that the greatest possible evil was approving an unsafe though possibly efficacious substance. In part this understanding lay in an institutional memory of colossal and highly public failures, such as those of thalidomide and Elixir Sulfanilamide, and in part it lay with the historical knowledge that few "breakthrough" drugs were in fact that. But more important, it lay in the psychological profile of the agency's scientists, who viewed themselves not as incubators of brilliance and innovation, but rather as guardians of the public.[46]

The FDA's intransigence reached a zenith with the gancyclovir episode, in which a nonapproved drug broadly prescribed on a compassionate use basis to fight the blindness caused by CMV retinitis was effectively pulled off the market once it actually entered formal clinical trials. The drug's effectiveness in treating CMV was so obvious to most clinicians that its maker, the drug company Syntex, applied for FDA approval with the intention of using the existing data to speed it through its treatment IND protocols. So overwhelming was the evidence for gancyclovir's effectiveness that a traditional clinical protocol would have been simply unethical.

When the drug's application came before the FDA, however, the advisory committee rejected it. Citing the data as too fragmented, anecdotal, and unscientific, the committee voted by large majority to disallow the drug's continued use on compassionate basis, and to demand traditional three-phase clinical trials. But such trials were ludicrous in the face of broad understanding that the drug worked, and that without the drug CMV sufferers would lose their sight. The oft-criticized Tony Fauci used his position in the NIH to fight for the drug's approval, suggesting that the FDA was ignoring common sense in deference to orthodoxy.[47] And GMHC attorney Jay Lipner noted, "Whatever the FDA was doing, it was doing wrong."[48]

The combined weight of the myriad rejections and road blocks proved too much for ACT UP. In October 1988, the organization staged a large demonstration at the FDA's headquarters, in which hundreds of protesters blocked the entrance to the building, chanted slogans, and held placards accusing the agency of murder. The demonstration garnered national press coverage, and seemed to have some effect on the agency. Commissioner Young began to streamline the treatment IND protocols, and within a year's time the period required to approve most INDs for AIDS drugs had shortened considerably.

PARALLEL TRACK

By 1989, at least four drugs were producing promising results in AIDS victims. AZT, the old standby, was proving most effective in reducing the viral load itself, but when used in conjunction with dideoxycytidine (DDC) seemed to work more quickly and consistently. Another antiviral drug, didanosine (DDI), was also proving effective in early clinical trials. And aerosolized pentamidine was showing itself to be effective enough against PCP pneumonia that the CDC was recommending that it be used prophylactically in AIDS patients. All in all, the pharmaceutical armament, while still imperfect, was growing in strength.[49]

The promise offered by the new drugs, though far from absolute, prompted renewed calls from the HIV community for streamlining approval processes for getting the drugs to market. These four drugs all demonstrated clear efficacy in early trials, and almost all infectious-disease physicians agreed that they worked some of the time. While all had potentially toxic side effects (AZT suppressed bone marrow production, and DDI caused peripheral neuropathy and pancreatitis, for example), all held out the promise of prolonged life for those very likely to die. Patients clamored for access.

The FDA had two different paths to getting experimental drugs to desperate patients by this point. The compassionate use method was informal and poorly defined, and relied on the drug maker itself to release the experimental compound to certain prescribing physicians. Compassionate use had been largely superseded by treatment INDs, which allowed desperate patients to become subjects within clinical trials so that they could be getting treatment while allowing necessary research to proceed. But many people could not qualify for participation in the treatment INDs, whether because of geographic inaccessibility or of complicating medical conditions that precluded their inclusion in clinical trials. In desperation, a number of these non-eligibles began to create "purchasing clubs" in the late 1980s in an effort to pool funds and illegally import AIDS drugs that were available in other countries.[50] Although the FDA had stated in 1988 that it would allow importation of small amounts of drugs for personal use, such purchasing cooperatives were clearly beyond the intention of the earlier FDA ruling.

The pressure to develop a new vehicle for making experimental drugs available more quickly increased as DDI proved itself to be a crucial new tool in battling AIDS. The drug was one of only two effective antiviral medications then available, and often worked in patients who proved incapable of tolerating AZT, or for whom AZT had briefly worked but now no longer did. With the backing of nearly all senior health officials, including Young and Secretary of Health and Human Services Secretary Louis Sullivan, drug maker Bristol-Myers began in 1989 to distribute DDI through a uniquely expanded treatment IND program, which allowed over 2,500 people emergency access to the drug.

Fauci pressed for a generalized parallel track that would allow all needy patients who failed to qualify for treatment INDs access to all unapproved experimental drugs. Rather than make ad hoc decisions on each drug through a laborious committee-centered process, Fauci understood that the clinical trial process was simply flawed in the face of the uniquely tragic AIDS epidemic. Combining forces with an array of AIDS activist organizations, Fauci pressed administration officials to formalize the track, and have it approved through the standard rule-making procedure.

But a variety of researchers both in and out of government resisted Fauci's efforts. One group of scientists, personified by Harvard's Jerome Groopman and Martin Hirsch, feared that the parallel track would undermine the ability of scientists conducting clinical trials to enroll patients in their studies. One reason that people enrolled in the dangerous phase II trials was to gain access to necessary drugs, and the existence of an unregulated parallel track would negate the need of those patients to enroll. "What is it going to do to the efficacy trials?" asked Dr. Howard Liebman of Boston City Hospital.[51] And noted Groopman: "There really are conflicting issues here. If the philosophy is that anyone can decide at any point what drugs he or she wants to take, then you will not be able to do a clinical trial."[52]

Other scientists expressed concern about protecting the public. While the AIDS epidemic demanded uniquely extraordinary measures, a parallel track for drugs for nonfatal diseases invited disastrous outcomes for the sake of appeasing vocal constituencies. Drugs often had unpredictable effects in interaction with other drugs, or unexpected long-term toxicities, or exhibited diminishing efficacy after several years of use (AZT fell into this last category). The only way to discover these various effects was to study the drugs in controlled trials over lengthy periods, and then conduct follow-up research once the drug was approved. Parallel tracks threatened to thwart this type of research, and in so doing expose the general population to unforeseen dangers.

Larry Kramer, of course, was unconvinced by these arguments. Eager to expand access to any and all potential treatments, he dismissed critiques of the parallel track as mundane bureaucratic griping. "They don't like the Parallel Track because they don't have control of it," he wrote.[53] Other AIDS activists agreed, viewing opponents of the parallel track as officious meddlers who would sacrifice the lives of thousands of young men for the sake of their own professional authority. G. Steven Rose of Boston's AIDS Watchdog Group wrote in January 1990, "That smaller models—the CRI projects—are carrying out trials at a fraction of the cost is a threat to the old-boy system."[54] In a sense, the debate was a classic standoff between citizen activists, who brought both passion and impetuousness to the situation, and professional civil servants, who viewed all radical changes skeptically.

Demonized throughout this process by all sides was National Institute of Allergies and Infectious Diseases (NIAID) director Anthony Fauci. Despite his championing of the parallel track and concern for the limitations of compassionate use protocols and treatment INDs, Fauci was attacked by both AIDS activists and the president's AIDS commission for misusing the funds deeded to him to run the AIDS Clinical Trials Group (ACTG) program. Despite investments of nearly $450 million by 1990, the ACTG program had failed to produce a single breakthrough antiviral medication, or even a substantially innovative drug to treat opportunistic infections. Moreover, racial minorities and women were grossly underrepresented in the trials that were going forth, suggesting that ACTG directors were not recruiting aggressively enough from those patient groups.[55]

Fauci responded with several programs designed to mollify his accusers. The Community Program for Clinical Research on AIDS (CPCRA) invited primary care doctors to help design research protocols "appropriate to community settings." If clinical trials were facing difficulties recruiting appropriate numbers of women and minorities to their ranks, and if parallel track programs and treatment INDs were failing to provide experimental drugs to the desperately ill, then perhaps a "bottom-up" program would prove more constructive. At the same time, the NIAID awarded $1.2 million in grants to the Association of Minority Health Professions Schools to support an "AIDS Consortium Center." And last, the institute sought to bring ACTG testing programs to community health centers, AIDS clinics, and drug treatment centers, all in an effort to facilitate AIDS drug distribution. Despite being hindered by interagency squabbling and tightly written federal regulations, Fauci was attempting to both accelerate and accentuate the work of the parallel track and of the ACTG, in an effort to maintain research standards while being as broadly compassionate as possible.[56]

Fauci was the tragic hero of the episode; he heaped praise on those who had hated him most, crediting them with humanizing the epidemic and bending the rigid federal bureaucracy to a more malleable stance.

For his tormenter, Kramer, he had nothing but praise, stating in an interview years later: "Larry, by assuring consumer input to the FDA, put us on the defensive at the NIH. He put Congress on the defensive over appropriations. ACT UP put medical treatment in the hands of the patients. And this is the way it ought to be."[57] Faced with the daunting tasks of identifying a new virus, developing an effective and nontoxic vaccine, creating and testing a new class of antiviral molecules, and sanctioning medications for opportunistic infections, all under the pressures of ongoing activist harangues and a reluctant administration, Fauci looked to new pathways and systems to revive a tradition-bound research and testing system. If the results were less than breathtaking, it was not for lack of innovative thinking.

POSTMORTEM ON ACT UP

Even as ACT UP was effectively applying pressure to various agencies, it was antagonizing so many individuals that it threatened to commit organizational suicide. Demonizing Mayor Ed Koch as a murderer, closeted homosexuals as traitors, and highly professional public officials as incompetent homophobes did little to help the cause, and ultimately possibly hurt it. "He [Kramer] blames *me* for the deaths of his friends," a furious Koch related. "I just looked at the figure today. It's something like forty or fifty million people have HIV. I'm responsible? I mean, people who know they shouldn't fuck without a rubber and nevertheless do—*I'm responsible for that?*."[58] Conservative and openly gay writer Andrew Sullivan queried, "If you call someone who is not doing enough in some bureaucracy a murderer, what do you do when somebody is stabbing someone in the street?"[59] And San Francisco–based gay columnist T. Vollmer noted: "There is a fine line between, on the one hand, street theater, civil disobedience, and the right to demonstrate, and on the other, undo behavior and brown-shirting. . . . Many fear that the politics of anger is causing the community to abandon its commitment to the freedom of expression and the right to privacy."[60]

In late 1991, several chapters of ACT UP began a strategy of "outing" closeted gay politicians in an effort to force them to identify more closely with the community's suffering. The move, while drawing press, also drew widespread condemnation from both gays and straights, and underscored a growing rift between young radicalized gay activists and older, more stalwart community leaders. "Now every closeted gay man has to fear the animosity of his fellow gays as much as straights," wrote Sullivan.[61] Despite its policy successes and colorful reputation, the organization began to lose support among more established gay groups, particularly those that concerned themselves with issues beyond AIDS. Lesbians looked askance at some of ACT UP's tactics, as did older, wealthier gay men, and homosexuals in committed monogamist relationships. "The fissures are many," reported the British newsmagazine *The Economist*. "Between younger and older gays; between liberationists and assimilationists . . . between those who defiantly call themselves 'queer' and those who do not."[62]

Kramer began withdrawing from ACT UP the following year. A brilliant innovator and organizational entrepreneur, he had founded two of the most successful and influential AIDS groups on the planet, and yet in both cases proved too incendiary to remain a constructive member after his initial contribution. ACT UP would rapidly lose power and prestige over the coming half decade, as breakthrough drugs and treatments rendered its confrontational style obsolete and irrelevant. As it diminished in size and authority, few but its original adherents would mourn its passing. Even as it had accomplished a great deal, it had left in its wake bruised and insulted individuals who would work for change through more established channels. The shining star in the activist firmament would burn out quickly.

CHAPTER 7

THE SHOOTING GALLERIES

SHIFTING DEMOGRAPHICS

Gay men had dominated the demographic mix of the epidemic from the beginning. Constituting approximately 4 percent of the adult male population (and thus only 2 percent of the entire population), gay men had accounted for nearly 80 percent of all recorded AIDS cases in the early 1980s, and even as that proportion fell they continued to personify the public face of the epidemic.

Toward the end of that decade, however, the case mix began to shift. Intravenous drug users, who made up only 15 percent of new AIDS cases in 1983, began to make up a quarter or more.[1] As AIDS permeated the drug-using population, the epidemic shifted from middle-class white gay men to poor minority men and women. Male drug users quickly infected their female partners, increasing the number of women with AIDS as well as the number of heterosexuals. By 1991, although heterosexuals still constituted less than half of all new AIDS cases, they were the fastest-growing portion of the epidemic, increasing by 40 percent in a single year.[2]

The drug-using population seemed more capable of transmitting the virus through heterosexual intercourse. While studies by Nancy Padian and her colleagues had shown that the virus had a very difficult time breaching the vaginal lining (resulting in male-to-female heterosexual transmission rates as low as 1 per each 50 episodes of intercourse), among drug users the virus traveled with greater facility. As the numbers of infected women rose to nearly 1 in 3 of all new cases, the proportion of those newly infected women who had not taken intravenous drugs rose as well, to nearly 35 percent by 1991.[3] Women were contracting the virus through needle-sharing, but also through sexual relations with their needle-sharing partners.

As the epidemic moved to IV drug users, it began to disproportionately affect racial minorities, who were themselves disproportionately represented among IV drug users. African Americans, who constituted 12 percent of the U.S. population, made up 27 percent of all AIDS cases by 1988, and over half of pediatric AIDS cases. Hispanics, although smaller in absolute numbers, were even more overrepresented in the epidemic, claiming 13 percent of all AIDS cases while making up only 6 percent of the U.S. population. The two groups posted different infection patterns: more women and children among blacks, more men among Hispanics. This may have been caused by differing social mores regarding gender distinctions and drug use, or it may have reflected differing levels of condom use or of education among the IV drug users in each minority group.[4] While numbers of new infections were growing in both groups, the Hispanic epidemic was growing fastest of all. For both groups, the percentage of new AIDS cases spread through homosexual intercourse was half that as among whites: 40 percent rather than nearly 80 percent.[5]

The shift showed up starkly in Army recruiting, the single most extensive screening forum in the country for a large pool of randomly selected young men and women. In the two years between 1985 and 1987, the numbers of white male recruits infected with HIV (per 10,000 screened) dropped from 28 to 19, while the number of infected blacks rose from 131 to 140. Among black women, the rate of infected recruits rose nearly 30 percent during this period, even as the infection rate among white women dropped from 5 to 2. Hispanic recruits were somewhat healthier than their civilian counterparts, although still infected at triple the rate of whites.[6]

Although the IV epidemic had been slowly growing throughout the 1980s, 1988 was a "watershed year" in the words of New York City health commissioner Stephen Joseph.[7] In that year, in New York, Los Angeles, and other large cities, the total number of new AIDS cases spread through drug use or through heterosexual relationships with drug users exceeded the number of new cases spread through homosexual activities. The newly infected were disproportionately uninsured or received indemnity through public programs such as Medicaid. Far more than their gay counterparts they were uneducated, unemployed, and homeless. And more and more, as the disease spread to women, they were children, who had contracted the disease either *in utero* or through breastfeeding. One stunning statistic that came to light at this time was that 9 percent of all street children ("runaways") were HIV-positive by 1988, having contracted the disease through either childhood prostitution, drug use, or some combination thereof.[8]

The new demographic profile of the epidemic meant a heavier burden for public agencies. The federal government reported that while it covered at least partial costs for 40 percent of all AIDS patients, it bore the costs for 70 percent of IV-drug-using patients, and 90 percent of pediatric patients. The trend toward public financing of the disease was further exacerbated by the growing tendency of private payers to exclude certain types of AIDS-related coverage, or to disallow experimental new AIDS drugs whose cost could easily run to $10,000 per year. Impoverished, sickly, and unemployed patients had no choice but to appeal to their state's Medicaid program or special uncompensated care fund for relief, or simply check themselves into the local public hospital. "The outlook is very bleak," noted GMHC legal affairs director David Hansell.[9]

The new group was also sicker than had been the previous group, with systemic illnesses, infections, compromised immune systems, and weakened constitutions *before* contracting AIDS. A growing number of the new victims were homeless, and a growing number of the homeless were infected with antibiotic-resistant strains of tuberculosis.[10] Consigned to homeless shelters or the street, they were more susceptible to widespread infection, physical abuse, or general mental breakdown.

"A shelter destroys your mind quicker than any disease ever could," reflected one AIDS patient who had experience in the system.[11] Upon contracting the virus, these compromised and weakened patients were less likely to respond well to the few antiviral medications available, less likely to be able to consistently comply with a medication regimen, more likely to quickly wind up in a hospital for treatment of opportunistic infections, and less likely to possess the comprehensive social and community ties needed to fortify them in their battle with the disease. "It's hard to imagine a more devastating double affliction: to suffer from AIDS and to have no place to call home," wrote one reflective journalist.[12]

Europe, too, experienced an epidemiological shift, as AIDS spread into drug-using denizens of the continent's capitals and major cities, and then spread among users through contaminated needles. Dublin and Edinburgh reported a "leapfrogging" of the American epidemic, skipping the homosexual stage to directly infect young heroin addicts.[13] In Ireland the epidemic, although small to begin with, was expanding at 50 percent per year by 1989, while in Scotland the disease jumped from negligible levels to a full-blown epidemic between 1986 and 1988. In a slightly different pattern, Caribbean nations began to exhibit greater numbers of women victims, who had caught the disease from shared needles or through engagement in prostitution with infected heterosexual clients.[14] Everywhere, the epidemic was moving out of its initial ensconcement in the gay communities.

THE SHOOTING GALLERIES

America's heroin users in the late 1980s constituted an isolated and reasonably stable population of some half million, the majority of whom used heroin at least once per day. The size of the group had neither grown nor shrunk appreciably in the preceding decades, although the shortened life of users coupled with the appeal of the drug to the newly disenfranchised dictated a constant churning in the broad pool of addicts. The pool had grown slightly in recent years, most likely owing to an influx of high-grade inexpensive Mexican heroin (known as "black tar"), and overall heroin use among the pool had risen as the available product became more potent and less adulterated.[15]

In addition to heroin, another 600,000 people in the United States regularly injected some other drug or combination of drugs, usually cocaine but often cocaine mixed with heroin. This pool was growing more rapidly than was the heroin-using pool, primarily because of the newer, more potent forms of injectable cocaine then becoming available. Additionally, the mixture of cocaine and heroin together was proving irresistible to many longtime drug users, who relished the euphoric calm of heroin when mixed with the libido-enhancing high of the cocaine.[16] The combined allure was so potent and compelling that all other concerns, including infection with a deadly virus, faded to near imperceptibility once the addiction took root. AIDS commission chairman Admiral James Watkins called the combined threat of drug use and AIDS "the most serious and potentially most expensive medical problem the U.S. has ever known."[17]

Intravenous drug users were a derelict and pathetic group. Nearly 80 percent lived below the poverty line, almost half had failed to complete high school, and over half received welfare assistance. The addicts' extreme lack of income and resources, coupled with an insatiable demand for expensive drugs, caused them to make horrific life choices leading them to conditions of near total degradation. Over 90 percent, for example, regularly shared needles in an effort to save the $3 cost of a new one, and nearly three-quarters repeatedly drew their own blood into the syringe and reinjected it in an effort to exploit every ounce of stimulus afforded by the drug.[18] The combined effect, of course, created near-perfect conditions for the spread of blood-borne diseases.

The "shooting galleries" where the needle sharing took place were not places where drugs were generally sold. Rather, addicts bought the drugs on the street and retreated to the galleries—often abandoned apartments in derelict buildings—where they could prepare the drug for injection, rent "works" (drug preparation and injection equipment), and relax to enjoy their drug-induced high or stupor in relative safety, all for a modest fee. Shooting galleries were most common in the poorest areas, where users could neither afford fresh needles nor rent a private home or apartment, and thus sheltered the most desperate and impoverished of the AIDS epidemic's victims. In such an environment, AIDS spread easily through virtually all regular clients, to the extent that by 1986 a user sharing a needle with 10 people stood nearly zero chance of emerging from the experience uninfected.[19]

The drug-using AIDS epidemic was most pronounced in New York City and the northern New Jersey cities of Newark (with the highest density of AIDS cases in the country), Jersey City, and to a lesser degree Paterson. In those cities, HIV infection "spread like wildfire" through the drug-injecting population in the early 1980s.[20] New York City health commissioner Stephen Joseph later estimated that in those cities the spread of HIV into the drug-using population had happened earlier than most people supposed, paralleling rather than following the spread in the gay community. The general invisibility of this community, however, as well as its myriad other afflictions, rendered the looming AIDS epidemic less compelling, and led early researchers to assume that this subepidemic lagged behind the gay epidemic.[21] In other cities, where shooting galleries were less popular (particularly San Francisco and Los Angeles), HIV penetration into the IV-drug-using population did not escalate until the late 1980s.

Concurrent with the spread of drug-transmitted AIDS was a growing epidemic among crack-addicted prostitutes. Crack, a smokable form of cocaine that became available in the early 1980s, gave an intense high, which, though short-lived, induced a ferocious addiction. Crack users quickly ran through their assets, and then frequently resorted to burglary or prostitution in order to support their habits. As crack use rose in inner cities, the number of women prostituting themselves rose, and prices for sexual services fell dramatically. In Newark, the epicenter of the nation's crack epidemic, the price for intercourse with a streetwalker plummeted from $40 to $5, meaning that women had to turn multiple tricks just to afford their next hit of the drug. In the process, they left themselves vulnerable to contracting AIDS.[22]

AIDS spread into the prostitute population in part through sheer volume—the vagina's natural defenses could thwart the virus to a point, but inevitably succumbed to the hundreds of exposures to HIV. But crack exacerbated the problem in a number of ways. Crack-addicted prostitutes, desperate for the drug, would take on violent, abusive, and sickly clients they might otherwise have shunned. In the crack houses themselves, women sold their bodies in exchange for the drug, often servicing men who were themselves high on crack. And although crack increased the libido, it delayed orgasm in men, lengthening the time and abrasiveness of the sex act, which further increased the chance of spreading the virus. "You see a woman with 20 men a day and you know she got to get the virus," noted a Newark denizen. "But people around here, they'll sell their mama to get the product. Especially cocaine—they got to be smoking it or poking it."[23]

Crack served as a conduit of the epidemic into women, but particularly into black women. In the poorer neighborhoods of Northeast cities nearly 90 percent of all women AIDS patients were black, and they in turn transmitted the virus to their babies.[24] The women most susceptible to the virus, the crack addicts themselves, lost nearly entirely their powers of judgment and discretion, offering oral sex for as little as 25 cents to customers with obvious venereal sores or who were otherwise clearly unwell. One woman reported, "I was sleeping while some friends were getting high in the room, and when I woke up I saw them crawling on the floor, picking up little white specks, taking lint off a sweatshirt— they were so desperate for coke."[25] And the victims of the drug, and the virus, seemed to show no age boundaries. Teenage prostitution, always present in poor urban areas, now included girls as young as 11 or 12, drawn into the trade by earlier crack addiction.

For nearly all the drug addicts at risk to AIDS exposure, the virus was of less concern than servicing their drug habits. Fear of death a half-dozen years or more in the future paled in comparison with the driving need to get a next heroin injection or crack hit. "I've got to come up with $400 each and every day, just to put in my arm . . . That's what I have to worry about, not some disease that may kill me in five years," related one addict.[26] In such an altered state of awareness, even a diagnosis of AIDS did little to alter behavior or impel greater care for bodily integrity. "They told me I got the virus and I've been shooting ever since," spoke one heroin addict. "There's nothing to live for. I'm going to shoot, shoot, shoot. Maybe I'll get lucky and get a heart attack."[27]

INTERVENTION

As the epidemic spread to IV drug users, public health officials and planners considered preventive steps they could take. One clear path was to try to reduce the numbers of people using drugs. In 1988, out of some 1.3 million IV drug users, fewer than 150,000 were in a treatment program, and of those only a fraction were receiving the complex mixture of social and medical support services that most experts considered necessary for ending an addiction. One director of a methadone center noted that the efforts of his and other centers constituted but "a drop in the bucket" in the sea of drug use affecting the nation.[28] For the remainder, the chance of defeating their addiction on their own was nearly nil. Indeed, the best-trod route out of addiction had always been, and continued to be, death—often at an early age.

Methadone treatment, used in cases of heroin addiction to ease the cravings of the addict, had proven to be effective, and allowed addicts to maintain more normal, successful lives. Methadone treatment programs throughout the country were overtaxed, however, and were actually facing budget *cuts* just as the potential dangers of addiction were increasing. Much of the funding of methadone programs had come from the federal government either through Medicaid reimbursements or through special funds from the National Institute for Drug Abuse, but budget allocations to these program were cut under Reagan budget adjustments in 1981. To compensate for the cuts, states needed either to supplement the programs from general revenues, charge patients themselves, or simply shrink the programs. New Jersey, with its extensive urban drug abuse epidemic, reduced its methadone treatment capacity from 8,700 to 3,000 patients between 1980 and 1984, prompting the medical director of the state's AIDS programs to designate the drug treatment programs as "overwhelmed."[29]

Although both Presidents Reagan and Bush created special cabinet-level positions in their administrations dedicated exclusively to fighting the "war on drugs," their administrations' efforts focused far more on stemming the supply of drugs (often through intervention in Latin American drug cartels) than on stemming demand. Most drug policy experts criticized the strategy, noting that the profits to be wrung from producing and distributing narcotics were so great as to induce extraordinary levels of creativity and tenacity from drug lords.[30] The better approach, they suggested, was thwarting demand, through drug education, expanded rehabilitation and treatment programs, increased capacity of methadone programs, and general community health efforts. Although such efforts would be expensive, they would ultimately prove cheaper and more effective than either the aggregate cost of drug abuse, or the mounting cost of the paramilitary war on drugs. Rising AIDS cases among IV drug users made the cost analysis even more persuasive. The Institute of Medicine in 1986, for example, estimated that while each AIDS patient would incur between $75,000 and $150,000 in treatment costs—drawn almost entirely from the public trough in the case of IV drug users—drug treatment programs of all types averaged less than $3,000 per year in costs per patient.[31] In response to such compelling analysis, the Reagan administration increased funding for drug treatment by an additional $160 million in 1987 and 1988.[32]

A related though largely discredited option was legalization of all narcotics, albeit in a controlled and regulated format. Proponents of such a move suggested that legalization would bring drug use out of the shooting galleries and guarantee a level of purity to both the drugs and the needles, thwarting both the spread of AIDS and the social dysfunction that accompanied drug use.[33] Most scholars of addiction and drug regulation rejected this argument outright. Switzerland, which had briefly legalized heroin, had been unsuccessful both in preventing the creation of new addicts, and in assimilating existing addicts into productive, socially acceptable lifestyles. As for the argument that "prohibition continues to fail miserably and tragically, at an unbearable cost," historical data showed otherwise.[34] Medical historian David Musto, for example, had found that despite all arguments to the contrary, alcohol prohibition in the 1920s and 1930s had reduced per capita consumption by at least a third, and that there was every reason to believe that laws against narcotics use were similarly squelching hundreds of thousands of potential users from embarking on the path of narcotics abuse.[35]

More feasible, and sensible, was the idea of legalizing not the drugs themselves, but rather the hypodermic needles. Advocates of legalized "needle exchanges" suggested that while the street cost of illegal needles was prohibitive to many addicts, the true cost of the needles to a legal purchaser was trivial. If a municipality or county purchased needles in bulk and doled them out to addicts (in a one-for-one exchange of used needles), addicts could be assured a supply of clean noninfected needles at no cost to themselves. The idea took root among health planners and academic epidemiologists, who argued that the public savings in treatment costs of just one or two prevented HIV transmissions would more than cover the cost of a year's supply of needles in an average municipality. Moreover, early needle exchanges in Tacoma, Washington, and New Haven, Connecticut, succeeded; a well-regarded study of New Haven's exchange conservatively estimated that it reduced HIV transmission by 33 percent in one year among drug users.[36]

The problem with such a program was its perceived endorsement of illegal narcotics use by the state. Such a program was "abhorrent," protested one New York state assemblyman. "Giving addicts government-approved needles will exacerbate the drug abuse problem and offer little benefit for confronting the AIDS epidemic."[37] Black politicians, in particular, opposed such programs, suspecting that if the programs resulted in an increase in drug use, the increase would disproportionately harm the black community. Black New York City councilman Hilton Clark called a proposed New York program "genocide," and the New York City police commissioner warned, "As a black person we have a particular sensitivity to doctors conducting experiments, and they too frequently seem to be conducted against blacks."[38] In Boston, Congregationalist minister Graylan Ellis-Hagler railed against a proposed program: "First they push drugs in the community. . . . Then someone hands out needles to maintain the dependency. Meanwhile, grandmothers live in fear of their own children because of what white society made them become."[39] And black New York City mayor David Dinkins vociferously opposed the creation of a program, fearing particularly that his endorsement would send a destructive message to young blacks who already used IV drugs in disproportionate numbers. "We have a conceptual problem with the concept of teaching people how to poison themselves more safely," offered mayoral spokesman Leland Jones."[40] The opposition resonated with the electorate; while a few cities, notably New Haven and Boston, tentatively inaugurated experimental exchanges, most large cities—notably New York and Los Angeles—resisted them at first.

Advocates of the programs argued that data did not suggest that the presence of free and available needles promoted drug use, and that in fact the presence of the needles helped suppress drug use as the addicts were given anti-drug messages when they came to exchange their needles. Several European cities had begun to experiment with programs starting as early as 1984, and none had discovered a marked increase in the numbers of drug users.[41] Public health researcher June Osborn suggested in the *New England Journal of Medicine* that the programs deserved a try, and that in the conservative-tilting war on drugs the forgotten victims were the "prisoners of war," those relatively harmless addicts who found themselves untreated, AIDS-infected, and imprisoned for lack of treatment, needle exchanges, and compassionate drug laws.[42] The New York state health commissioner admitted, "Frankly, I'd be willing to do just about anything to try to stop this disease."[43] And when New York State finally passed its own needle exchange program to be implemented on an experimental basis in New York City, the left-leaning *Nation* magazine wrote, "The administration of Governor Mario Cuomo has apparently decided that doing something about AIDS is more important than avoiding charges by the church, the law-enforcement community, and the Reaganites that it is soft on drugs."[44]

Another possibility was simply expanding condom education aggressively into the IV-drug-using community. Safe-sex campaigns had been very effective among gays, sharply cutting the rate of infection-disease spread over the half decade since the program's large-scale adoption. While condom use would not stop the virus from spreading among drug users, it would stop the virus from jumping to the sex partners of IV drug users (including prostitutes), and thereupon into the general population. Skeptics suggested that individuals imprudent enough to share needles, or even use IV drugs to start with, were unlikely to take precautions in their sexual relations, but advocates pressed on.

Opposing this campaign, much as it had opposed all safe-sex campaigns (as well as needle exchanges), was the Catholic Church, which saw the path to controlling AIDS as abiding by the Church's proscriptions against adultery, extraconjugal sex, homosexuality, and drug use.

Bishops and archbishops uniformly opposed all condom education efforts, and eschewed needle exchange proposals. "We don't say, 'Smoke carefully,' " noted New York City monsignor John Woolsey. "We say, 'Don't smoke.' A huge campaign could work to stop kids from having sex. We don't water down principles."[45] Similarly, Boston archbishop Bernard Law responded to that city's needle exchange program: "The answer to drugs must be an unequivocal no. It is difficult to say that convincingly while passing out clean needles."[46] The Church faced a formidable adversary in British billionaire Richard Branson, principal owner of Virgin Records and Virgin Airlines, who, in clear violation of Irish law, began to sell condoms in his Dublin record shop in an effort to prevent the spread of AIDS in Ireland. "In this case, the law is clearly an ass," commented Branson, after being taken to court.[47] "I want to make condoms in Ireland as common as sliced bread." But the Church cleaved to the rectitude of its high moral standards, insisting that moral depravity as much as anything else had caused the AIDS crisis, and that a return to moral propriety would be the most direct path to its ultimate resolution. In a stunning rejoinder to pro-condom protesters, chief Vatican spokesman Joaquin Navarro-Valls noted in 1988, "From the Church's point of view, saving a life is not the foremost value on a moral issue."[48]

Navigating the treacherous shoals of public opinion, religious fundamentalism, and general social squeamishness, several AIDS groups began educational outreach programs, not to end drug use, or promote condom use, but simply to try get IV drug users to wash their needles with bleach between uses, in order to kill off any live virus clinging to the equipment. Distributing cartoon-illustrated pamphlets featuring Bleachman and other whimsical characters, these AIDS consortiums and foundations disseminated information on the power of bleach and hygiene. "If you use the drug, you gotta use the jug [of bleach]," preached the cartoon character with a jug-shaped head.[49] Other cartoons featured handsome men sharing their needles, preaching the gospel of bleach-clean "works," and happily injecting themselves with heroin.

Advocates of needle exchanges and bleach education failed to seriously consider the magnitude of public disgust with their proposals. Intravenous drug use was considered by many Americans to be among the most depraved, self-destructive, and self-polluting activities

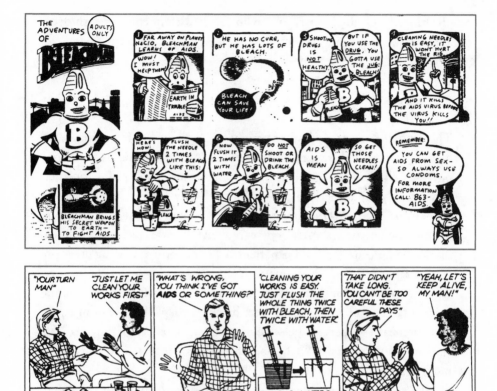

Cartoon campaigns featuring "Bleachman" were effective in reaching target audiences, but proved to be controversial. (San Francisco AIDS Foundation and Haight Ashbury Free Clinic)

imaginable—a refuge of the truly desperate and pathetic who showed scant interest in life and little potential for salvation. In the minds of many observers, AIDS might not be a just desert for these souls, but it was hardly a substantial diminishment of their life conditions. Investing efforts in protecting the integrity of their drug-shooting habits seemed bizarre to many, if not wholly immoral. Even drug-abuse professionals who had spent their professional lives working to aid drug users questioned the rectitude of the formula. "The day we teach someone to sterilize needles is the day we close down," stated Robert Galea, president of Spectrum House, a drug abuse treatment center in Westboro, Massachusetts.[50] And although Galea ultimately changed his mind on the issue of needle exchanges, he remained troubled by its implications. For most Americans, who recoiled from contact with drug addicts, the proposal was that much more difficult to accept.

BLACKS

The group of patients who had caught AIDS mainly either through IV drug use or through sexual relations with an IV drug user, was disproportionately black and Hispanic. Although these two groups together constituted only 19 percent of all Americans, by 1990 they represented 80 percent of all AIDS patients who had caught the disease through drug-related activities, and 38 percent of AIDS cases overall.[51] Among blacks, 35 percent of all AIDS patients were heterosexual drug users (in contrast with 5 percent of whites), and a growing percentage were women and children. Indeed, of all children with AIDS in the United States in 1988, fully 80 percent were black or Hispanic, and of infected women, nearly 70 percent belonged to those groups.[52] Not only was the epidemic no longer primarily one of gay men; increasingly it was no longer one of white people.

HIV's spread among blacks was facilitated by the paradoxical social norms of that community. While blacks remained the single most liberal voting block in the country, their attitudes toward homosexuality, and sexuality in general, were conservative. Gay black men were more reluctant than were their white counterparts to publicly acknowledge their homosexuality, and black community organizations were decidedly uncomfortable recognizing the gay individuals in their midst. At the same time, gay black men faced hostility, or at least indifference, when trying to join the larger white gay community, resulting in an unusually isolated and alienated social group. "Black gay men often feel little desire to come out of the closet, fearing rejection from straights without having access to the support systems that form the pillars of the white gay community," noted black gay editor Charles Stewart in 1991.[53] Surgeon General C. Everett Koop was more succinct in his assessment of blacks' attitudes toward homosexuality. "They don't want to deal with it," he noted at a 1989 luncheon meeting.[54]

Black rejection of homosexuality largely stemmed from conservative black clergymen. Heavily black denominations, particularly Southern

Baptists and African Methodist Episcopalians, were more likely to view homosexuality as sinful than were the more progressive white denominations, and less likely to embrace their stricken members.[55] Black pastors preaching in poor urban areas were reluctant to acknowledge the growing scourge in their midst, and even more reluctant to preach compassion and forgiveness. "The church does not necessarily see itself as in the business of rescuing people who go outside its teaching," reflected New York black AIDS leader Ronald Johnson.[56]

Black homophobia and pastoral unease discouraged black homosexuals, infected or not, from establishing their own self-help groups like the ones that had been created by their white counterparts. Throughout the country, black AIDS organizations faced difficulty raising money, recruiting members, implementing programs, and educating the community. The concomitant invisibility undermined the nascent organizations' efforts to win grant money, which could advance their visibility and further outside fund-raising efforts. "For every $500,000 in funding [white groups] get, a black organization might get $5,000," reflected Chicago AIDS activist Kenneth Allen.[57] And New York leader Johnson noted with sardonic remove that his own Minority Task Force on AIDS could not mention condoms or anal sex when holding education workshops in black churches, and indeed refrained from even putting the word "AIDS" on its office door. One black activist reflected angrily, "Our white allies drive us crazy, but they're still our allies, and our racial compatriots don't give two shits about us."[58]

Black clergy were not the only black leaders who abnegated responsibility; black political figures did too. Such eminent grises of black society as NAACP president Benjamin Hooks and past presidential hopeful Jesse Jackson eschewed mention of the disease, or at least of its homosexual roots, with Jackson taking care to stipulate in his eulogy of black newscaster Max Robinson that the AIDS that had killed him had most assuredly been a result of "heterosexual promiscuity."[59] Highly visible mayors such as Washington's Sharon Pratt Dixon and New York's David Dinkins tended to follow, rather than lead, the national discussion on minority AIDS, as did Harlem congressman Charles Rangel, the senior member of the congressional black delegation and chairman of the House of Representatives Subcommittee on Narcotics. Alexander Robinson, executive director of Washington's Inner City AIDS Network, explained the national reticence: "I get real concerned when I hear people talk about denial in the black and Hispanic communities because, while that's true, it's also true that we're just further behind. . . . You're adding another burden to an already overburdened people."[60] One black social worker illustrated the denial with this chilling description:

> There are sections where the epidemiologists can go block by block in central Harlem and say, "This block will no longer exist in ten years because of AIDS." And the community-board leaders in Harlem are saying, "AIDS is not a problem for us. AIDS is a white man's disease."[61]

Black reluctance to confront AIDS aggressively extended to eschewing needle exchange programs. Controversial even among the most progressive of policy thinkers, needle exchanges insulted black sensibilities on many levels, from resurrecting fears of genocide, to normalizing narcotics, to simply recognizing that black IV drug use was a special problem that demanded unique attention. The program recalled one of the most infamous and abusive episodes in racial medicine, in which (white) public health physicians studied untreated black syphilis patients at the Tuskegee Institute in Alabama for decades, maintaining the surveillance long after antibiotics could have rendered the disease harmless.[62] Black leaders feared that needle exchanges would further encourage young black men to inject narcotic drugs, exacerbating a problem that already affected the community disproportionately. In October 1988, responding to Health Commissioner Stephen Joseph's proposal for a needle exchange program in New York City, 14 influential black leaders wrote a letter to the *Amsterdam News* condemning the proposed program as a "very serious mistake," representing "the first step in legalizing intravenous drug abuse, thereby encouraging an additional number of addicts, and even enticing addicts currently in treatment, to drop out."[63]

So great was black skepticism around public health efforts that even mention of racially explicit statistics was cause for condemnation. Joseph recalled a "very uncomfortable half hour" while taping *Tony Brown's Journal*, a television talk show aimed predominantly at a black

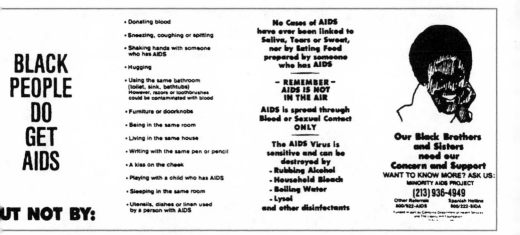

BLACK PEOPLE DO GET AIDS

UT NOT BY:

- Donating blood
- Sneezing, coughing or spitting
- Shaking hands with someone who has AIDS
- Hugging
- Using the same bathroom (toilet, sink, bathtubs) However, razors or toothbrushes could be contaminated with blood
- Furniture or doorknobs
- Being in the same room
- Living in the same house
- Writing with the same pen or pencil
- A kiss on the cheek
- Playing with a child who has AIDS
- Sleeping in the same room
- Utensils, dishes or linen used by a person with AIDS

No Cases of AIDS have ever been linked to Saliva, Tears or Sweat, nor by Eating Food prepared by someone who has AIDS

— REMEMBER — AIDS IS NOT IN THE AIR

AIDS is spread through Blood or Sexual Contact ONLY

The AIDS Virus is sensitive and can be destroyed by
- Rubbing Alcohol
- Household Bleach
- Boiling Water
- Lysol
and other disinfectants

Our Black Brothers and Sisters need our Concern and Support
WANT TO KNOW MORE? ASK US:
MINORITY AIDS PROJECT
(213) 936-4949
Other Referrals   Spanish Hotline
800/922-AIDS   800/722-SIDA

Public health educators attempted to reach African Americans with poster campaigns designed specifically for that audience. Cultural sensitivity in such efforts proved to be critical for their success. (Minority AIDS Project)

middle-class audience. "The host accused me of spreading a racist doctrine because I insisted that black women in New York City were at risk of AIDS," Joseph wrote later in his memoir about the epidemic. At that time, the incidence of AIDS among black mothers was several times that of white mothers, raising legitimate concerns for the health commissioner, and the integrity of the statistic was beyond reproach. Brown, however, insisted on emphasizing that only black women who had sex with IV drug users were at risk: technically true, but unnecessarily picayune. "My response that women didn't always know the drug histories of their current or former partners cut absolutely no ice with either host or audience," recalled Joseph.[64]

Black sensitivities dictated that any public health education efforts targeting the community be handled with the utmost discretion. Public health poster and pamphlet campaigns aimed at the community took care to use only clearly identifiable African Americans as models and used a message of caring and brotherhood. "People of Color: Because We Care, Let's Talk" read one poster. Another said: "Our Brothers and Sisters Need Our Concern and Support," while still another portrayed five individuals of varying ages, tied together with a band of ribbons, and read, "Break the Chain of Ignorance."[65] All such efforts eschewed images of condoms, needles, and other drug paraphernalia, which had been used to good effect in educational efforts targeting vulnerable white individuals. Humor, intimidation, and graphic portraits of sex were avoided. Rather, the campaign drew on a black sense of community, brotherhood, and shared values.

HISPANICS

Hispanics, like blacks, were disproportionately affected by the migration of AIDS to IV drug users. Disproportionately poor, uneducated, and vulnerable to narcotics abuse, Hispanic America injected drugs at rates far higher than did white America in the late 1980s, and thus contracted AIDS through needles at similarly high rates. By 1987, Hispanics, who constituted only 8 percent of all Americans, represented 15 percent of all AIDS cases, with the epidemic likely to worsen. Hispanic women were 11 times as likely to contract AIDS as non-Hispanic white women, and in some cities Hispanic children represented over half of all pediatric AIDS cases.[66]

The Hispanic epidemic, unlike the white and black epidemics, differed significantly from city to city. While in western cities the majority of Hispanic AIDS patients were gay men, in the upper Midwest and Northeast most were IV drug users, and a growing portion were women and children. And to an even greater extent than was true with blacks, Hispanic AIDS was almost exclusively an urban problem. New York, Miami, Los Angeles, and San Francisco registered the preponderance of Hispanic AIDS cases, with New York in particular posting an incidence of Hispanic AIDS 10 times that of the rest of the country.[67]

Hispanic vulnerability to AIDS rested on a number of cultural mores and values, in addition to the general poverty and unemployment so closely tied to IV drug use. Needle use was unusually prevalent in parts of the Hispanic immigrant community, possibly due to widespread use of injectable vitamins and medications in parts of the Caribbean and Latin America.[68] At the same time, many Hispanic men strongly resisted using condoms, viewing them as insults to cultural visions of masculinity, or simply as uncomfortable. Even as AIDS firmly established itself in Hispanic neighborhoods, many men refused to acknowledge the risk it posed, or the value of wearing condoms. Related one

Hispanic Chicago teenager: "After the drugs, people were going into rooms for sex, but I told my buddies, hey, we should go across the street to the gas station and get some condoms. They told me I was crazy, like I was acting like some kind of woman."[69] And reflected an AIDS counselor in a Hispanic neighborhood in that city: "Guys around here aren't going to watch out for these kinds of things. They sleep with whomever they want."[70] Such observations were confirmed by the 1982 National Survey of Family Growth, which found that a substantially lower percentage of Hispanics than non-Hispanics had ever used a condom: 39 percent as opposed to 53 percent.[71]

Part of the problem was simple ignorance. Even after targeted Spanish-language AIDS awareness campaigns, Hispanics demonstrated higher rates of ignorance about the epidemic than any other group. Pamphlets, brochures, posters, and call-lines were largely ineffectual in raising AIDS awareness within the community, owing to either general distrust of public health authorities, illiteracy, or apathy. Surveys of youths in San Francisco schools, and of communities elsewhere showed that Hispanics were far less knowledgeable about the disease than were blacks or non-Hispanic whites, and that into the late 1980s they continued to harbor misconceptions about the disease's spread. In one 1989 study, over half of all surveyed Hispanic respondents claimed that they knew nothing of AIDS, and only 5 percent were deemed to be "properly informed."[72]

At least part of the epidemic of drug use (and the concomitant AIDS infections) among American Hispanics had been imported. Puerto Rico was festering at that time with twin epidemics of heroin and crack use. A 1990 Puerto Rican government report estimated that IV drug use on the island had increased 13 times faster than it had among the general population, and Puerto Rican émigrés to mainland American cities brought these social plagues with them. Ensconced in the local "hospitalillos" (little hospitals, the local vernacular for shooting galleries) young Puerto Rican men shot up with "speedballs," injectable solutions of cooked heroin and crack (known locally as "la cura," the cure).[73] And while it was unclear if the drug culture was being exported from the island to expatriate Puerto Rican communities on the mainland, or being imported by returning émigrés, Puerto Rico by 1989 led all states and territories in the nation (save only Washington, D.C.) in

AIDS infection rates, with incidence among women five times the national average.[74]

As on the mainland, drug use (and the spread of AIDS) was concentrated in the cities, with the densely packed streets of old San Juan marking the disease's epicenter on the island. Coupled with a cultural unwillingness to acknowledge homosexuality, Puerto Rico's drug problem primed the AIDS pump, spreading the virus into condom-averse young men who thereupon spread it to prostitutes, gay hookups, and wives and girlfriends. And while this pattern was hardly unique, cultural rejection of condoms and safe-sex education increased the spread of AIDS infection to levels unknown on the mainland. One San Juan public health nurse testified before a government AIDS commission about San Juan streets "littered with used hypodermic needles" and "lines of cars going to La Perla to openly buy drugs."[75]

Nothing about the Hispanic AIDS epidemic was unique. Rather, it represented a variety of social plagues and disfunctionalities on a worse scale than existed elsewhere. While ignorance about the disease's spread existed in all pockets of America, among Hispanics it was more pronounced. Where other ethnic groups might eschew condom use, among Hispanics the reluctance was more heartfelt and consistent. And while Americans of all types, races, colors, religions, and income groups used injectable groups, Hispanic men used them far more frequently. Suspicious of institutional authority, and often unwilling to heed the lectures of public health educators and high school sex education teachers, Hispanic men placed themselves, and their partners, at grave risk, which would soon be transmuted to their children. "San Juan is a beautiful city that is slipping into decay—moral and physical," opined a pessimistic observer, and nobody "was willing to take responsibility."[76] The reflection was merely anecdotal, but anchored in statistics nonetheless.

PRISONS

As AIDS migrated from gays to IV drug users, it found a sizable perch in prisons. Inundated with thousands of drug offenders, the nation's prison populations had swelled in the 1980s. From 1977 to 1987, state prison populations increased an average of 7 percent annually, with many state's prison populations growing substantially faster. In the seven years after 1980, 18 state prison systems doubled their inmate populations, while New Jersey, Alaska, New Hampshire, and California nearly tripled theirs. New York City's prison system alone grew from 7,000 inmates in 1977 to 20,000 ten years later. In the words of one social researcher, corrections was "a growth industry."[77]

Much of this growth could be traced to drug-related arrests and crimes. Mandatory federal sentencing guidelines, along with harsh "Rockefeller"-type drug laws in New York and elsewhere, meant that a large portion of the nation's heroin and crack users found themselves spending substantial portions of their lives in jail. Reacting to a perceived crisis of criminality on the streets in those years, several large U.S. cities elected as mayors or district attorneys "law-and-order" candidates, who pledged themselves to reducing street and drug crimes, and restabilizing public space. The result of these various policies was an expanded prison population swollen with nonviolent drug offenders who often brought HIV with them as they entered the corrections system.

AIDS in prisons increased substantially through the 1980s, but not equally in all prisons. While in New York's penal system, the nation's most infected, 13 percent of prisoners were HIV-positive, systems in many western states posted infection rates of 0.[78] Women inmates varied even more in their HIV status, with the nation's cleanest systems boasting infection rates of, again, 0 percent, while the nation's worst-hit systems claimed infection rates of over 20 percent.[79] Overall, by 1989, 2 percent of all inmates in state prison systems were HIV-positive, while just over 1 percent of those in the federal system were so. Although the percentage of HIV-infected prisoners nationwide was quite small, it was still 10 times larger than the percentage of infected persons in the population at large.[80]

AIDS-infected prisoners faced a variety of challenges, ranging from the merely humiliating to the life-threatening. Many reported being abused by guards who, unsure of the exact threat the prisoners posed, handled them as if they were a deadly threat to all. Guards protected themselves with rubber suits, riot helmets, and plexiglas shields, and restrained AIDS-infected prisoners with equipment intended for use on superviolent inmates. Prisoners reported being bound, gagged, thrown into solitary confinement, and handcuffed to their beds. In at least one incident, an inmate was so heavily restrained and forcefully gagged that he died of asphyxiation.[81] Others reported being fed through trap doors in their cell doors, and kept from any human contact.

The guards' fear was in part justified, as stories emerged about HIV-infected prisoners purposefully biting guards in an effort to infect them, or throwing beakers of their own blood, or spitting. Many of the guards, possessing no expertise in the nature of HIV infection, were incapable of distinguishing truly hazardous behavior from the merely odious, and began to treat all encounters with AIDS prisoners as potentially lethal. While the American Civil Liberties Union's (ACLU) National Prisons Project objected to the harsh reprisals meted out for nonlethal behavior (such as spitting), judges tended to side with the guards. One judge upheld a harsh punishment imposed on a prisoner who had tried to spread AIDS to a guard by biting him. The ACLU had defended the prisoner, claiming that it was highly unlikely that the prisoner could have spread the virus through biting, and that furthermore the guard in question emerged from the incident uninfected. The prosecution argued that the prisoner had *intended* to kill, and thus should not be excused simply because of his ignorance of molecular biology. "Impossibility is no defense to a charge of attempted murder," argued the prosecutor.[82] Prison guards, not surprisingly, sided with their violated comrade.

More common was segregation. Prisoners testing positive for AIDS were marked and separated from their fellow inmates in a variety of ways, violating their right to medical privacy. Inmates reported being placed in separate cell blocks, being made to wear distinguishing clothes, and being placed in separate areas of the mess hall for meals. AIDS patients often ate off paper, disposed of their garbage in specially marked red bags (bearing the encryption "AIDS" in large lettering), and even had their laundry separated out. Some AIDS inmates had signs placed on their doors warning those around them to avoid bodily fluids. "It was made clear that we were a people not to be around, like lepers," wrote one prisoner.[83] Alexa Freeman of the ACLU related that at least one prisoner reported being required to scrub out his shower stall and toilet with bleach after each use, and then being required to scrub the floor with bleach as he returned to his cell.[84] One prisoner in Alabama, upon being placed in a separate AIDS unit, wrote of the experience: "I felt like an animal on display at the zoo. There is this double fence with razor wire atop separating HIV+ inmates from the general prison population."[85] Other prisoners reported being barred from regular prison activities, such as the recreation yard, trade or GED courses, and hobby areas.

Noninfected prisoners responded to their infected comrades with disgust and fear. AIDS prisoners reported being told by their fellow inmates not to share their toilets, nor to sit with them at meals, nor to participate in contact sports with them. A few related that they had been physically threatened, and warned not to come out of their cells into the general indoor recreation area. Although technically a prisoner's medical status was supposed to be confidential, news of a diagnosis of AIDS generally spread quickly through the prison community, sometimes accelerated by gossip from guards and administrators. "There is the attitude here that you can get AIDS from mosquito bites," related one Minnesota prisoner. "Each time I get in line for dinner, it just kills me. You've got people saying stuff, people who won't come near me."[86]

Harsh and humiliating treatment was not always malicious or punitive—sometimes it resulted simply from guards' efforts at managing an uncertain situation. In Massachusetts, prisoners at the Framingham state prison reported being strip-searched and shackled together naked en route to medical visits at nearby Shattuck Hospital. For routine doses of AZT, AIDS patients were made to stand in line three or four times per day, even after their physical integrity had deteriorated and their strength had ebbed. While prison medical personnel argued that they were simply taking reasonable precautions against a deadly disease that they did not fully understand, the effect on the prisoners was demoralizing and detrimental. "Sometimes they are so weak, they refuse medical care just not to go through the ordeal of being shackled," commented Nicholas Parkhurst of the Multicultural AIDS Coalition.[87]

And yet, even as prison administrators resisted providing appropriate care for the infected prisoners, and supported their security staff's often inappropriate precautions, they were equally resistant to letting the prisoners go. Across the country in the late 1980s, sporadic reports described patients being involuntarily tested for HIV before release or parole, and then refused release if they tested positive. Prison administrators suggested that the tests were not punitive, but either were required by law (in the case of the federal prisons) or were simply a means of providing proper counseling to the soon-to-be ex-convicts and their partners and families. "The bureau's policy provides for testing, treatment, and counseling for inmates, as well as education for staff and inmates. We believe that the policy is a well-balanced approach to a complex issue," wrote an official with the Federal Bureau of Prisons.[88] Prisoners argued, to the contrary, that if they resisted being tested, they were automatically denied parole.[89] "Many are denied parole for the first time, due to [the] fact that they are not ready for the 'free world,' " wrote one frustrated inmate.[90] Off the record, prison administrators admitted succumbing to political pressure not to release the infected prisoners. "If we parole too many with the virus, we're accused of paroling people to get them out of prison," stated Massachusetts Parole Board director Edward Dolan.[91]

Shortcomings in the prison medical system exacerbated the plight of AIDS-infected prisoners. Long an object of reformist critiques, the atrocious state of prison medical care had been illuminated following the Attica Prison uprising in upstate New York in 1971. Reformist investigators reported on the inhumane conditions they observed: "prisoners performing surgery on fellow inmates; inmates left to die with wounds covered with maggots and encased in their own filth; and systems that separated sick and disabled inmates from medical caregivers by two locked sets of doors and no means of communication across them."[92] A 1973 American Medical Association study had found that the vast majority of prisons (82 percent) had neither full-time medical personnel on-site nor reasonable medical facilities, and that 16.7 percent lacked any medical facility whatsoever.

Medical facilities had improved in the intervening years, but remained inadequate for the care of AIDS patients. Despite the availability of full-time nursing staff, part-time medical staff, and reasonable infirmaries, AIDS-infected prisoners faced ignorance of their disease, lack of appropriate pharmaceuticals, and an absence of sensitivity and discretion from medical personnel. Prisoners described being "treated like a leper" by medical personnel, and being "refused hands-on treatment."[93] Others described waiting in line for hours for AZT, when available, or having to describe their symptoms to medical personnel in front of other prisoners, or having their medical records divulged to prison guards. Described one Attica inmate: "Sick-call here at Attica is held at the front of the 'company' (gallery) where there is no room which allows for privacy and usually, where officers congregate. Not only is there an officer breathing down the nurses' neck, at times you might also find him/her actually handling medical records."[94]

When medical care was provided, it was often simply inadequate. Prison observers reported an absence of AZT, aerosolized pentamidine, appropriate antibacterial medications, and painkillers for the cancers that frequently occurred. T cell counts were rarely, if ever, taken, and prisoners continued to be treated on an outpatient basis long after hospitalization was required. "Our medical experts testified that every single case of AIDS and symptomatic HIV disease was mishandled," testified the ACLU's Alexa Freeman in 1990.[95] Physicians and other medical personnel within the prison systems, often lacking specialized training in infectious-disease medicine, were unaware of current studies of AIDS treatment, or uninformed as to the availability of the latest generation of drugs. At times, simple ignorance resulted in near-lethal treatment decisions. One prisoner reported seeing AIDS-infected prisoners housed in the same cells as those suffering from tuberculosis, posing extraordinary risk for prisoners with compromised immune systems.

Along with inadequate medical treatment, prisons provided inadequate medical prophylaxis. Despite reports that 10 percent or more of all prisoners engaged in sexual intercourse while in prison, most prisons refused to distribute condoms, or make them available through the prison commissary. Similarly, despite reports that a significant minority of prisoners continued to use intravenous drugs while in jail (and that 60 percent of those users were sharing needles), prisons refused to make needles available, or create adequate treatment programs for drug users. As late as 1992, only 8 percent of all inmates in U.S. prison systems had participated in prison-based drug abuse programs, despite 52 percent of all inmates having had drug abuse problems, and 70 percent of all inmates having committed drug-related offenses. In the federal prison system, the General Accounting Office estimated in 1991 probably fewer than 1 percent of all inmates with persistent drug addictions were participating in substance abuse programs.[96]

Prison administrators faced the same dilemmas over needle exchanges as did elected officials. Taking appropriate prophylactic measures required tacitly endorsing certain illegal activities, or even acknowledging that they existed. If prisons distributed condoms and needles, they would be acknowledging that forbidden sex and drug-use were continuing, despite the constant presence of guards and cameras. Either the security systems were inadequate or the prison guards themselves were complicit in the activities. Such admissions were politically problematic for prison administrators and legislators alike. Nonetheless, denying the extent of the problems promised that AIDS would continue to spread in the system. "The fact is that this activity is going to continue whether condoms are provided or not," wrote one incisive inmate. "The question is, will the DOC recognize that homosexuality is a fact of prison life and provide or sell condoms? Or will they deny the fact and allow unsafe sex to continue?"[97] In fact, if the black market cost of clean needles was any indicator, the demand was very high. Researchers estimated the cost of needles in one Canadian prison at $34 in 1994, and even then the needles came with no guarantee of being sterile.[98]

CHILDREN

As AIDS spread to users of IV drugs and their sex partners, it also spread to their children. By 1989, nearly 1,500 children under 13 had been diagnosed with AIDS in the United States, and over 800 had died.[99] Epidemiologists estimated that as many as half of all infants born to HIV-infected women were themselves infected, and that of these nearly 85 percent would develop AIDS by their sixth birthday. Although a few children would prove to be highly resistant to the virus (owing in part to perinatal transfer of antibodies), the majority would die by age 12.[100] And the pediatric epidemic was growing rapidly; Public Health Service physicians estimated that by 1991 over 20,000 U.S. children would be infected.

AIDS traveled from mother to child primarily during birth, but also *in utero* as well as through breastfeeding. Women who were themselves unaware that they had AIDS could unknowingly transmit the virus to multiple children, and in at least one case a woman contracted the virus after giving birth, and thereupon infected her child through her breast milk.[101] As the infected women were often drug addicts or prostitutes, they proved stubbornly resistant to outreach and education campaigns, either because of their distrust of authority or because of simple apathy. Counselors reported cases of women who had lost a child to AIDS and promptly gotten pregnant again to replace the lost child, despite the high chance that subsequent children would be born infected. "A child filled her need for love and affection," explained a social worker of one such mother. "She knew her daughter would die, and she hoped to replace her."[102]

The pediatric epidemic was disproportionately minority, with over half of all childhood cases afflicting black babies, and another quarter afflicting Hispanic ones (despite populational representation of 13 and 7 percent, respectively). It was concentrated in cities, and heavily affected single-parent households living at near-poverty levels. In Newark's Children's Hospital, physician James Oleske pioneered a variety of aggressive pediatric interventions during the late 1980s, but admitted ultimately that he wished only to "make a difference" and that the "worst was yet to come."[103] Furthering the horror was the growing number of orphans among the infected children. Social service agencies strained to adequately care for children who were virtually impossible to place in foster homes and required extensive medical attention.

In some sense, the pediatric epidemic was self-limiting. Children could only catch AIDS from infected mothers, who themselves could only produce infected children so long as they were alive. The pediatric epidemic was horrifying, but could never spread beyond the limited confines of the adult epidemic. In light of this reality, dispassionate policy dictated that the preponderance of resources should target potential adult patients, with the understanding that they actually had the prerogative to alter their behavior in a way that children did not. Advocates of children, however, violently rejected such a coldhearted approach. University of Michigan public health professor June Osborn demanded far more aggressive drug intervention programs, testing and treatment programs, and a richer safety net of counselors and therapists. "What's being done is pitiful compared to what needs to be done," she complained.[104]

More pragmatic planners questioned if any of these efforts would make a difference. Drug prevention and treatment programs had proven to be only partially successful where implemented, and parents of infected children, as a group, were proving to be among the lowest-functioning of all patient subgroups. Resistant to education, desperately poor, often drug addicted and subject to the violent whims of boyfriends, pimps, and husbands, they stood little chance of taking anti-drug lessons to heart. The pediatric epidemic appeared to be an ugly appendix to the growing AIDS epidemic in IV drug users.

CHAPTER 8

WHO PAYS?

Who would pay for the enormous cost of the growing epidemic? By 1989, with 90,000 cases having been recorded, AIDS was costing the United States some $6 billion per year in direct medical costs, with such costs growing fast. Various epidemiologists and health-care economists estimated that this figure would continue to rise to possibly $9 billion by 1991, with aggregate medical costs by the end of the century of $50 billion or more. With patients accruing $75,000 in medical expenses over the course of their expected 15-month lives with AIDS, and no cure, vaccine, or effective treatment in the offing, there was little reason to believe that the trend would taper off.[1] Of course, the nonmedical costs of the disease in lost wages and productivity were anybody's guess, but at least one economist estimated them in aggregate at $168 billion, even as early as 1991.[2]

The disease's gargantuan appetite for funds threatened to overwhelm various payers and agencies. In 1989, for example, AIDS-related programs and grants consumed 9.6 percent of the Public Health Service's budget, and this would rise to 13 percent within two years. Likewise, it consumed 40 percent of the budget of the Centers for Disease Control, and 50 percent of the budgets of the National Institute on Drug Abuse and the Food and Drug Administration.[3] Urban hospitals and hospital systems were devoting an increasingly larger share of their beds to treating the disease's victims, with New York and San Francisco devoting 8 and 12 percent, respectively, of all beds to AIDS patients by 1991. The portion of beds in the public, municipal hospitals being used to treat AIDS by that time was several times larger.[4]

The bill fell at first disproportionately on private health insurers. With few elderly among the afflicted, the huge national Medicare program was largely shielded from medical liability for AIDS, forcing other payers to assume an unusually large share of the cost of the disease. Private payers estimated that by 1989 they were paying nearly 50 percent of all medical costs associated with AIDS (versus the usual 34 percent),[5] driving most to cut benefits for AIDS, exclude those who had the disease, or in the absence of information about disease status, find proxies by which they could exclude probable AIDS victims. Companies hard hit by the disease purchased policies that capped AIDS-related benefits at $5,000 per year, or lower.[6] One small company in Alaska found its monthly insurance premiums *quadrupled* after 1 of its 20 workers was found to be HIV-positive.[7] Workers at the Gay Men's Health Crisis, ironically, found themselves with inadequate coverage for AIDS, having failed to find a provider willing to underwrite the risk of insuring a gay men's health services organization. "We were turned down everywhere," recalled GMHC executive director Timothy Sweeney. Only Blue Cross/ Blue Shield would take on the risk, at less-than-ideal benefit levels.[8]

Insurers, unable to ask explicitly about sexual orientation, used proxy indicators such as marital status, neighborhood of residence, and even profession, to try to identify gay men, who posed much higher risks for the disease. States responded by attempting to police these illegal practices, but often had little success. Sorting by disease state was perfectly legal, and indeed was the essence of risk assignment in the insurance industry. Insurance spokesmen argued that they were not antigay, simply anti-AIDS, and thus were protected from antidiscrimination suits brought by individuals and state attorneys general. The distinction, while legally significant, produced the same results, however, as gay men found themselves locked out of group policies, or excluded for certain diseases or conditions crucial to proper coverage. Moreover, a study by the Congressional Office of Technology Assessment challenged the validity of the claim after finding that over a fourth of surveyed companies admitted to considering sexual orientation when underwriting policies.[9] "Insurers are betting that people with AIDS will be too demoralized, too ill, too frightened to fight them in court. Either that, or they hope the life span of the suit will be longer than the life span of the person with AIDS," speculated National Gay Rights Advocates lawyer Benjamin Schatz.[10]

Filling in much of the remainder of the payment gap were the 50 assorted state Medicaid plans designed to cover acute as well as long-term care for the impoverished of each state, as designated by that state. Owing to the largely impoverished state of the IV-using AIDS patients, and the increasingly impoverished state of the gay AIDS patients, Medicaid programs were forced to shoulder an ever-larger portion of the AIDS bill as the decade progressed. By 1989, Medicaid programs were covering between 25 and 30 percent of all AIDS-related medical costs, despite the programs covering less than 9 percent of health-care costs as a whole. For AIDS hospitalizations, Medicaid covered as much as 50 percent of total costs (in the worst-afflicted states), and nearly 65 percent of AIDS-related costs in public hospitals (versus 28 and 38 percent, respectively). And on pediatric wards, Medicaid picked up as much as 85 percent of all costs in some areas.[11]

Hospitals generally, and public hospitals in particular, struggled with the burden. Medicaid tended to reimburse at substantially less generous rates than did private payers. In Connecticut, for example, Medicaid reimbursed $45 for AIDS testing versus $185 from private payers, while in New York an intermediate office visit was reimbursed $78 by Blue Cross, but only $7 by Medicaid.[12] At such reimbursement rates, hospitals lost $2,000 per AIDS-related admission on average, and the problem was only getting worse as greater numbers of AIDS patients lost their jobs with their private health insurance benefits, and descended into the ranks of the Medicaid-covered, or even worse the wholly uncovered.[13] President George H. W. Bush's AIDS commission reported that casting hopes on Medicaid as a source of payment for impoverished AIDS patients was simply a "Medicaid fantasy," and a George Washington University research study reported that by 1991 the states were spending $170 million per year on AIDS in non-Medicaid money in an effort to close the reimbursement gap.[14]

Yet even with the growing coverage and concomitantly lower reimbursement levels, many people were barred from qualifying for Medicaid. Each state set its own qualification standards for the program (within established federal ranges) and in some states the maximum allowable income level was low indeed. In New York, for example, any individual earning more than $5,700 in 1989 failed to qualify for the program, despite employed but uninsured AIDS patients being able to accrue $75,000 in annual hospital billings.[15] And even when patients reached qualification standards, they often collided with bureaucratic barriers and general malaise in their quest for health insurance. Recounted one exasperated patient of his experience at New York's Saint Luke's Hospital:

> My Medicaid hadn't gone through and my second admission was about a month after the first one, so you know, it wasn't enough time anyway. So I had this $10,000 bill that was unpaid. And I was wheeled into the admitting office in a wheelchair with a 104 fever, you know, gasping for breath and this administrator from behind the desk said that I couldn't be admitted because I owed them $10,000 and that I would have to pay the $10,000 before they could possibly admit me, and kept me there for three hours. Finally, the friend who was with me *lost* it and raised holy hell and they sent me to the emergency room.[16]

Public hospitals shouldered an increasing share of the burden, and those in the worst-hit cities shouldered the preponderance of the cost. Nationwide, public hospitals treated twice as many AIDS patients per hospital, on average, as did private hospitals. One-third of all AIDS patients were treated by just 10 hospitals (all in the five worst-hit cities), most of which were public. And the public hospitals lost more on each AIDS patient than did private hospitals, averaging losses of $218 per day, versus only $92 in losses per day for the private institutions. Public hospitals, always money-losers for municipalities, were turning into money sinks whose appetites far exceeded the capacity of their urban tax bases to provide for them. Yet as rural AIDS patients flooded the nation's cities seeking specialized AIDS care, the problem could get only worse. The patients, for the most part, would be neither insured nor Medicaid-eligible, and would draw upon the resources of municipal hospital systems and uncompensated care funds.[17]

Frustrated AIDS patients turned to other government programs for help, particularly the disability benefits of the federal Social Security program, but here again their aspirations were frequently blocked. Despite the disabling effects of advanced AIDS, many AIDS patients found that their diseases failed to fall into easily qualifiable disability categories, and were forced to repeatedly appeal benefits refusals, or even sue, to gain access to funds. Waits of 20 months and more were not uncommon, and frequently patients died before seeing the first of their disability checks, despite having been unable to work for two years or more. Overwhelmed administrative judges tried hard to dispense justice, but the backlogged system was simply ill-equipped to handle the deluge of applications. One weary supplicant, after waiting for 5 months, found that his file had been sent to Omaha for a decision, and to Wilkes-Barre, Pennsylvania, for typing, and thereafter to parts unknown. He died one week before receiving the first disability check, 15 months after initially applying.[18]

RYAN WHITE

The federal government, already investing a great deal of its public health and CDC funds into the AIDS crisis, responded with new funds to help the beleaguered states and municipalities. Its initial effort, a 1988 measure to raise funding levels for research and drug approval, avoided controversy by eschewing support of clinical services and testing. The $1 billion law did provide funds for home health care for AIDS patients, but left the strapped public hospitals and city clinics, as well as stretched state Medicaid programs, untouched. While far from ideal in the minds of AIDS advocates, the bill was an important first step in federal support for the epidemic, and demonstrated that even stalwart conservatives could support an AIDS program under the right circumstances. "The bill is better than none," noted Connecticut senator Lowell Weicker Jr.[19]

More critical was the Comprehensive AIDS Resource Emergency (CARE) Act of 1990, later renamed for Ryan White, an Indiana boy who received substantial media attention after contracting AIDS from a contaminated blood transfusion. The bill, cosponsored by Senators Edward Kennedy (D-Massachusetts) and Orrin Hatch (R-Utah), as well as Henry Waxman (D-California) in the House of Representatives, provided substantial funds for a variety of purposes, including emergency assistance to the states and cities, early intervention, and health services research. The section of the bill drawing the most attention was the Title I provision for providing hundreds of millions of dollars to the worst-afflicted cities and metropolitan areas in the country (later termed eligible metropolitan areas, or EMAs). These 13 cities contained over 65 percent of all diagnosed AIDS cases in the country, and were facing dire shortfalls in funds for emergency medical care, public hospitals, clinics, private hospital reimbursement, and emergency social services for AIDS patients and their families. In defending his bill, Kennedy noted that the death toll for AIDS was already "a hundred-fold greater than any natural disaster to strike our nation in this century," and constituted a crisis "as devastating as an earthquake, flood, or drought."[20] Waxman was less diplomatic. "The sins of the Reagan prevention policy are now visited on the Bush payment plans. Having missed the opportunity to get the ounce of prevention, we now have to pay for the pounds and pounds of cure."[21]

Opponents of the bill expressed concern that it set a precedent of singling out specific diseases, and provided targeted funding to them rather than releasing general funds to Medicaid, the CDC, the NIH, and the PHS to disseminate as those agencies saw fit. Such a move invited future interest groups to lobby for extraordinary funding for their own "diseases of the month," and opened up Congress to potential emotional blackmail. Moreover, the application of special federal funds to state medical care budgets (outside of Medicaid) created an odd precedent, with the potential for reimbursement abuse and exploitation by qualifying providers. This "unorthodox funding mechanism," in the administration's words, would create confusion in payment to providers, while allowing private insurance companies to renege on their existing payment obligations.[22] But despite misgivings, the Bush White House agreed to support the bill if passed in Congress, and refused to support the opposition voiced by Senator Jesse Helms (R-North Carolina), who decried the "hysteria that has been whipped up and verges on terror."[23] The bill passed overwhelmingly in August 1990, and named 16 cities to initially qualify as EMAs.*

Within two months, however, AIDS advocates would face disappointment. Although the Ryan White bill had passed, separate funding legislation was necessary to fully fund all of its provisions, and on this Congress balked. In October, the Senate Appropriations Committee slashed funding for the program from $875 million for the first year to $159 million, of which only $49 million was available for new city-based programs. Senators who had supported the initial bill refused to cut alternate social services programs to free up funding for AIDS, and the Bush White House was ill-disposed to support new taxes to pay for the program. Senator Arlen Specter (R-Pennsylvania) defended his decision thus: "There has been an enormous increase in other AIDS funding this year. Now we are talking about taking money away from cancer, heart disease, childhood immunization, diabetes, arthritis."[24] The president's own National Commission on AIDS urged the president to support full funding for the program, and AIDS advocates termed the cuts a disaster. New York City mayor David Dinkins was "deeply distressed" over the decision.[25]

Despite its initial compromised state, however, the program grew over the following three years to become a nearly $600-million-per-year program. By 1994, the initial 16 EMAs had grown to 32, and the Title I funds that directly benefited these heavily affected urban areas had grown to over half the total program. Services purchased with these funds included direct primary care, case management, housing, medication, transportation, dental services, and mental health services. The EMAs created AIDS planning agencies to determine funding priorities, and directed the money accordingly.[26] As befitted the congressional vision of the program, the Title I funds allowed the cities substantial latitude in allocating funds according to local need, with Newark, for example, allocating a third of all funds to case management, while At-

---

*The original EMAs were Atlanta, Boston, Chicago, Dallas, Fort Lauderdale, Houston, Jersey City, Los Angeles, Miami, New York City, Newark, Philadelphia, San Diego, San Francisco, San Juan (P.R.), and Washington, D.C.

lanta invested nearly three-fourths of its funds in primary care. Notably, all 50 states used their Title II funds in part for medication programs, which were quickly bankrupting Medicaid programs and exhausting existing emergency charity care programs.[27] Although far from a panacea, the Ryan White funds had been a godsend to the worst-hit states and cities.

TESTING AND OUTREACH

After money, the most pressing AIDS-related issue facing the federal government was testing. The country was divided on the subject, with those fearful of catching the virus balanced almost equally by those fearful of surrendering their right to privacy to the government. President Bush himself had come out quite forcefully in favor of mandatory national testing, albeit with strong guarantees of confidentiality ("It is absolutely *imperative* that those records are kept appropriately confidential," he had stated to an international AIDS conference in 1987).[28] Practicalities aside, a number of prominent epidemiologists and public health experts supported the stance, including the usually liberal editor of the *New England Journal of Medicine,* Marcia Angell. "I believe that, on balance, systematic tracing and notification of the sexual partners of HIV-infected persons and screening of pregnant women, newborns, hospitalized patients, and health care professional are warranted," she wrote in a controversial 1991 editorial.[29] With similar finesse, Stephen Joseph, the former health commissioner of New York City, argued that the civil rights of the infected were not "absolute," nor could they "supersede the rights of noninfected people."[30] A number of conservative politicians rejoiced at the endorsement.

Many people, including virtually all active members of AIDS activist organizations, gay community groups, and civil rights groups, rejected the proposal, suggesting that such an erosion of civil rights and privacy protections could simply not be justified. However, the rationale for such a stance was strangely inconsistent with the thrust of the pro-testing advocates' argument. While those who supported testing suggested that the move was justified on the grounds of protecting the noninfected public from a uniquely toxic disease, those who opposed testing often suggested that the *infected* individuals would have little to gain from such a move. David Rogers and June Osborn argued in the *New England Journal* that testing would "work against the desired outcome of finding and treating the maximal number of infected women and children," while antitesting congressman Ted Weiss (D–New York) expressed his concern that testing was not adequately leading to treatment and counseling for infected persons.[31]

Such an argument missed the basic concern of the pro-testers, which was that while treating the sick was all well and good, protecting the well ought to be the overarching concern. While testing might drive some infected persons to shun the medical establishment and reject treatment, it might expose many more who were ignorantly walking around infected, and prevent them from spreading the epidemic still further. Bush emphasized that while testing was a "complex" issue, it was the responsibility of political leaders to "decide among competing principles." "Ultimately," he warned, "we must protect those who do not have the disease."[32] More blunt was Palm Beach infectious-disease physician Sanford Kuvin, who decreed it "unconscionable that a lethal infectious disease is nonreportable."[33]

In September 1991, the bizarre case of Kimberly Bergalis, a 23-year-old woman infected with AIDS by her dentist, David Acer, in the course of having two teeth removed, drew national attention to the issue. Bergalis herself intensified the focus on her case when she testified before Congress about the need to prevent future such mishaps. "I did not do anything wrong, yet I am being made to suffer like this," she told a rapt congressional audience, and urged them to pass a mandatory testing bill for health-care workers.[34]

But Bergalis was perhaps the person with the least perspective on her own illness, providing a poor pretext for legislative activity. The Acer case had been unique, and those who followed AIDS saw the danger in using it to spur broad testing legislation, whether for the general public or exclusively for health-care workers. Former surgeon general C. Everett Koop pointed out that Bergalis's death was the first in 187,000 known AIDS cases in the United States in which the disease was transmitted from an infected health-care worker to a patient, and that even that case suggested possibly depraved motives on the part of the dentist.[35] Congressman Gerry Studds (D-Massachusetts) spoke out against the Bergalis backlash, condemning those "snake-oil" salesmen who were willing to "pacify—and exploit—our fear." "Compared to the HIV virus, the risk of contracting hepatitis from your dentist is 100 times greater," he argued.[36] The snake-oil salesmen to whom Studds referred were none other than his conservative congressional colleagues Jesse Helms and William Dannemeyer (R-California), who had invited Bergalis to testify in the first place.[37] And GMHC policy director David Barr argued that one insidious result of forced testing of health-care providers could be to make those scarce physicians and nurses willing to treat AIDS patients even scarcer. "The average wait to get T cell test results in a public hospital in the Bronx is three to six weeks. It is common for people to wait up to ten days in emergency rooms before getting hospital beds. Every day we face a crisis in providing basic health care, yet the CDC is advocating the restriction of workers from treating people," he declared that November.[38]

Alongside calls for testing for health-care providers were calls for testing a variety of other groups. Prisoners, immigrants, and even prostitutes all came under the gaze of vigilant legislators in federal and state bodies. Utah and Wyoming both passed laws in 1989 to mandate HIV testing for all state prisoners, while a dozen states passed "duty-to-warn" regulations giving physicians the discretion to "warn or inform" individuals at risk.[39] In Washington, Senator Helms successfully introduced a bill to make AIDS one of the grounds for denial of entry to immigrants or legal aliens.[40] And the concerned lawmakers of Nevada enacted a "buyer-beware" program in 1991 forcing brothels to post prominent warnings to patrons that sexual activity might result in AIDS.[41]

Along with the mandatory testing of certain subpopulations in some states, was the widespread refusal by the states to prohibit testing by insurance companies. By 1989, 43 states had no laws or regulation prohibiting in any way AIDS testing by insurance companies of applicants seeking policies, and 33 states allowed insurance companies to exclude AIDS coverage from comprehensive sickness policies.[42] Americans, generally, seemed comfortable with relatively broad mandated testing, and discounted the possible erosion of civil rights.[43] Although the federal government in the end resisted mandating testing for either the general population or select health-care workers, many

Americans quietly wished for more, rather than fewer, inroads into their privacy.

More acceptable than mandated testing to federal lawmakers and regulators was spending on education and outreach, which had been funded at increasing levels through the 1980s. By the end of that decade, the CDC was spending $400 million on its AIDS programs, much of it directed at education and prevention, and the Public Health Service as a whole was spending another $100 million.[44] And although President Bush had repeatedly stated his preference that education remain a purview of the states and municipalities, he wholeheartedly backed education and information as broad general strategies for fighting the epidemic. "We've got to put into the hands of parents and students and people throughout America essential facts about AIDS," he insisted repeatedly while campaigning in 1988.[45] Despite the hand-wringing over the federal government's reluctance to act, the government was slowly bringing its enormous might and wealth to bear against the disease in all aspects: clinically, biologically, epidemiologically, and pedagogically.

HOUSING

One unexpected consequence of the strange patterns of AIDS was a housing crisis for patients. AIDS patients died slowly, often living two years or more after contracting the disease. During this time, they usually had to stop working at some point, and often soon exhausted disability benefits, ran through private health coverage and COBRA benefits, and spent down their personal assets. As a result, AIDS patients frequently found that they ran out of money before they ran out of their time on earth, and periodically lost their homes in the process.

Exacerbating this phenomenon was the large and increasing number of AIDS patients who were homeless, or nearly so, to start with. As the epidemic moved into the IV-drug-using community, it afflicted the single most disenfranchised group of people in America. Those who were not homeless to begin with frequently had sought shelter with friends or relatives, or shared a bedroom in an inexpensive apartment. After AIDS hit, their ability to generate even a meager income was eradicated, as was the generosity of their friends and families. AIDS patients found themselves on the street, and frequently even beyond the help of local shelters, which refused to allow them in. Their Orwellian plight seemed beyond the reach of social service safety nets.

The problem was growing. Although no reliable numbers existed for the nation, New York City estimated in 1990 that it had between 8,000 and 11,000 homeless AIDS patients, with only 230 AIDS-appropriate beds available for them.[46] The American Hospital Association estimated that possibly 30 percent of all hospitalized AIDS patients were being held longer than necessary owing to inadequate housing and long-term facilities for postdischarge care.[47] Among other problems with these prolonged stays were the extra costs with which they burdened Medicaid and charity care programs: a day for an AIDS patient in the hospital cost nearly $700, versus $80 or less for a day in a nursing home.

Cities responded by placing at least some of the homeless AIDS patients in shelters or SRO hotels, but both were inappropriate venues for care. AIDS patients frequently soiled their beds with blood and pus (from skin ulcers), vomit, and diarrhea. They might cough incessantly, or be racked with cold. Frequently they needed assistance simply eating, drinking, or using the bathroom, and at advanced stages of the disease they were unable to cook, clean, or maintain their own possessions. Given their terrible physical condition, their placement in shelters was decried as "the equivalent of putting a Band-aid on a shotgun wound," by one AIDS advocate.[48] The shelters were usually large open floors with beds for several hundred people, and dining, bathroom, and recreation facilities were all open, shared, and devoid of privacy. Petty crime was rampant, as was the fear of nighttime attacks. And while the SROs offered a bit more privacy, they were equally inappropriate. Wrote one frequent denizen: "Many of the SROs are infested with bedbugs, roaches, and rats. Drug use is rampant and is ignored by many of the security personnel. . . . The strong will steal from the weak, those not able or too scared to fight back."[49]

What the patients needed was a cross between a halfway house, a long-term-care facility, and supervised public housing. Beyond simple rent subsidies, they needed some sort of medical or paramedical supervisory presence, a transportation service, and a grocery delivery service, all designated specifically for AIDS patients lest the noninfected recoil at their presence. Cities were hardly prepared to offer such services, and given their already stretched domestic resource services, they were hardly in a position to start.

At least part of the gap between need and supply began to be filled by the community service AIDS organizations that had been started originally with more medical intentions. Organizations like Washington's Whitman-Walker Clinic and Seattle's Northwest AIDS Foundation began to devote more of their resources to housing starting in the mid-1980s, insofar as their finances would allow. In 1990, the Northwest AIDS Foundation described its multitiered housing effort as a "continuum" of options that included a "rental subsidy program, emergency housing, independent housing, private houses and apartments, adult family homes, long-term care facilities, and hospice services."[50] Similarly, Boston's AIDS Action Committee maintained its own rental subsidy program, lobbied private developers to set aside some new housing for AIDS patients, and ran free-standing facilities to house a limited number of AIDS-infected adults and children.[51] And the Whitman-Walker by 1990 controlled eight residences housing 40 individuals, as well as six group homes and a six-unit apartment building to house AIDS patients with a range of different caretaking needs.[52]

Besides providing sanctuary and shelter for the afflicted, these housing programs actually saved a great deal of money. While hospital care cost $800 per day for most AIDS patients (whether or not it was ultimately reimbursed), Whitman-Walker found it was able to run its residence program for just $60 per day per patient. And while hospitals were ill-equipped to provide the supportive living structure so necessary for substance abusers, Whitman-Walker and the AIDS Action Committee committed themselves to maintaining on-site counselors and support groups. Testified Barry Bianchi of the Northwest AIDS Foundation, "The only successful housing program for persons with AIDS is the program which provides counseling and referral, maintains a plurality of housing options and is cost-effective."[53]

The efforts of the community groups, while laudable, were costly. In one 12-month period, Whitman-Walker provided nearly $150,000 in emergency rental assistance beyond maintaining its residency and halfway houses. And while cities, and a few states, began to contribute to the cost of these programs, the amounts they contributed were dwarfed by the true needs of the population. In Boston, for example, despite all of the efforts of the AIDS Action Committee, over 50 percent of all AIDS patients by 1992 were still homeless or in "imminent" danger of being so. The programs repeatedly sought funds from the federal Department of Housing and Urban Development (HUD), but their pleas were largely ignored. "There is an acute shortage of resources available for creating housing for PWHIVs," proclaimed the committee's legal adviser Robert Greenwald in 1992, "and this is largely the result of the fact that the federal office of Housing and Urban Development has largely ignored the AIDS crisis."[54] As if to lend credence to the complaint, HUD prioritized AIDS housing that year as 31st in a 33-item list.

Greenwald's pronouncements had not been exactly correct. The federal government had funneled some money toward AIDS housing, albeit far less than was called for given the magnitude of the problem. The National Affordable Housing Act of 1990 had established the Housing Opportunities for Persons with AIDS program, which received $50 million per year over its first several years. The dedicated funds went almost entirely to the same EMAs that qualified for Ryan White money, and could be used for a variety of AIDS-related housing needs. In addition, the Section 811 program within that bill, dedicated to providing housing for people with disabilities, could be used in part for AIDS-related housing as well. Both programs were slated to increase over the coming years, and HUD secretary Jack Kemp appeared capable of making his case with the Bush White House.[55]

The numbers were misleading, however. Although they appeared large compared with the budget of any single community housing provider, in fact the two programs together could probably not purchase more than 1,000 units of housing per year, in an effort to alleviate a problem that affected some 30,000 or more people. Moreover, many of the units being built with the funds would not be available for some time, and local agencies had to establish programs that heeded federal protocols. The federal government was not ignoring the program, but its effort fell short of the challenge. AIDS patients were barred from the majority of HUD programs, and even those programs that were made accessible to them seemed to require long waits and endless bureaucratic barriers—always unpleasant, but positively absurd in the context of a disease that killed most of its victims within two years of diagnosis. "You name the program and HUD had denied us access," testified Greenwald before the National Commission on AIDS.[56] It was no wonder that so much of the Ryan White money, when it was finally distributed to the desperate municipalities, was ploughed into housing rather than medical assistance.

BUSH IN RETROSPECT

In fact, the debate over federal involvement in Medicaid, Ryan White funding, and housing programs, was part of a larger discussion over the appropriate role of the federal government in paying for AIDS. The United States had never had a comprehensive national health insurance program in the manner that most other industrialized nations did, yet between Medicare, Medicaid, the Indian Health Service, and the Veterans Administration, the federal government paid for nearly 40 percent of all clinical services purchased in the country (not including the CHAMPUS military health-care program). Moreover, through the agencies of the Surgeon General's Office, the Public Health Service, the Environmental Protection Agency, the Centers for Disease Control, and the National Institutes of Health, the federal program provided many billions of dollars more in research support, statistics keeping, health-care education, and disease prevention. Even during times of budget trimming, the federal government's role in the production and provision of health-care services was immense.

Liberals had objected strenuously to President Reagan's offhand approach to AIDS. The 40th president had avoided public association with the illness: resisting addressing it in formal speeches, shunning the afflicted, and generally denying the prestige and power of his office to those in need. President Bush, superficially, appeared to reverse this trend. Throughout his 1988 campaign and during the first years of his presidency, he called for antidiscrimination laws for AIDS victims and offered sympathy to victims and their families. In a moving speech before the National Leadership Coalition on AIDS, he declared his unity with the cause of the victims:

Once disease strikes, we don't blame those who are suffering. We don't spurn the accident victim who didn't wear a seatbelt. We don't reject the cancer patient who didn't quit smoking. We try to love them and care for them and comfort them. We don't fire them, we don't evict them, we don't cancel their insurance.[57]

President Bush's public support of AIDS funding reached its apogee with his appointment of basketball star Earvin "Magic" Johnson to the National AIDS Commission, which had continued over from his predecessor's watch to his. Johnson, one of the most beloved and accomplished athletes of his time, stunned America with his announcement in the fall of 1991 that he was HIV-positive. Claiming to have caught the disease through heterosexual contact, the athlete urged responsibility and testing for all Americans, and declared his intentions of fighting the disease in any way possible.[58] Millions of heterosexual Americans responded by calling AIDS hot lines, local clinics, and physician's offices demanding information, testing, and counseling. The CDC's own AIDS hot line immediately went from fielding 3,000 calls per day to answering 40,000, while a local clinic in Hollywood, California, had 200 AIDS-related visits in the afternoon of the Johnson announcement, when it normally had 700 each *month*. Somehow Johnson had trumped years of apathy and indifference, if not total ignorance. A sort of national epiphany followed in the wake of Johnson's announcement, and millions who had seen AIDS as beyond their purview and concern suddenly regarded the disease as a legitimate threat. Noted one college nursing administrator, "Here is a virile, healthy male, such an idol, and, my God, he got it too."[59]

In such an environment, Bush's decision to place Magic Johnson on his National AIDS Commission signaled to many Americans the president's highest commitment to combating the epidemic. He was willing to align himself with its victims, publicize its threats, and centralize its challenges. If AIDS policy before had simmered in the margins of public life, it was now moved to center stage, where the federal government could flood it with funds, brains, and legislative muscle. It was now everybody's concern.

Opponents of Reagan's AIDS policies, however, were unassuaged by Bush's more open rhetoric, and continued to see an absence of leadership and tangible commitment in the administration's actions. Gadfly congressman Henry Waxman noted bitterly that the president had had "his picture taken with people with AIDS, but his budgets are business-as-usual."[60] Similarly, Waxman's House colleague Gerry Studds, who represented one of the nation's greatest concentrations of gay constituents in his Provincetown precinct, called the president's tepid AIDS-education advertising campaign "somewhere between exasperating and insulting."[61] A special Institute of Medicine panel recommended immediately raising AIDS research funding by 25 percent,[62] while the president's own National AIDS Commission saw so many gaps in the administration's AIDS policies that it termed them, as a whole, "woefully inadequate."[63]

Everywhere, the watchword within the administration seemed to be "leadership," or lack thereof. National Commission on AIDS chairwoman June Osborn harshly critiqued the president and his cabinet for not meeting his obligations in "leading the national response," while the commission itself called upon the president to exercise his "leadership potential."[64] Waxman claimed that what was missing was "leadership from the top,"[65] and even Magic Johnson called on Bush to throw his "moral leadership" behind the campaign, before resigning from the AIDS commission over disgust at having been exploited for his name.[66] Administration critics somehow believed that when all was said and done, Bush was little more than an old-fashioned conservative striving toward political expediency.

But the numbers simply did not support these harsh judgments. Whatever Bush's personal feelings may have been toward gays, drug users, or AIDS victims generally, his policies had favored AIDS to an unprecedented degree in the history of U.S. health and research programs. By 1992, the administration had raised its funding of AIDS-related research by some 170 percent since 1988, with a projected $2.1 billion to be spent in the coming year on AIDS research, prevention, and treatment. On research alone, the administration's AIDS allocations were double its heart disease disbursement, quadruple that spent on diabetes, and nearly equal to that spent on all cancer research combined. When prevention and treatment were thrown into the mix, AIDS spending topped all other diseases, despite affecting only 120,000 patients annually; by contrast, a combined 50 million Americans suffered each year from heart disease, stroke, and cancer.[67] If one examined the research investment, per death, for varying diseases, AIDS funding led the pack with $20,000 spent per each death in 1992, versus $5,000 for diabetes, $4,000 for cancer, and $1,000 or less for heart disease, stroke, and diabetes.[68] As of 1992, AIDS spending comprised 10 percent of the NIH budget, 38 percent of the CDC budget, and 9 percent of the FDA's.[69] If money was love, the Bush administration was stricken.

In the sea of anti-AIDS conservatism lived a few activists who rose above regressive rhetoric to familiarize themselves with the White House's budget allocations and the CDC's statistics. Doing so buttressed their anti-AIDS arguments, and laid open the defenses of their opponents. The most articulate and forceful of the anti-AIDS scholars, Michael Fumento, deemed the National Commission on AIDS a "propaganda unit" for the disease, and refuted the doomsday predictions about AIDS becoming a disease of the middle class, of straights, of women, and of the preponderance of Americans. Responding to the commission's calls for national health insurance to deal with the coming AIDS-induced financial Armageddon, he queried why AIDS, at 50,000 deaths per year, would bankrupt a health system that seemed perfectly able to withstand 500,000 cancer deaths per year. As for Magic Johnson's claim that he had been exploited for his name, Fumento pointed out the hypocrisy of such words from a man who annually accepted $12 million in endorsement money. "Perhaps he was under the impression that he had been appointed to the NCA because of his expertise in retrovirology and epidemiology," wrote Fumento sardonically.[70]

Ultimately, the AIDS commission bowed to fiscal reality, and issued a restrained set of final recommendations to President Bill Clinton in early 1993. Resisting calls for yet more funding for the already over-funded research program, it called for the president to do little more than "discuss" the crisis with the American people, remove those immigration and employment restrictions that were clearly tangential or superfluous to fighting the epidemic, and to establish an AIDS coordinator's office. It did call for fuller funding for the provisions of the Ryan White Act, but Congress had already been moving in this direction. And while it called for better treatment for substance abusers, the thrust of its recommendations centered around developing a strategic plan with interoffice cooperation mechanisms, coordinators, and articulated goals. In the face of the deluge of Bush-released research and treatment funds, there was little more to say.[71]

CHAPTER 9

MYTHS

If there was a prevailing orthodoxy in the late 1980s concerning AIDS, it was that the disease would inevitably spread into the general population. While the American epidemic may have started with gays, and spread to IV drug users (so proclaimed the dogma), it must ultimately come to roost in the broad middle range of heterosexual Americans. The orthodoxy was perpetuated through media accounts of non-drug-using heterosexuals contracting AIDS, and intensified by liberal public health groups, gay advocates, and well-meaning bureaucrats. *U.S. News* editor Mortimer Zuckerman, for example, editorialized in 1989 that it was a "delusion to think AIDS is confined to homosexual men and intravenous drug users," while Army physician and AIDS authority Robert Redfield warned that the spread of AIDS into heterosexuals, while possibly slow, would be "implacable."[1]

The orthodoxy seeped into popular culture, with movies, television sitcoms, and talk show hosts illustrating the presumed reality of middle-class American heterosexuals dying of AIDS. On the popular NBC drama *Saint Elsewhere,* the fictional plastic surgeon Bobby Caldwell contracted AIDS from a lady friend, while on *The Oprah Winfrey Show*, the talk show host predicted that possibly one-fifth of heterosexuals could be dying of AIDS within a few years' time.[2] Los Alamos

National Laboratory statistician Stirling Colgate predicted, based on mathematical modeling, that the disease would infect 10 percent of the U.S. population by 1997, pronounced "the safety of the heterosexual population is largely an illusion," and called for the declaration of a national AIDS emergency.[3] National AIDS Commission chairwoman June Osborn chimed her assent, predicting: "By the end of the 1990s, people will be shaking their fists and saying, 'Why didn't you tell us?' "[4] Statisticians and epidemiologists across the country agreed with the prognosis, or predicted worse.

College campuses proved particularly susceptible to the dogma. Starting in the mid-1980s, college health services across the country offered safe-sex clinics for all undergraduates (sometimes as required freshmen orientation courses), distributed condoms and dental dams throughout campus dorms and bathrooms, and promoted peer education networks and sex information films and pamphlets. The University of Wisconsin held a "condom Olympics" hosted by mascot "Pat the Prophylactic," while dorms on other campuses displayed candy bowls of condoms, free for the taking, labeled "love jugs" or something similar.[5] The Dartmouth College AIDS information group ("RAID") ran workshops in which students practiced slipping condoms onto plunger handles.[6] Indeed, many college students seemed to feel that taking seriously the risk of AIDS defined a sort of adult sexuality, as distinct from the irresponsible gropings of an adolescent.

The most extreme statement of the orthodoxy was articulated by famed sex researchers William Masters and Virginia Johnson, who, along with researcher Robert Kolodny, published *Crisis: Heterosexual Behavior in the Age of AIDS* in 1988. The book, based on a study of 400 sexually active and 400 monogamous individuals, labeled the view that AIDS affected primarily gay men and IV drug users "extraordinarily erroneous," and asserted that the current estimates for the prevalence of AIDS were off by 100 percent or more.[7] The authors doubled the estimate of AIDS carriers in the United States from 1.5 million to 3 million, suggesting that most did not know that they were infected. "The AIDS virus is now running rampant in the heterosexual community," they concluded.[8]

The Masters, Johnson, and Kolodny study was based entirely on interviews with 400 self-proclaimed "sexually active" adults, who had been recruited through a series of posters and ads placed in singles clubs and bars. The adults recruited, however, were unrepresentative of the general population, claiming 11.5 and 9.8 different sex partners per year, on average, for women and men respectively.[9] But such levels of promiscuity placed the sample group on the margins of American sexual practices; the authors themselves acknowledged that their previous sex research indicated that the individuals were more promiscuous than 95 percent of the nonmonogamous U.S. population.[10] As a result, the authors' conclusions were grossly exaggerated, despite being supported by analysis of their own data. Given the statistical sophistication of the authors, the methodological mistake was inexplicable, and reflected, perhaps, the authors' desire to shock their readers rather than conduct sound analysis. Despite initial broad publicity, the book faded from the public debate quite quickly.

GROWING SKEPTICISM

By 1988, a growing skepticism concerning the popular orthodoxy had begun to take hold in certain scientific circles, and even liberal-minded researchers began to admit that evidence pointed to the epidemic being contained in high-risk groups for the foreseeable future. Studies of 3 million military recruits produced an infection rate of .03 percent nationally, rather than the 6 percent asserted by Masters and Johnson.[11] Even staunch advocates of AIDS research and treatment voiced their skepticism of the more alarmist figures. AmFAR founder Mathilde Krim decreed, for example, that Masters and Johnson had "no credentials to justify their recommendations concerning public health policy," and that their book was "needlessly alarming," and an attempt at "exploiting the public fear in order to sell a book."[12]

Skepticism of the stated dogma trickled in from a growing number of sources. As early as 1987, CDC AIDS chief Harold Jaffe had admitted, despite all of his dire warnings concerning promiscuous sex, that data simply did not indicate that AIDS was spreading beyond the primary risk groups and their immediate sex partners.[13] That same year, physician and columnist Charles Krauthammer decreed that AIDS was "not the pandemic its publicists would like us to believe," but rather a "relatively small public-health problem."[14] And New York psychiatrist Robert Gould precipitated a firestorm of controversy the following February when he wrote in a widely read *Cosmopolitan* article that there was "almost no danger of contracting AIDS through ordinary sexual intercourse."[15] That same year, MIT researcher Jeffrey Harris estimated that the chance of an individual contracting the disease in a random sexual encounter in the United States was approximately 1 in 1 million—one-twentieth the risk of dying in a car crash in any given year.

In fact, a growing number of researchers and policymakers began to understand by 1988 that the extraordinary aspect of heterosexual AIDS was not its ongoing movement into the general population, but rather its high rate of containment in the minority population. Staid *Time* magazine admitted in 1989 that despite having placed the disease on its cover two years previously, it was "increasingly clear that much of the panic and scaremongering was not justified."[16] Heterosexual AIDS simply spread much more quickly and easily between drug users and their partners than between two non–drug users, and the IV-drug-using population in the United States in the late 1980s was heavily immigrant and minority.

The great divide between alarmists and naysayers involved the willingness, or lack thereof, to tease out the risk factors in those who tested positive for the virus. The investigative process, consisting of interviews, perusals of medical records, and letter writing, was timely and expensive, but invariably resulted in greatly diminished numbers of infected individuals outside of the risk groups. The Army, for example, found that such interviews indicated that over 90 percent of all recruits testing positive for HIV were members of high-risk groups, while studies of infected blood donors produced results nearly as high.[17] Everywhere researchers looked they found AIDS accompanied by high-risk behavior, or by sexual coupling with a high-risk partner. The broad incursion into the American heterosexual heartland simply did not exist.

Nowhere did this become as clear as in New York City. Almost alone among the nation's urban areas, New York found almost no recorded heterosexual AIDS cases beyond the parameters of the high-risk groups. In one study of AIDS-infected patients in Queens, all 19 infected women and

61 of 63 infected men turned out to be either active homosexuals, drug injectors, or partners of drug injectors, and even the 2 exceptions were suspect.[18] In another citywide study, the 1 infected subject with no initially known risk factors turned out to be an actor in gay pornography films.[19] And in Health Department studies conducted in 1987 and 1988, viral transmission from prostitutes to heterosexual male customers appeared to be extremely low, except in cases where the clients were already infected with other venereal diseases. Through mechanisms not entirely understood, heterosexual intercourse accompanied by drug use (even smokable crack) or preexisting sexually transmitted diseases facilitated HIV transmission. In the absence of these factors, the virus failed to jump.[20]

THE MYTH OF HETEROSEXUAL AIDS

Increasing skepticism found its true voice in the acerbic and iconoclastic lawyer-turned-reporter, Michael Fumento. A self-described "Burkean conservative," Fumento had first raised hackles on both sides of the AIDS debate with a 1987 *Commentary* article stating that AIDS would largely miss heterosexuals, and did not merit the conservative monogamy-mission emanating from the Reagan White House.[21] The gadfly followed his *Commentary* article with a piece in the *American Spectator* entitled "The Incredible Shrinking AIDS Epidemic," and thereafter enlarged his ideas into a 1991 book, *The Myth of Heterosexual AIDS*.

Myth was written in a combative style, generously delegating blame for misinformation and fear-mongering to journalists, college officials, left-wing activists, gay leaders, liberal politicians, and irresponsible scientists and epidemiologists. Indicting the "worried well" along with general alarmists, Fumento listed the litany of doomsayers and their varied horrific prophecies about the impending heterosexual epidemic of 1987. "But a funny thing happened on the way to the apocalypse," he wrote in response. "By the end of the year, heterosexuals still were not dropping like flies, and it was looking more and more as if they were not about to start."[22]

Bellicose he may have been, but Fumento buttressed his arguments with copious facts and statistics. According to his data, only 4.5 percent of the 106,000 AIDS cases reported to the CDC by 1989 had resulted from heterosexual intercourse, and of these cases nearly a third had been born in either Haiti or central Africa. Of the remaining 3 percent (3,300 cases), only 960 were white, and probably fewer than a third of these had contracted the disease through intercourse with a nonbisexual non-IV-drug-using partner. That is, as of 1989 only .5 percent of AIDS patients—about 1 in 200 cases—were white, heterosexual, non–drug users.[23]

Furthermore, some of the patients in this .5 percent were probably lying about their sexual pasts. Fumento cited the careful New York City investigations into the lives of HIV-positive individuals, and noted the many patients who could be placed into high-risk groups upon close examination. Anna Lekatsas, who had led the investigation, noted of the 8 men who fit into no known risk group: "I have doubts about seven of them, but we couldn't prove anything."[24] Similarly, Army medical testers found that only 2 in 10,000 HIV-positive recruits fell into the no-risk category.[25]

Although Fumento positioned his exposition as an attack on irresponsible journalism and science, at heart he was a moralist. The heterosexual myth seemed to bother him not so much for the wasted educational efforts it incurred (the collegiate outreach efforts particularly offended him), but for the equating of heterosexual and homosexual mores. Besides the fact that the mechanics of anal sex simply led to far greater transmission rates than that of vaginal sex (a point on which Fumento discoursed at length), gays in the early 1980s had simply behaved in ways wholly at odds with virtually all of heterosexual America. While even nonmonogamous Americans tended to have fewer than a half-dozen different sex partners per year, promiscuity among gays, wrote Fumento, "would boggle the imagination of the most lusty heterosexual male."[26] Epidemiologists had firmly established that early gay AIDS victims had had an average of 1,100 lifetime sex partners, and nearly a third of all white gay men claimed over 1,000 lifetime sex partners. That the media and public health leaders had failed to grasp the significance of these statistics bothered Fumento greatly; both for its moral implication and for its analytic sloppiness.[27]

Moreover, Fumento took offense at gay mobilization efforts, which he considered thuggish and irresponsible. Gays, for example, consistently cited the 10-percent-of-the-population homosexuality rate conjectured by sex researcher Alfred Kinsey, but more recent scientific studies had put the rate far lower—possibly less than 4 percent.[28] Such exaggeration was understandable—greater numbers meant greater political influence—but Fumento saw the gay claims as more than run-of-the-mill political posturing. By demanding that such extraordinary efforts be made on their behalf by researchers and clinicians, gays had forfeited their right to privacy. "None of this intrinsically says anything about the morality of homosexuality or homosexual practices," he wrote in an article two years after *Myth*. "But to the extent that homosexual activists believe it is very important for the world to know that they constitute 10 percent of the population—and therefore, by inference, 10 percent of the electorate or of the military—it seems that it ought to be important to know if they do not."[29]

Much of Fumento's argument was ultimately proved true, but in one crucial area he was fantastically wrong. Based on his understanding of the differential risks posed by anal and vaginal sex, Fumento posited that the African heterosexual epidemic, while worse than that in America, would also peak early for the same reasons that bounded the virus's spread in the United States. Noting that the World Health Organization was predicting 8 million AIDS cases in Africa by 1990, Fumento triumphantly noted that the actual number of reported cases was little more than 150,000.

Here Fumento's skepticism misled him, for underreporting in Africa was rampant, and the disease was far more embedded in central and southern Africa than anybody understood. While Fumento conjectured that the African epidemic would peak soon ("There has been no heterosexual breakout, and probably there never will be," he wrote in 1992), in fact within a decade prevalence rates in the worst-hit African nations would top 30 percent.[30] The African epidemic had in fact already broken out (unbeknownst to Western epidemiologists), and its transmission patterns would soon prove to be radically different than those in the West.

Fumento's book, while path-breaking in the meticulousness of its data, did not so much foster a revolution as give voice to existing opposition. Many Americans had either known, felt, or somehow intuited that AIDS was not really touching them, and had been skeptical of the claims that they were but one step removed from infection. Individuals who lived their lives in the heterosexual heartland found that they knew nobody suffering from AIDS, and that AIDS victims always seemed to be two or three steps removed from their lives—"my son's college roommate's friend." Fumento's book validated the perceptions of this class, without really challenging the orthodoxy of those who differed.

The book received a few positive reviews, mostly in conservative newspapers (New York's *Newsday* seemed particularly enamored), as well as in conservative periodicals and newsletters.[31] Politicians latched on to the message, and without specifically lauding the book propounded its message of sexual exclusion. AIDS, more than anything, was a *behavioral* problem, emphasized a group of congressional Republicans, and as such demanded not a biomedical response but rather a social response. "We need to send out a loud and clear message that we want our teenagers to abstain from practices that endanger their health," wrote the lawmakers. "Teens are seeking to belong, to be given a sense of community with shared values, and we are giving them a hall pass to see the school nurse."[32]

Very few in the gay community ventured to support the book, but one who did—the conservative gay writer and editor Andrew Sullivan— paid a heavy price. Writing and preaching that HIV remained "remarkably confined to those groups of people it has always affected: homosexual men, intravenous drug users, and their sexual partners," Sullivan drew near-universal ire and condemnation from his fellow gays.[33] One acquaintance would scream, "Collaborator !" at Sullivan upon seeing him in public.[34]

Opprobrium to Fumento was the far more common response. Gays, civil libertarians, AIDS activists, epidemiologists, public health experts, and liberal intellectuals rejected the book outright as gay baiting, homophobic, and possibly fascist. Many independent bookstores across the country refused to stock the book, as did the large Waldenbooks discount chain. General interest magazines refused to publish profiles of Fumento, or op-ed pieces or articles sympathetic to the book's thesis.[35] Fumento, noting that the same chain that refused to stock his book had taken on fundamentalist Christian groups for attempting to bar sales of pornography, suggested that the book might have proved to be more acceptable had he "included some dirty pictures."[36]

The book was largely condemned by book reviewers and critics, and even scientific journals rejected its premise. Both *Nature* and *Science*, two of the most prestigious scientific journals in the world, handed the book off to humanities scholars to review (rather than experts in epidemiology or infectious disease), and both subsequently published highly negative reviews. Across the country Fumento was vilified, tarred as a homophobe, racist, and fascist, and generally consigned to the ranks of kooks and hatemongers. When he attempted to fight these allegations with letters or op-ed pieces, his submissions were usually rejected. And even when critics could find no obvious evidence that Fumento was wrong or misguided, they fell back on the circular argument that Fumento must be wrong about claiming that most Americans were misinformed about the AIDS epidemic, because most Americans thought he was wrong. An ACT UP protest against Fumento's conclusions started with the assertion that they were invalid because "a vast majority of Americans said that addressing AIDS should be our #1 national health priority."[37]

THE SCIENCE

By the time that Fumento penned his philippic, the preponderance of data lay in his favor. Despite the pervasiveness of the established orthodoxy, the "everybody-is-going-to-get-it-especially-your-grandmother" syndrome (in the words of the conservative *National Review*),[38] almost all of the research trickling out of the nation's epidemiological and infectious-disease laboratories supported the model of a far more limited heterosexual epidemic in America. By 1989, for example, the U.S. military reported that only 6,200 active duty personnel out of 2.3 million were infected with HIV, and the AIDS epidemic had had only "a minimal impact on overall DOD operations," according to the General Accounting Office.[39] The National Research Council, a branch of the National Academy of Sciences, reported in 1993 that while AIDS would continue to grow, large portions of the population were "virtually untouched" by the epidemic, and would probably continue to escape its ravages into the foreseeable future.[40] And in 1992, despite all pessimistic prognoses to the contrary, the number of teenage AIDS cases had actually dropped 5 percent. In response, the *National Review* pronounced that the myth of pandemic heterosexual AIDS was "collapsing."[41]

One of the problems with the ongoing debate over heterosexual AIDS was in defining who constituted the "typical American." Richard Nixon had famously asked if his policies would "play in Peoria" some 20 years earlier, indicating that a midsized midwestern American city still represented the archetypical American majority—predominantly white, almost entirely heterosexual, married, and neither very wealthy nor very poor. It was precisely to this America that so much of the AIDS awareness campaign of the past half-decade had been directed, and it was the misdirection of this campaign that had so enraged Fumento.

In an attempt to target this population, a team of researchers investigated sexual mores in exactly this population in the early 1990s by surveying the sexual practices of 334 randomly chosen households in two upper midwestern communities. Their results suggested that Americans were having less sex than most public health educators had assumed: a lifetime median of five partners for men and three for women. Indeed, only 17 percent of men and 9 percent of women reported having had more than one sexual partner in the previous year.[42] The data, even if underreported, suggested that projecting homosexual practices on the heterosexual population of Middle America was absurd, as was developing AIDS infection models based on homosexual norms.

The second leg in the tripod supporting Fumento's conjecture was the data on the intransmissibility of HIV from women to men coming out of San Francisco researcher Nancy Padian's laboratory. Padian had been exploring the rates at which HIV passed heterosexually since the mid-1980s, and her work on the specific modes of transmission of the virus from women to men lent credence to the Fumento hypothesis. Padian had found that the virus traveled from women to men with great difficulty—only 1 percent of monogamous male partners of infected women in her cohort tested positive for HIV after several years of study (versus close to 20 percent for female monogamous partners of infected men).[43]

Virologists struggled to understand why the rate of transmission from women to men so greatly differed from that of men to women. The virus existed in vaginal secretions, but at much lower concentrations than it did in ejaculate. Also, certain portions of the cervix appeared particularly vulnerable to the virus. Last, Padian and her colleagues noted that transmission rates were significantly affected by vaginal and penile bleeding, as well as by certain types of vaginal inflammations. In short, any condition that brought the blood supply closer to the surface of the skin or epithelial tissues, or that breached the circulatory system entirely, seemed to be highly correlated with greater HIV transmission.[44] In addition, Padian advanced the theory that one man's semen, still harbored in a woman's vagina, could infect a subsequent male sex partner. This might explain the high incidence of spread through prostitutes, particularly in Africa.[45]

And speaking of Africa, why were heterosexual transmission rates there so vastly different than they were in the United States? In Africa, AIDS had turned to a full-blown heterosexual epidemic early, without the exacerbating factor of IV drugs. Padian's prostitution theory was one plausible explanation; most AIDS researchers agreed that prostitution and extramarital sex was more common in most sub-Saharan countries than in the United States, and thus the sex industry might be acting as a transmission nexus.

But more persuasive was the evidence produced in studies by Francis Plummer of the University of Nairobi and the NIH's Thomas Quinn. Both men, along with teams of researchers, had found very high rates of correlation between ulcerative sexually transmitted diseases (particularly syphilis) and HIV transmission. Open sores on both male and female genitals, visible or not, vastly increased the chance of the virus spreading.[46] Moreover, uncircumcised men appeared to be particularly vulnerable to HIV, which would explain the different incidences of AIDS in (circumcised) west Africa and (uncircumcised) east. Noted Plummer at a Tanzania AIDS conference: "I think that we can now explain a lot of the African heterosexual AIDS dilemma. Ninety percent of the cases were due to either genital ulcer disease or lack of circumcision."[47] In fact, one Kenya-based study showed that circumcised men with no genital ulcers who were exposed to AIDS-infected partners posted a 2 percent HIV infection rate, while uncircumcised men with present genital ulcers posted a 52 percent rate. While other factors may have been operating, the relationship among ulcers, circumcision, and AIDS was too apparent to be denied.[48]

Condom use, despite having been much touted in the nation's colleges and high schools, did not seem to be the answer. Studies conducted in the early 1990s, by the University of North Carolina's Michael Rosenberg along with colleagues, showed that condom use declined in the United States almost precisely in relation to the risk profile presented by the individual. That is, the people who were most consistent in using condoms regularly and correctly were married couples at least 30 years old—precisely the cohort at the lowest risk for contracting AIDS. Condom used dropped in a linear fashion depending on how many sex partners a male had each year. Teenage males who posted only one partner in the previous year used condoms 63 percent of the time, but males with two partners over the previous year used condoms only 56 percent of the time, and those who had had three, 45 percent. Teenage males who claimed four or more partners used condoms only 37 percent of the time, and Rosenberg estimated that the rate for higher-risk groups was 30 percent or lower.[49] Observed *New Republic* writer Malcolm Gladwell: "When it comes to personal risk reduction, there is a growing divide along the lines of income and education. There is a class of Americans who eat well, see their doctors regularly and attend aerobics classes. And there's a class for whom these things make little or no sense."[50]

OTHER MYTHS

Although infectious-disease specialists, epidemiologists, and public health engineers had struggled mightily in the opening years of the epidemic to understand what the mechanism was by which thousands of otherwise healthy gay men were falling sick and dying, the 1985 discovery of HIV by Montagnier and Gallo had persuaded almost everybody that AIDS was a specific disease, viral in etiology, and spread through direct exchange of body fluids. While HIV infection did not inevitably lead to full-blown AIDS, it did much of the time, and untreated AIDS usually resulted in death within a fairly predictable time range.

Aberrations existed, of course, and not all had been well explained by 1990. A small group of people appeared able to live with the virus seemingly indefinitely, without getting sick or showing symptoms. Others showed symptoms but survived for many years, long past the time when physicians would have predicted death. Still others seemed oddly immune to infection at all, sleeping with countless infected partners, unprotected, for years on end, without contracting the virus. Most of these cases fell within the expected range of human responses to a specific pathogen, yet they continued to gnaw at the integrity of the HIV theory of AIDS.

Despite the broad acceptance of viral causation, a small cohort of scientists questioned the pathogen model. These theorists came from a variety of backgrounds—some were Ph.D. scientists, others were self-taught hacks—but all suspected the scientific establishment, if not the entire U.S. government, of somehow fabricating AIDS, or fabricating the explanation for AIDS, or some combination thereof. While most were dismissed as kooks fairly quickly, a few found a positive reception in various communities of like-minded conspiratorialists, or general skeptics. These "myth-makers" did not ever jeopardize the AIDS research program, but they did attract enough attention to force mainstream researchers to expend time and energy debunking their alternative theories.

By far the most persuasive of these alternative theorists, and one possessing impeccable mainstream scientific credentials, was Berkeley microbiologist Peter Duesberg—a well-published cancer researcher who wrote a series of scathing dismissals of the HIV hypothesis starting in the late 1980s. Claiming that the HIV theory was untenable because it violated the basic tenets of virology, the biologist hammered at the unusually low levels of virus frequently found in AIDS victims, at the irreproducibility of AIDS in laboratory monkeys injected with HIV, and at the lack of toxicity demonstrated by HIV in laboratory Petri dishes of healthy cells.[51] But most of all, Duesberg rejected HIV as the cause of AIDS because in his extensive experience this was simply not the way that retroviruses behaved. Most retroviruses promoted cell growth, while HIV promoted cell death in T cells.

But what of the millions of people dying of AIDS? This was simply misdiagnosis in Duesberg's mind. Virtually all were dying of other infections, of overdoses of drugs and of ancillary contagions, and HIV simply happened to be found in their blood in low levels. Duesberg particularly emphasized the dangers of recreational drug use, and conjectured that the sexual revolution had greatly increased incidences of syphilis, gonorrhea, and various other STDs. The epidemic raging in Africa was in fact multiple epidemics, all of them completely predictable in a continent ravaged by malnutrition, unhygienic water and food supplies, sexually transmitted disease, and a dearth of modern medical interventions. That HIV existed he did not deny. That it caused AIDS was, for Duesberg, a myth constructed in the interest of "careerism . . . job security, grant money, financial benefits, and prestige."[52]

Duesberg's hypothesis met with limited approval in scientific circles. While most considered him a kook, his reputation at least guaranteed him the respect of being taken seriously and of being rebutted in major scientific journals. Moreover, at least a few credentialed colleagues actually agreed with him, either in whole or in part. Harvey Bialy, editor of *Biotechnology*, for example, dismissed HIV as a red herring. It had produced only "a vaccine that doesn't exist; AZT, which is iatrogenic genocide; and condom use, which is common sense."[53] Duesberg's own Berkeley colleague, Harry Rubin, shared the skepticism.[54] And Michigan State University physiologist Robert Root-Bernstein, while avoiding the vituperative accusations of malfeasance, did suggest that the HIV thesis was premature and incomplete. It was quite possible, in Root-Bernstein's reckoning, that AIDS was really a collection of different maladies, some of which might be caused by HIV, and others rooted in alternate pathogens or behaviors, or some combination thereof. Mostly Root-Bernstein pleaded for humility—for the recognition that the scientific community was still "ignorant of the causes of this disease."[55]

Duesberg's theory attracted some attention from both mainstream media and renegade researchers, but most AIDS investigators were quickly able to dismiss both his theories and his purported facts. HIV did destroy T cells in the laboratory, argued Harvard Medical School professor Jerome Groopman, and thus there was no reason to believe it would not do so in a human being. People who were irresponsible with neither drugs nor sex but became infected with HIV—through blood transfusions and needlesticks—did get AIDS and did die. While HIV did not propagate itself in monkeys, the closely related SIV did, and did weaken the simian immune systems. And people infected with HIV who were treated with the nascent protease inhibitors then on the market did get better.[56] On virtually every factual assertion, Duesberg was simply incorrect.

Duesberg found positive reception among several African nationalists who claimed, as he did, that AIDS in Africa was a chimera being used to draw attention away from Western doctors, aid agencies, and drug makers who were making their fortunes treating the putative "epidemic." Among the most extreme of these charlatans was medical journalist Joan Shenton, who traveled to Africa to debunk the myth of African AIDS. Not surprising for a researcher of such tendentious orientation, she emerged from the continent convinced more than ever that AIDS simply did not exist. In her observation, most people dying of AIDS were simply being misdiagnosed; careful blood work would probably reveal that most were being struck down by hunger.

Along with her colleague, Bialy, Shenton made a documentary of the nonepidemic, with Bialy's narrative voice-over intoning, "From both my literature review and my personal experience over most of the so-called AID centres in Africa, I can find no believable, persuasive evidence that Africa is in the midst of a new epidemic of infectious immunodeficiency."[57] Unfortunately, several prominent media outlets gave voice to these absurd claims, usually under the banner of "objective" journalism, or wishing to present "both sides" of an issue. No less a newspaper than the *Times of London,* for example, ran a series of articles in late 1993 quoting Duesberg and suggesting that the idea of nonexistent AIDS was a perfectly acceptable theory among the scientifically informed.[58]

Equally absurd, and perhaps more malicious, were countertheories being put forth by African nationalists to rebut the widely held notion that AIDS had originated in Africa. In this line of thinking, AIDS had not only originated in the West, it had actually been created intentionally by Western scientists and governments with the specific goal of killing black people, both in the United States and in Africa. Various theorists postulated that AIDS had been brought back from the moon by American astronauts, that AIDS had been genetically engineered, or that AIDS had emerged from U.S. military germ warfare labs. Whichever theory one chose to espouse, all concluded that the widely held theory of AIDS originating in central Africa was a symptom of ubiquitous prejudice.[59] "Racism, like AIDS, is not a very selective disease," wrote Richard and Rosalind Chirimuuta. "It infects liberal academics and fascist scholars alike."[60]

The most vocal and outwardly hostile of these propagandists was philo-African Los Angeles physician Robert Strecker, who wrote and produced a series of articles and videos in the late 1980s. Strecker posited that AIDS had been created by the United States government explicitly to kill black people, and in colloquia and pamphlets warned America's blacks that they were the target of an ongoing genocide in which all doctors were potentially culpable. Strecker claimed to have traced the origins of AIDS to the Army's Fort Dietrich biological warfare complex, and to have found that the virus had been initially disseminated to Africans through bogus smallpox vaccinations. While he did not deny that thousands of homosexuals had died of AIDS (contrary to Duesberg), he did claim that homosexuals had been infected in a deliberate effort to "draw attention away from the true objective which is to wipe out the black, brown, and yellow races of the world."[61]

Strecker's hypothesis was either more or less insidious than Duesberg's, depending on which goals were being compromised. On one hand, the accusation of genocide was vicious and obscene. On the other hand, in not denying that AIDS existed, Strecker could at least give his audience some reasonably sound advice on protecting themselves, particularly with regard to condom use, monogamy, and dirty needles. Such advice had its limits, though, as Strecker also recommended that blacks avoid all white doctors, white vaccination clinics, and Western medicine in general. In one informational pamphlet he wrote:

> If you have small children you should think twice about letting them receive vaccination shots especially in public hospitals in Black neighborhoods and from white doctors. Remember that white people tricked 50–75 million Africans into receiving smallpox vaccinations that had been infected with the AIDS virus. Rest assure [sic] that what they did in Africa they are doing right here in the U.S. Consult a Black wholistic [sic] doctor about natural alternatives to vaccinations. As a last option consider having the vaccination in a predominately

[*sic*] white neighborhood. Vaccination shots there will probably not be contaminated.[62]

Strecker's brightest acolyte, Alan Cantwell Jr., viewed the AIDS-as-genocide theory as simply one component of a general conspiracy carried on by government scientists for decades, using putative "bions" to "infect" people with cancer. Cantwell cited the accomplishments of Royal Rife and Wilhelm Reich, who had discovered these bions and other assorted microbes, and related the savagery and murderousness visited upon them by the federal government. Rife, for example, had been driven to alcoholism by relentless government agents, while Reich had been arrested and imprisoned, and had lost all of his instruments and lab journals to FDA officials who had maliciously destroyed his laboratory and all of its contents. "The destruction of Wilhelm Reich's laboratory by the U.S. government was like a scene out of Nazi Germany, but it happened in America," wrote Cantwell.[63] The creation of AIDS was the "ultimate horror story of all time," he wrote, "the most frightening and diabolical deed ever perpetrated on this planet."[64]

Tony Brown, a popular black talk show host, preached a similar message, but sparked further controversy by claiming that AZT, like AIDS, was a pernicious creation of white doctors, the "medical cabal," and the "$25 billion AIDS industry." Stopping short of accusing these interests of genocide, he accused them of the lesser crime of "triage for fame and fortune," and wrote at length of the death of his friend, tennis great Arthur Ashe, whom he was certain had been killed not by AIDS, but by "AIDS treatment." AIDS was a "scientifically dishonest construct," and a "poorly masked attempt to marginalize blacks," while the viral model of the disease was no more than "theory,"[65] Brown wrote. "The medical establishment would have us believe the bizarre theory that 'AIDS' originated when a monkey bit an African on the butt . . . [who] then went home and engaged in debauched sex and seeded the human species with a modern plague."[66] The mechanics were correct, but the overtones hardly so. Virtually all mainstream virologists and geneticists understood by 1991 that AIDS had originated in central Africa, having jumped species from monkeys as it mutated from SIV to HIV. If debauchery existed in the history of AIDS, it was more appropriately associated with the American gay epidemic of the early 1980s than the original species transposition of the 1930s.

While the various myths under consideration concerning AIDS in the early 1990s ranged from the reasonable to the absurd, all represented efforts by individuals or groups to exploit the epidemic to their own advantage. At their most benign, the myth-makers' agenda included the laudable goals of increased research funds and greater treatment options. At their worst, the propagandists consciously exploited the epidemic to strengthen resentments and hostilities between Africa and the West, between black and white, and between modern medicine and alternative healing. The war on AIDS had attracted, as had all wars, its share of charlatans and profiteers. Strecker used his infamous video "memorandum" to boost his own prominence in the black community, while Duesberg seemed intent on exploiting his iconoclasm to draw attention to his own eccentric genius.

Ultimately, the myths did little damage to progress in seeking a cure for the disease. Few government and scientific leaders took the accusations seriously, and they seemed to have no effect on research funding decisions, and little effect on the distribution of Ryan White funds and international aid efforts. The myth-makers were perfidious and outrageous in their accusations, but ultimately ineffective.

CHAPTER 10

AFRICA

Africa, most experts agreed, was the point of origin for AIDS. Theories diverged on details, but by 1990 most AIDS researchers agreed that the disease had jumped species in central Africa sometime in the past half-century, had festered in relative isolation, and then had spread to Haiti through the conduit of Haitian mercenaries and guest workers resident in Zaire. From Haiti, gay American vacationers carried the virus to San Francisco, Los Angeles, and New York, whereupon it spread into the American megalopolis, to Europe, and beyond.[1]

The African epidemic was probably more advanced at an earlier time than most researchers initially understood. As early as 1980, French researcher Françoise Brun-Vezinet found that 7 percent of serum samples collected from Kenyan prostitutes carried the HIV antibody, and by 1984 the portion had risen to 51 percent. By that date, 13 percent of men visiting an STD clinic in Nairobi carried the antibody, as did over 90 percent of prostitutes in Butare, Rwanda. A broader Rwandan study of blood donors in 1984 produced a general population infection rate of 10.5 percent, and an urban population rate of 17.5 percent. Notably by that time, no central African country had officially reported a single case of AIDS.[2]

By 1986, the Panos Institute projected that possibly 1 million Africans could die of AIDS over the following decade, and that the prevalence of HIV in major urban areas in Uganda, Rwanda, Zambia, Zaire, and Tanzania was at least three times that of New York.[3] The disease appeared to be spreading through heterosexual intercourse. Half the patients were female, and both governments and populace seemed unaware of the need for monogamy, prophylaxis, and education. "We prefer to talk about malaria, diarrhea and parasitic disease and malnutrition," admitted Rwandan health minister Francois-Xavier Hakizimana.[4] More ominous were the jarring demographics of the African epidemic: most victims were members of the middle and upper-middle class—the core of the educated and professional workforce.

By 1989, the epidemic was so far advanced in certain heavily affected towns in central African countries that wholescale depopulation appeared to be taking place. In some towns, a fifth of the population was either dead or dying, and virtually every family had lost a member. "It started in January, 1987," recalled Joseph Kowamele of Kanyigo, Tanzania. "First died the baby, my granddaughter. Then on May 15, 1987, I lost another one. The in June '87 another died. A daughter. And another daughter gave birth to three children, all died of AIDS. Then this June my other daughter died."[5] By that point, the World Health Organization estimated the number of infected people worldwide at 6 million to 8 million, with the rate of spread still increasing, and the first evidence appeared that the disease was spreading into the west African nations of Nigeria, Ivory Coast, and Senegal.[6] In Ghana, Gambia, and Togo, as many as one-third to one-half of prostitutes were testing positive for HIV. The continent seemed unwilling to yet reveal the extent of its epidemic, however, and the official AIDS statistics reported by African nations to the World Health Organization totaled just under 6,000.[7]

Complicating matters was the discovery of a second AIDS virus, dubbed HIV-2, which predominated in the far west African nations of Guinea-Bissau and Ivory Coast. The new virus, while closely related to the more common HIV-1 of central Africa and the United States, appeared to have circulated in west Africa since the early 1960s and was now, similarly to HIV-1 in central Africa, spreading through the vectors of prostitutes and bar girls. And as in central Africa, the west African epidemic seemed to be spreading most rapidly in middle-class and professional men, who had the means and necessity to travel widely, and the discretionary cash to purchase sex services. "If I am traveling outside Nigeria, what care should I take?" queried one informational pamphlet at the Lagos Airport. "Avoid indiscriminate sexual contacts," it advised.[8]

AFRICAN LIFE

What was causing the extraordinarily high rates of heterosexual transmission in Africa, particularly in central and east Africa? Although some epidemiologists had speculated that the African epidemic was simply more advanced than was the American epidemic, growth models indicated otherwise. While the American epidemic was clearly becoming more deeply ensconced in drug users and their partners and skirting the broader heterosexual population, the African epidemic was becoming ubiquitous in the worst-affected countries, spreading into heterosexuals without regard to poverty, drug-using status, or sexual preference. In fact, the African epidemic appeared to be spreading most aggressively into those portions of the population least affected in the United States: educated, employed, married, middle-class heterosexuals. The poorest of the poor, as well as rural denizens, seemed to be slightly less vulnerable to AIDS than were the remainder of the population: a phenomenon at odds with the Western experience.

Sub-Saharan Africans lived very different lives than did Western Europeans and Americans, and disease watchers began to consider whether some of these "lifestyle" differences affected the manner in which HIV spread. Female circumcision was still quite common in a number of countries in west Africa (as well as in the Arabian Peninsula and the horn of Africa), and logic dictated that the accompanying mutilation could facilitate the spread of the disease. At its most severe, the procedure involved total removal of the clitoris, and excision of large parts of the labia majora and minora (the vulvular "lips"), and the suturing closed of the vagina. The procedure, often performed with crude implements in a nonsterile environment, created extensive vaginal scarring, which left women prone to bleeding during sexual intercourse. Since all evidence in the West associated such bleeding with enhanced infectious spread of HIV, it seemed reasonable to suppose that the procedure was facilitating the spread of AIDS.

Yet geographic overlays of areas with widespread practice of female circumcision and areas of the worst HIV infection simply did not mesh. AIDS was spreading fastest in central and south-central Africa, as well as in southern Kenya and Tanzania, while circumcision was practiced predominantly in west Africa, the Sudan, Somalia, Ethiopia, and northern Kenya. In fact, in a bizarre etiological turnabout, female circumcision might be supposed to have a protective effect against AIDS, if one looked only at the overlays. Nobody supposed that this was such, but numbers simply did not support the female circumcision theory.[9]

Some people speculated that homosexuality was actually more widespread in Africa than was supposed. Central African societies generally denied the existence of homosexuality or relegated it to the most marginal of activities, yet there was little reason to believe that rates of homosexuality (or bisexuality) for central Africa significantly diverged from the 4 percent found most everywhere else in the world. Certainly that part of the world was homophobic; most countries outlawed homosexual acts, the local churches preached vociferously against it, and cultural mores disallowed its expression. "Why should we discuss something that is not a priority for us," queried Densen Mafinyani, general secretary of the Zimbabwe Council of Churches. "It is like me coming to your country and discussing how to eat a dog. That is not something you do."[10] Less provocatively, *Newsweek* African correspondent Lynn James related that African society generally did not tolerate "an alternative lifestyle." Even self-admitted homosexuals felt "compelled to have children," as not to do so marked one as an "outcast, dependent on others who never forget that the man or woman without a child is shamed."[11] Yet no evidence suggested that rates of homosexuality were unusually high, or could explain the rampant spread of HIV. Cultural mores aside, central Africa did not appear to harbor a hidden gay subpopulation gestating and spreading the virus.[12]

Public health advocates looked at the more chauvinistic attitudes of central African males, which created somewhat different patterns of sexual activity, as well as handicapping the adoption of prophylaxis. African men, for example, shunned condoms even more forcefully than did their

Western counterparts. Some viewed government condom education efforts as surreptitious efforts at genocide, while others associated condom use with homosexuality.[13] Many men simply did not like the feel of condoms, or associated them with emasculation. "They say, 'Unless it's flesh on flesh, it's not real sex,' " reported one young South African woman.[14] Or more trenchantly noted one young man, "Sex with a condom is like eating a sweet with the wrapper on."[15] And some rejected condoms simply for financial reasons, as they could cost as much as 30 cents in central Africa—a substantial sum in an area where daily wages hovered at around $2. "The guy would rather buy a beer than a condom," noted South African epidemiologist Nicky Padayachee.[16]

Whatever the reasons, condom use among virtually all Africans trailed that of the West. Fewer than 5 percent of sexually active teens in Tanzania admitted to regular condom use, while only a fifth of Zairian prostitutes interviewed admitted to using condoms with clients (versus nearly 90 percent of American prostitutes by 1990).[17] And even aggressive public education campaigns accompanied by distribution of subsidized or free condoms failed to significantly alter behavior. One South African nurse recalled that when she requested her husband start using condoms, she was confronted at knifepoint with accusations of infidelity. A male educator, who might have been expected to understand the need for prophylaxis in the face of a growing scourge, responded with contempt to the query of whether he would consider wearing a condom. "That question is nonnegotiable," he remarked to the reporter.[18]

Moreover, traditional gender roles dictated that women had less control, generally, over their sexual prerogatives than was true in Western countries. African women reported that they had little latitude to refuse their husbands' or boyfriends' sexual advances, regardless of their fears of infection or concerns about prophylaxis. Women who questioned their husbands' fidelity faced violent repudiation, and sometimes outright rape. And low rates of female literacy, employment, earning power, and land ownership served to further disenfranchise many wives.[19] Recalled one long-married woman in Tanzania: "Our customs demand that a wife be faithful to her husband and accept whatever comes from him. Even if it means he comes home one evening in the company of a young lady and proudly announces to you that she—the young lady—will be your co-partner!"[20]

But lack of condom use alone did not explain the extent of the epidemic, or the speed of its spread. American condom use, while higher, was not enough higher to explain the great disparities in infection rates, and American adolescents' condom use was nearly as low as that of their African counterparts. And while the prostitution nexus appeared to be contributing to the spread of the African disease, higher condom use compliance among African prostitutes could not be expected to curtail an epidemic that seemed to be infiltrating all walks of African life—not just the clients of prostitutes. The African epidemic differed from the Western one in ways so profound that it seemed to indicate an almost wholly different mechanism, rather than just a facilitated Western path. What were they doing differently?

Part of the answer seemed to lie in the high levels of rootlessness and transiency of much of the central African population in the 1980s. As in all parts of the developing world, central and east African nations had experienced high levels of rural to urban migration over the preceding two decades, as impecunious farmers and farm workers sought out higher-paying work in the quickly growing cities. Such migration created hordes of extremely impoverished urban dwellers who crowded shantytowns that lacked running water, sewers, and basic public health protections. In South Africa, to cite one of the most extreme examples, 25 percent of the black population "squatted" in cardboard and corrugated iron shacks, adjacent to urban areas but essentially homeless. While technically designated "informal settlements," the U.S. Public Health Service deemed the term a "ludicrous euphemism" for the slums in which only 1 child in 40 attended school.[21]

A great many of the men able to find reasonably remunerative work in this changing economy had to leave their families to do so, disrupting traditional familial bonds and social structures. Miners, soldiers, truckers, and builders constituted a disproportionate share of the continent's middle-class wage earners, and all were spending large portions of their lives away from home. The situation catalyzed promiscuity and adultery, as lonely travelers sought the companionship of girlfriends, barmaids, "second wives," and prostitutes. It was this population of men, with disposable income and an inclination toward extramarital fornication, who appeared to be the main victims of African AIDS.

Statistics bore out this hypothesis. A 1987 study of Ugandan soldiers indicated that one in three was infected with HIV.[22] Other studies found almost the same portion of truck drivers infected, and in some towns along heavily traveled truck routes, as many as 80 percent of all barmaids were infected.[23] A study of Carletonville, South Africa, miners found that a third admitted to having used the services of sex workers, and that one in eight women whose husbands worked in the mines was HIV-infected. By contrast, the same study showed that no woman whose mine-employed husband slept more than 10 nights per month at home was infected.[24]

Truckers seemed to be a particularly potent vector, as they tended (unlike soldiers) to have wives in rural areas to whom they promptly passed the virus after having picked it up from a barmaid, girlfriend, or prostitute in their travels. Truckers interviewed in the late 1980s seemed to take extramarital sex as a right of employment, regardless of the risk of disease. "I been away two weeks, madam. I'm human. I'm a man. I have to have sex," explained one confident driver. "Sex is natural. Sex is not like beer or smoking . . . unless you castrate the men, you can't stop sex."[25]

Most drivers eschewed condoms, and some indulged in particularly dangerous practices such as "dry sex," which required a woman to apply astringent herbs or bleach to her vagina to dry it out and afford more friction during sex. Dry sex was far more conducive to vaginal bleeding during intercourse, and moreover seemed to kill some of the vagina's naturally protective bacteria. Some public health researchers estimated that dry sex doubled the risk of contracting AIDS during the course of any one sexual encounter, but the inflated fees for dry sex proved too attractive for many sex workers to forgo. Dry sex paid triple that of the normal kind: as much as $7.00 per encounter.[26]

Dislocation of wage earners was exacerbated by what many outside observers described as a culture of promiscuity. No matter how carefully public health experts worked to avoid stereotypes and irresponsible generalizations, they were left to conclude that Africans simply had more sex than Westerners, and with greater numbers of partners. Moreover, promiscuity was generally socially accepted. Remarked the former American adviser to the Kenyan Ministry of Health, "It was my impression that sex was as natural as feeding (as opposed to eating or dining) and without the ego involvement and acceptance-rejection that plagues our culture . . . the western view of sex, permeated with our ideas of right and wrong, just doesn't compute."[27]

Africans had a variety of names for their extramarital partners, ranging from the "city wife," to the "second wife," to the "permanent girlfriend." Men spoke of heading to *"le deuxieme bureau"* (the second office) after work—the local hotel that rented rooms by the hour. While firm statistics were elusive, one study of married men in Zimbabwe found that 40 percent admitted to extramarital sex in the previous year—and the true percentage was undoubtedly higher. In a Nigerian survey, the portion was over half of married men, and over a third of married women. Related one Lusaka businessman, "Yes, I've got a wife, but sometimes I go to a girlfriend for a night. That's very usual for most men—it's very easy to find a girl."[28] Ruefully noted one Africa watcher, "The educated elite painfully built up from nothing over the last twenty years, will be especially hard hit by AIDS because it is they who can best afford to run around with many women, and having many women is a status symbol, part of the image of the successful African male."[29]

And for AIDS victims, the numbers were even higher. A 1985 study revealed that the median number of sex partners in the previous year for African men testing positive for HIV was 32, versus 3 for the noninfected.[30] One Ugandan businessman testing positive for HIV admitted to sleeping with possibly 100 women over the previous year.[31] Coupled with the high degree of dislocation in the middle class, and disruption of the traditional ties of rural communities, the promiscuous norms were supercharging the epidemic and spreading it deep into the population of central and east Africa. Concluded Africa scholar Sanford Ungar in 1989: "The disease has followed the path of the heavy trucks that haul food and other material from Indian Ocean ports into the interior of the continent. . . . To the extent that this urban disease has reached small towns and rural areas, those places invariably lie along or near the truck routes."[32]

VECTORS

The peripatetic workforce, while destabilizing, could not have fomented such explosive epidemic growth without catalytic vectors, and in all of Africa the most volatile of those vectors was prostitution. Prostitutes throughout central and east Africa caught AIDS at the onset of the epidemic, and as early as 1986 were already displaying tremendous rates of infection. That year in east Africa, for example, 66 percent of prostitutes of "low socioeconomic status" were found to be infected with HIV, while in Nairobi the rate approached 90 percent.[33] A year earlier, over a quarter of "barmaids" in Matonge, a class of women who did not quite consider themselves professional prostitutes yet who engaged in sexual activities for money, were infected.[34]

Changing economic conditions promoted high levels of participation in the sex trade. Married women engaged in prostitution as *femmes libres* or second wives in an effort to increase family income, or to purchase independence from domineering or abusive husbands. Increasing divorce rates in postcolonial Africa induced women with few economic choices to dabble in prostitution. And peripatetic students, desperate for sustenance, engaged in the sex trade through their student years in an effort to offset tuition. Explained Brooke Schoepf, a medical anthropologist working in Kinshasa:

> The colonial power kept the women out of town and broke up the families because it didn't want to pay a family wage. The women had to stay and work in the fields to feed the colonial labor force. There was tremendous displacement and social disruption. After independence many women escaped to the towns because the drudgery of forced cultivation was so unbearable and became second or third wives or *femmes libres*.

The infected prostitutes proved remarkably facile at transmitting the virus to their clients, particularly those with preexisting ulcerative sexually transmitted diseases (STDs), and most specifically those with preexisting STDs who were not circumcised. Nairobi researcher Francis Plummer, for example, found that among Nairobi men who admitted to frequently patronizing prostitutes, incidence of HIV was 2.5 percent for circumcised men without genital ulcers, 13.4 percent for circumcised men with ulcers, 29 percent for uncircumcised men without ulcers, and 53 percent for uncircumcised men with ulcers.[35] And ulcerative STDs were ubiquitous in Africa, with over 15 percent of all women and 40 percent of prostitutes infected with syphilis throughout the subcontinent—rates 20 to 30 times those found in the United States or Western Europe.[36]

But even these rates did not tell the magnitude of the problem. Owing to widespread availability of inexpensive antibiotics, most men and women who contracted syphilis, gonorrhea, or chlamydia were able to heal themselves fairly rapidly with pharmaceutical intervention. Yet because of low rates of prophylactic medical visits, infected individuals tended to wait until advanced symptoms developed—itching, pain, urethral or vaginal discharge, or visible sores and chancres—before getting treatment. Thus, the number of people at any one time infected with an STD was far below the number who had contracted an STD at some point in their lives. While numbers were hard to pin down, one South African medical team estimated that over a third of men and as many as three-quarters of women in certain mining towns had been infected with syphilis at some point in their lives.[37]

The circumcision phenomenon was a puzzle, for researchers initially did not understand the mechanisms by which circumcision might afford protection from HIV infection. Yet the difference was profound, in both vulnerability to HIV and vulnerability to other STDs as well. In one study, researcher Francis Plummer found that uncircumcised men were eight times as likely to have had a genital ulcerative disease as circumcised ones, and that uncircumcised men infected with an STD had a 50 percent chance of contracting HIV after just one sexual contact with an infected partner. The correlation was so marked as to account for virtually the entire difference in HIV prevalence between Africa and the United States. In one of his many studies of the phenomenon, Plummer concluded that "lack of circumcision and genital ulcers could explain up to 90 percent of the difference between American and African heterosexual transmission of the AIDS virus."[38]

Early circumcision appeared to induce changes in the skin on the glans of the penis making it substantially less likely to suffer microlesions and abrasions that in turn thwarted the contraction of STDs (including AIDS). One team of medical researchers found that men who were circumcised later in life—at the onset of puberty or after, as was common in some tribes—possessed lower levels of protection from AIDS and other STDs than was true of men who had been circumcised earlier. In a study of men of the Basotho and Shangaan tribes, men who were circumcised between ages 15 and 20, for example, had similar AIDS rates as their uncircumcised tribe-mates, in contrast with those who had been circumcised before age 15, who had AIDS rates a third lower than the uncircumcised individuals in the sample.[39]

The elements of promiscuity, infected prostitutes, preexisting STDs, and low circumcision rates all built on each other, and each exacerbated the infectious tendencies of the other cofactors. But further amplifying the effects of the toxic combination in Africa was an accompanying epidemic of highly virulent tuberculosis whose spread appeared to be facilitated by HIV, while in turn facilitating the further spread of AIDS. The tuberculosis bacillus was common around the world, but fewer than 1 in 15 people infected with the bacterium ever exhibited symptoms. When accompanied by HIV, however, the bacillus's virulence escalated some thirtyfold, weakening the infected individuals while at the same time making them significantly more infectious toward others. "TB and HIV are feeding off each other at an alarming rate," noted WHO researcher Arata Kochi. "When they're together, they multiply each other's impact."[40]

As AIDS advanced through central Africa, it created a new TB epidemic, which in turn further facilitated the spread of AIDS. By 1993, HIV prevalence among tuberculosis patients in sub-Saharan Africa ranged from 30 to 50 percent. The presence of HIV limited the number of patients who could be effectively treated, and even those who could be treated relapsed more frequently than did TB patients without AIDS.[41] The combined effect both heightened AIDS and reignited a worldwide epidemic of tuberculosis: a disease that had been on the wane for some four decades. By mid-decade, the U.S. Public Health Service would warn that new outbreaks were threatening Eastern Europe, Asia, and parts of the Americas, while the World Health Organization would warn that the new outbreak of TB constituted a "global emergency." The predicted worldwide deaths from TB over the following decade, either accompanied by AIDS or not, was approaching 100 *million*.[42]

DENIAL

The African epidemic would have posed a daunting challenge to even the best-prepared of government agencies. Unfortunately, in most African countries the growing epidemic was met with silence from government health ministries, and in some cases with outright denial. The impetus for the evasiveness came from a variety of sources: tourism ministries fearful of jeopardizing their nations' tourist industry; trade ministries fearful that produce and commodities exports would be tainted; and African nationalist politicians and assemblies who resisted saddling their nations' already shaky public images with yet another stigma.[43] Tiny Rwanda, for example, near the epicenter of the central African epidemic, required all AIDS information to be "channeled through appointed national committees" (in the words of one public health group) in an effort to preserve a positive image of the nation for would-be tourists. By 1988, Nigeria refused to admit to hosting any AIDS cases at all (despite harboring several thousand by international estimates), while Kenya's government threatened with expulsion any journalists or international agency employees who reported on AIDS without official permission.[44] And as early as 1985, a Ugandan health official lashed out at Western media for "conveying out of all proportion what is happening in Africa."[45]

The official reluctance to confront the epidemic in many countries was frequently exacerbated by certain norms of conduct and deportment, almost prudish in their outlook, which contrasted strongly with the realities of highly sexualized societies. A number of the African nations, for example, disallowed condom advertising and discouraged explicit educational materials. Religious leaders, both Christian and otherwise, eschewed mention of the epidemic at large, and forbade endorsing safe-sex techniques specifically, for fear of offending their parishioners. Wrote one frequent traveler to Africa: "I remember sitting in a church service in a village in the southern part of Zambia and hearing the preacher say that one in four Zambians had AIDS. A loud murmur moved through the congregation, indicating their distaste for even a mention of the subject."[46]

Africans who had AIDS often hid the disease from their neighbors and relations for fear of ostracism. Across the continent, AIDS patients spoke clandestinely with international health officials or investigating journalists about their fears for their children lest they die, or of their lack of options for shelter. Orphanages reported being deluged with young orphans who could find no home with uncles and aunts, according to the tradition in many African societies. And in some areas, observers reported seeing an increasing number of cases of infanticide as mothers chose to kill their infected children rather than allow their illnesses to jeopardize the entire family. "One little girl had been put in front of a truck by her mother; another had been thrown onto a fire and rescued by a neighbor who heard her cries," reported an American volunteer at a rural hospital in southern Africa.[47] In one horrific account outside Francistown in South Africa, an orphaned teenager fought off relatives who tried to appropriate the family homestead upon his mother's death. The relatives relinquished their claims, but retaliated by refusing to offer any help with the upbringing of the surviving younger siblings. "It's as if we don't exist anymore either," related the young scion.[48]

In South Africa, vestiges of apartheid exacerbated the political ineffectiveness. The creation of ethnic homelands during the apartheid years had produced tremendous social upheaval as blacks commuted out of their homelands to white-owned mining and factory jobs, from which their wives and children were barred. Such transitory migration facilitated the spread of the epidemic as it had in other parts of Africa, but here the problem was all the worse because of the utter distrust of the government by blacks, and a reciprocal distrust of blacks by the still white-dominated medical system. Such distrust barred the government from embracing the scope of the epidemic until years after it had become firmly embedded in the population, and left blacks weary of any government-backed condom distribution and medication programs. "At first the government didn't take AIDS seriously," recalled Natal doctor Nkosazana Zuma. "Then, during the state of emergency, it used AIDS for political games, saying things like 'Beware of the A.N.C., they come from outside the country and bring AIDS.' "[49] Noted one jaded South Africa correspondent, "In a migrant society, AIDS commutes."[50]

Further muddying the true dimensions of the African AIDS crisis was a stated opposition to the prevailing theory about the origins of the AIDS virus itself. While most epidemiologists by 1990 accepted the simian virus hypothesis, a number of African officials rejected the model as racist. One theory strongly supported by several African leaders was that while the epidemic may have begun in Africa, it had actually been released on the native population through a Philadelphia-based research institute distributing tainted polio vaccine. Another theory posited the idea that the virus had evolved in the West and only been brought to Africa much later by tourists, visiting soldiers, or foreign businessmen. Some leaders suspected outright biological sabotage by European governments wishing to undermine the independence of their former colonies, while others offered no alternative explanation, but simply rejected outright the central role of Africa in the disease's development. At a 1985 international AIDS conference in Brussels, representatives from 50 African nations signed a statement proclaiming that papers presented at the conference "did not show any conclusive evidence that AIDS originated in Africa."[51] And Uganda's health minister explained away the African-evolution theories as mere Eurocentric prejudice: "The AIDS problem has unmasked thinly veiled racism and fascism in some quarters where Africans are labeled the breeders of a scourge," he explained.[52]

In the generally unconstructive muddle of official African governmental response, a few leaders stood out for their foresight and candor. Malawi's president Bakili Muluzi, for example, repeatedly attempted to educate the public about AIDS at forums in which he had the opportunity to speak, while Uganda's president Yoweri Kaguta Museveni aggressively responded to that nation's early AIDS epidemic by cooperating with the World Health Organization to create a National Committee for the Prevention of AIDS. Nations in west Africa, who encountered the disease a half decade after their central and east African neighbors, tended to be more candid at the onset of infection, and confronted their pending epidemics more effectively. In Ethiopia, the Ivory Coast, Liberia, and Ghana, governments all established AIDS agencies long before the disease was widespread, and helped prevent its spread through education campaigns, antipromiscuity messages, and blood screening.[53]

MEDICAL CARE

Medical care, of course, was utterly inadequate across sub-Saharan Africa. Even in the United States, medical care was incapable of significantly altering the disease's trajectory; in Africa, it was so inadequate as to invite contempt. At a time when Americans were spending over $1,200 per capita per year on health care, virtually all Africans were spending less than $30 per year, and some significantly less. Zambians, for example, spent $5 per person on medical care in 1987; Malawians $3, and Ugandans an extraordinary $1. Physician and nursing availability followed concomitantly, with most sub-Saharan nations harboring 1 physician for each 7,000 citizens, the Sudanese 1 per 10,000, and the Rwandese 1 per 35,000. (The United States, by contrast, had 1 per 600.) Nursing ratios were slightly better, with most nations having about one-third to one-fourth the number of staff of the United States, albeit at substantially lower levels of training.[54]

Even before AIDS hit, the medical systems of these nations had been able to provide the majority of citizens only the barest essentials of primary care; after AIDS, the systems collapsed entirely. Most health systems quickly ran short of beds, syringes, blood products, antibiotics, blood-testing equipment, and personnel. In Bukoba, Tanzania, the hospital coped with its six-hour electrical shutdown every day by using flashlights to read monitors and by keeping refrigerated blood and drugs in darkened rooms. Across the continent, the frequent response to an AIDS diagnosis was the simple dismissal of the patient. "You've got AIDS. We can't help you. Go home and die," was the not uncommon directive to patients from rural hospital staffs, according to South African physician Tony Moll.[55] In virtually all hospitals and clinics, needles were washed and reused, sometimes so frequently that they had to be resharpened on whetstones.[56] Blood-testing equipment was so inadequate that AIDS diagnoses could take two weeks or longer, and this was for the small minority of infected individuals who bothered to be tested at all. And everywhere large swaths of the infected population eschewed interaction with the formal medical system.

Even so, enough AIDS patients entered the formal health system to swamp the existing facilities and resources. Under the onslaught of the legions of newly incurable patients, the continent's hospitals and clinics buckled. In Tanzania by the early 1990s, 40 percent of the already vastly inadequate public health budget was going to fighting AIDS, while in Rwanda over 65 percent of the nation's health funds were being expended on AIDS patients. One pessimistic health economist estimated that South Africa's AIDS budget by the year 2000 would need to be 10 times the nation's entire 1990 health budget for it to adequately serve the growing patient population.[57] And even those estimates presupposed that doctors and nurses would be willing to treat AIDS patients at all, which was not necessarily the case, as fearful medical personnel recoiled at the prospect of treating the deteriorating victims. "Many of our nurses do not even want to touch these patients, nor do our social workers know exactly what to tell them," related a Rwanda physician.[58]

Some of the burden was taken up by the parallel system of traditional healers, herbalists, and shamans who practiced widely across the continent. Long a hidden pressure valve for overburdened physicians and hospitals, the traditional healers were frequently able to assuage anxiety, and could periodically effect physiological improvement. Under the onslaught of AIDS, however, their powers of both healing and comforting proved inadequate. Reaching for such exotic herbal remedies and plant extracts as MM1, Kemron, UM-127, levamisole, and Fusidin, they found that none interrupted the progress of the disease.[59] Worse, certain traditional healing practices, such as ritual lacerating, actually served to expedite the epidemic's spread. In response, international organizations created educational programs to ameliorate the most harmful and ignorant of the alternative healers' practices. The Kampalan organization THETA (Traditional and Health Practitioners Together Against AIDS) taught traditional healers to cease "bewitching" AIDS sufferers, to stop sleeping with their patients in efforts to exorcize the pathogen, and to cease sacramental bleedings. Remarked one traditional healer after completing THETA education: "The training was useful. I can now diagnose HIV/AIDS related sickness without calling on the spirits."[60]

The virological ignorance of most traditional healers pointed to a larger treatment impediment in Africa: high rates of ignorance about hygiene, health, medicine, and nutrition. In many of the nations most affected by AIDS, general illiteracy rates approached 40 percent, and among women exceeded 60 percent. Ignorance of modern biology, physiology, and anatomy was profound, with such eminences as Kenyan president Daniel arap Moi insisting on the efficacy of such useless bromides as Kemron in AIDS treatment. Indeed, the British *Economist* reported Ugandan skepticism of the seriousness of the threat. "Many do not see why they should change sexual habits just because of another disease; arguments that would be compelling elsewhere can be weak in a society inured to death."[61]

Further exacerbating the dismal treatment picture was the fact that in sporadic cases doctors and nurses were themselves responsible for further transmission of the virus, albeit unintentionally. So inadequate was the supply of medical equipment that clinicians often resorted to using incompletely sterilized needles and scalpels. International public health experts actually feared the effects of a major vaccination program—should an effective vaccine ever become available—lest the vaccination process itself accelerate the disease's spread. One study of Zairian babies demonstrated that the AIDS-infected among them had received a mean of 44 lifetime injections versus a mean of 23 for the uninfected. The irony of the evidence could not be ignored: the children who had had greater access to modern medicine in that country were twice as likely to be sick with AIDS as those who had been too poor to receive routine childhood vaccinations.[62]

Yet even as the continent's medical systems strained to accommodate the expanding burden being placed on them, nationalist governments seemed intent on discarding one of the few functional components of their nation's health-care system—the white-dominated private hospitals and clinics that still pervaded ex-colonial outposts such as Zambia, Zimbabwe, and South Africa. In all of those nations, much of the white minority sought care outside the bounds of the state medical systems, in private facilities manned by mostly white and Indian clinicians who had completed Western or Western-style medical education and training programs. Despite the potential of these systems to play leadership roles in educating the public about AIDS, to train paraprofessionals or traditional healers in basic AIDS care, and to provide Western-quality health care to the elite of their nation's workforce, several African leaders seemed intent on dismantling the systems and ejecting the few Western-trained physicians. The African National Congress's new "National Health Plan for South Africa" called for dismantling the nation's existing system of tertiary care (which catered disproportionately to the white population) and focusing instead on primary care. While the goals were politically laudable, they threatened to undermine the one sector of biomedical excellence in an otherwise derelict system.[63]

COSTS

The costs were immense. Besides the catastrophic human cost—parents witnessing the deaths of their children, men and women losing their spouses and friends, and the innumerable truncated friendships, destroyed families, and attenuated social networks—and the tremendous medical costs, African nations faced cataclysmic macroeconomic disintegration. Rates of the growth of the epidemic were so great in many countries that they more than offset the naturally high population growth rate of the continent; demographers predicted population implosion and the eradication of whole towns and regions. One British scientist, modeling the Ugandan epidemic, estimated that by 2002 the country would be 20 percent smaller than it would have been in the absence of AIDS.[64] Zimbabwe, with possibly the fastest-growing epidemic on earth, faced a decline of life expectancy from 61 years in 1993 to 49 years by 2000.[65] And many employers began to seriously assess the wisdom of training people who might not live long enough to produce adequate returns on the cost of the education.[66]

Declining population created declining GDP growth, or even negative growth, as the undercapitalized continent faced widespread labor shortages. World Bank data and growth models indicated, for example, that Tanzania's average annual GDP growth would decline from 3.9 percent to 2.8 percent solely owing to the "AIDS effect," while Cameroon's might drop from 4.3 percent to 2.4 percent.[67] In agricultural regions, family farms facing the loss of the homestead's patriarch would be forced to either cut back production or pull children from school to exploit their labor on the farm. When women died, men were forced to spend time on child rearing, or dispose of their children with relatives or in orphanages.[68] And the traditional surplus labor pools of unmarried young men were sure to decline as those men in the prime of their sexually active years were themselves left debilitated, and ultimately dead, by AIDS.

As a result of the odd demographic nature of the African epidemic, all nations faced particularly harsh losses among their pools of educated labor, with scarce managerial talent being particularly diminished. These losses were extremely difficult to overcome, as the nation would lose not only its scarce technical talent, but the subsequent generation of middle-class children who themselves would provide skilled labor in the future. African correspondent John Barnes wrote pessimistically, "In countries that count themselves lucky to have a dozen qualified engineers, the loss of even one is deeply felt."[69] And empirical data produced in the early 1990s validated the growing suspicion that it was the most educated, the most talented, and the most successful members of Africa's workforce who were succumbing most frequently to AIDS. One *JAMA*-published study of 1991 showed that the rate of HIV infection among skilled workers rose directly in relation to the seniority of their positions, with 2.8 percent of workers in one particular textile factory being infected, as opposed to 4.5 percent of foremen and 5.3 percent of executives.[70] Such a trend was unprecedented, and ominous.

Most costly of all was the growing ranks of orphans, or children bereft of a parent, who promised to exhaust the states' resources while constituting a potentially disruptive and maladjusted social force. The United Nations estimated in 1990 that in parts of Uganda 14 percent of all children had lost a parent.[71] By 1995, several central and east African nations would see 2 percent of their children under 15 orphaned, and by the year 2000 this number promised to rise to 3 percent. Those numbers sounded modest, until one realized that in nations that were primarily youthful in their demography, they translated into staggering numbers of orphans: nearly 600,000 in Kenya, 700,000 in Tanzania, and 900,000 in Uganda.[72] No country in history had faced such orphan rates, and government officials feared for the social upheaval and human misery that might follow. The girls, for one thing, would lack a dowry, and thus faced almost certain spinsterhood; the boys would lack education, skills, or even basic literacy, and would be thus denied any work beyond the menial. And with extended families also diminished from the epidemic, the chance of those orphans being taken in by sympathetic relatives was all the less likely.

INTERNATIONAL AID

The world's response to the African epidemic came slowly, with most countries pledging only modest gifts through the late 1980s. In 1991, when the World Health Organization (WHO) estimated the African epidemic to be infecting six million souls, the United States pledged only $52 million—barely $8 per infected individual—and the United States was the single most generous donor in the world.[73] One Congressional Research Service analyst admitted that the amount was "a modest commitment," and yet it represented over one-fourth of all contributions to WHO's AIDS relief efforts from all nations.[74] And although WHO, the single largest conduit of funds to the afflicted countries, estimated that its AIDS budget would rise to $110 million within a few years' time, the sum was minuscule compared with the scope of the problem. In the United States, for example, AZT treatment alone was budgeted at over $13,000 per individual per year, which translated into an aggregate cost of $78 *billion* per year for Africa, without factoring in hospital or physician expenses.

The early international aid effort had its successes. WHO global AIDS director Jonathan Mann in 1989 pointed proudly to WHO's evolving "Global AIDS Strategy," which was implementing blood-screening programs and educational efforts around the world, and the United Nations Development Program announced in 1988 that it was in the process of creating agreements with various international and regional organizations throughout Africa and Latin America.[75] But these minor milestones could not hide the basically symbolic nature of the efforts.

One question posed by the tepid international commitment was whether greater funds could actually accomplish anything. By 1992,

AIDS was still untreatable. AZT could delay death for a year or so, but the principal difference between AIDS therapeutics in the West and AIDS therapeutics in Africa was one of treating the opportunistic infections, meaning simply that AIDS in Africa killed more quickly, and more effectively, than it did in the West. True, more funds could pay for more palliative and preventive care, including condom distribution efforts and general educational programs, but these were relatively inexpensive. Uganda, for example, one of the poorest countries in the world, was able to launch an effective antipromiscuity campaign in the late 1980s with relatively little international help. And even with the puny funds available, the Agency for International Development (AID) and WHO were able to saturate the continent with 270 million condoms in the late 1980s with funds to spare.[76]

The underlying systemic challenges—vast illiteracy, insalubrious sexual mores, pervasive ulcerative STDs, and a transient workforce—would all require decades of economic development to be thwarted, if indeed they ever could be.[77] In the absence of a vaccine or effective medical intervention, an increase of international aid to fight HIV promised few concrete results in 1992. In light of this reality, even wealthy Western nations were reluctant to commit money to a problem that seemed insurmountable and unsolvable. The real debates lay in the years to come, when new medications that could really cure, rather than merely assuage, would become available to Western patients but be denied to African ones—simply for want of money.

CHAPTER 11

BREAKTHROUGH

By 1995, good news was breaking out for AIDS in America. Infection rates were declining, as was the number of people actually living with AIDS. In San Francisco and New York the total population of AIDS-infected individuals had peaked in 1992, and in both cities had declined by 20 percent over the ensuing three years.[1] Safe-sex education programs, condom distribution efforts, and general word-of-mouth all seemed to be playing their part in reducing the numbers of new people contracting the virus. Rates of new AIDS infections among gay men fell fastest, but even among New York state prisoners prevalence had dropped from 26 percent to 6 percent in just six years. "It's certainly going in all the right directions," noted former CDC director James Curran.[2]

The Clinton White House had taken a moderate course in its approach to the epidemic, increasing research funding and public health efforts while generally associating itself with the disease more publicly and visibly than had either the Bush or Reagan administrations. In his first year in office, Bill Clinton increased research funding by 25 percent (to $2 billion), named a White House AIDS coordinator (Public Health Service veteran Kristine Gebbie), and empowered Health and Human Services Secretary Donna Shalala to create an AIDS task force to set research and treatment priorities for the administration. At the same time, the president used AIDS Awareness Day to speak about the administration's AIDS agenda at Georgetown University. Such actions provided moral support for an exhausted and somewhat demoralized AIDS advocacy community, and buttressed many AIDS leaders' resolve to continue their work. "Clinton at Georgetown, Gebbie on the stump, Shalala rejecting business as usual for AIDS—that kind of official rhetoric matters greatly," wrote Berkeley public policy professor David Kirp in the liberal *Nation* magazine in July 1994.[3]

The administration made errors as well. In June 1995, White House spokesman Michael McCurry apologized for "an error of judgment" after White House security staffers donned blue rubber gloves to check the parcels and personal affects of a group of visiting gay elected officials.[4] And six months before, in a nod to political pressure, Clinton had fired Surgeon General Jocelyn Elders after she had suggested that part of an expanded sex-education curriculum might include training in masturbation. Although Elders later suggested that her intention had been merely to *inform* adolescents about the role of masturbation in sexual life, rather than actually *teach* them masturbation techniques, the damage had been done. With Elders having previously accused the Catholic Church of having a "love affair" with fetuses, the White House deemed that her latest gaffe was "just one too many" and demanded her resignation.[5] And while conservatives in Congress celebrated her departure, AIDS advocates rued the loss of so staunch a supporter.[6]

Despite the waning press attention accorded to AIDS, it still remained the target of considerable conservative vitriol. Although by 1995 the disease had ceased to be one predominantly afflicting homosexuals in the United States (and hardly at all afflicting homosexuals abroad), debate over the 1995 Ryan White reappropriation bill attracted the usual screeds from the right, with Jesse Helms tarring the gay community for its "deliberate, disgusting, revolting conduct," and House conservatives inserting a provision into their version of the bill denying Ryan White funds to any state that did not require newborn testing for HIV.[7] And although the bill ultimately passed, the legislative battle, coming after a decade of attacks on gays and other AIDS victims, had weakened the AIDS lobby's standing, and left many gay and public health leaders feeling bruised and demoralized. Lesbian novelist Sarah

Schulman articulated the feeling of many when she noted, "Throughout the nation, gay and lesbian people are engaged in hand-to-hand combat against the religious right's ballot measures and stealth candidates."[8]

Accompanying the good news about declining infection rates was bad news as well. Among blacks and Latinos, the epidemic continued to grow into the mid-1990s, with over one-third of all new cases reported nationwide involving Latinos. Many of the infected individuals in this group were relatively young women who risked transmitting the virus to babies in utero unless careful precautions were taken during pregnancy and birth. At the same time, new mutations of the virus emerged that were largely immune to the antiviral action of AZT, weakening the one consistently useful tool that virologists could claim in their fight against the disease.[9] And, as in Africa, a new virulent strain of tuberculosis was emerging in the wake of AIDS that threatened to exacerbate the toxic effects of HIV while facilitating its spread. This last threat was so grave that some infectious-disease specialists actually considered it a more pressing public health concern than AIDS itself. "At no time in recent history has tuberculosis been of such great concern as it is now, and legitimately so, because tuberculosis is out of control in this country," pronounced CDC tuberculosis expert Dixie Snider.[10]

GAY LIFE

Despite a decade and a half of AIDS-induced gay baiting, and the rise of Christian conservatism during the late 1980s, gays enjoyed a delicate but rising social acceptance as the 1990s progressed. The establishment of gay community groups, gay synagogues and churches, and gay political clubs (including the gay Log Cabin Republicans), all indicated a wish by gays for more mainstream life patterns, and the American populace responded with a growing, if tacit, acceptance. In 1995, several of New York City's oldest and most powerful corporate law firms announced that they would cover gay partners with spousal health and pension benefits, marking a further step toward broader acceptance of homosexuality. "Within two years, firms not offering health benefits to gay employees will become the exception rather than the rule," predicted one partner at a prominent New York firm.[11]

The year before, Olympic diver Greg Louganis announced that he was gay, and followed his claim the next year with an admission of HIV infection. Although the announcement spurred some accusations of irresponsibility (Louganis had competed in the 1988 Seoul Games knowing that he was HIV-positive, and actually sustained a modest head cut without informing either the team physician or his fellow divers about his HIV status), in general the public responded supportively. Coming in the aftermath of admissions of AIDS by both Magic Johnson and tennis great Arthur Ashe, Louganis's announcement furthered a general perception by many Americans that AIDS could infect even the most accomplished and celebrated of the nation's citizens.[12]

Likewise, the arts and entertainment industries, after tentatively broaching AIDS in *Philadelphia* and *The Normal Heart,* seemed to become more comfortable with the idea, and AIDS was featured prominently in Paul Rudnick's *Jeffrey* and Tony Kushner's *Angels in America.* The *New York Times,* in reviewing *Jeffrey,* pronounced it a "consistently funny story of sex and romance in the age of AIDS," while *The New Yorker* magazine's review of the Kushner opus pronounced, "From its first beat, 'Angels in America' exhibited a ravishing command of its characters and of the discourse it wanted to have through them with our society."[13] *Angels* garnered a Tony Award and a Pulitzer Prize.[14]

But perhaps the best indicator of public acceptance of gays, and of AIDS as well, was the vocal and financial support given to the disease in a well-developed philanthropic circuit. As the 1990s progressed, expressions of support for AIDS became ubiquitous in certain liberal circles on both coasts. Hollywood and New York fund-raisers, hosted and sponsored by such celebrities and public figures as Elton John, Whoopi Goldberg, Madonna, Princess Diana, Elizabeth Taylor and Liza Minnelli, raised millions in support of basic research, and small red AIDS commemorative ribbons became commonplace. Pushing the bounds of taste, clothing retailer Benetton featured in its advertisements an apparent AIDS victim bedridden and skeleton-thin, and encouraged pa-

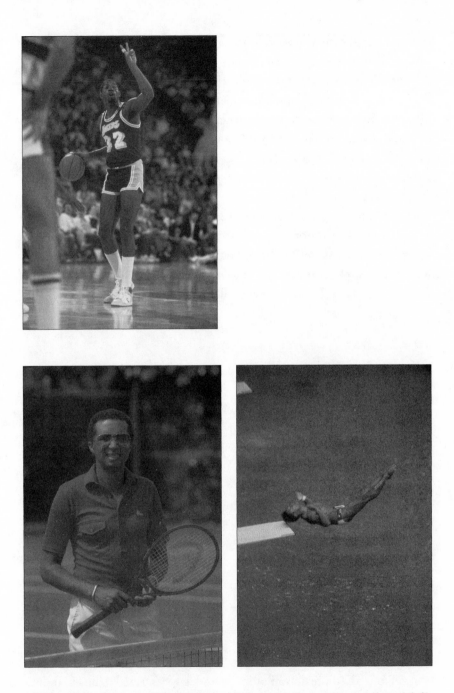

Athletes Magic Johnson, Arthur Ashe, and Greg Louganis were among the celebrity personalities who admitted HIV infection. Their announcements reinforced the idea that a broad swath of the American population might be vulnerable to AIDS. (Ashe and Johnson, Stockphoto; Louganis, Rich Clarkson/TimeLife Pictures/Getty Images)

trons to find the nearest store where they could shop and support AIDS research simultaneously. "AIDS may be the first disease to have its own gift shop," noted writer Daniel Harris in the summer of 1994.[15]

At the same time, empirical evidence seemed to lend support to the idea that homosexuality had a genetic basis rather than a behavioral one, and that as such homosexuals could not be blamed for the "choices" they had made, regardless of the discomfort they caused their fellow citizens. A series of investigations had shown that identical twins were far more likely than were fraternal twins, or regular siblings, to share homosexuality as a trait, and geneticists speculated that a specific gay-linked gene or series of genes might be discovered in the near future. "Homosexuality is not an illness, not a contagion, not a moral failing. It is simply a predisposition," asserted writer and commentator Hendrich Herzberg.[16] To an increasing degree, the public seemed to agree, or seemed, at least, to not disagree.

AZT

By 1994, the armament of anti-AIDS tools was still pitifully small. AZT remained the standard-bearer of medications, but it was proving to be even less effective than had been originally supposed. While AZT did retard the rate of CD4 cell decline (a reasonable measure of the disease's progress), it appeared to diminish in efficacy over time, and seemed to prolong life no more than a year on average.[17] Moreover, a large portion of AIDS patients found that the drug caused significant negative side effects, ranging from fevers to muscular atrophy to weight loss. Skeptical scientists and investigative journalists pointed out that many of the most optimistic studies of AZT's efficacy had been funded by its maker, Burroughs-Wellcome, and a comprehensive European study conducted in the early 1990s disclosed that patients who started earlier on AZT fared no better than those who began treatment after their symptoms advanced.[18]

AZT mirrored the action of many widely prescribed drugs in inducing extreme reactions in a small minority of patients. But unlike other drugs, AZT had no viable substitute. Moreover, the extraordinary fatality rate associated with AIDS compelled many AIDS victims to persist in AZT treatment through noxious and painful side effects. It was only after the ancillary effects became so severe that they actually outweighed the malignancy of the disease itself that people gave up on the drug. Three-year-old AIDS patient Lindsey Nagel, for example, suffered such severe leg cramps, appetite loss, and nausea while on AZT that her parents withdrew the medicine after a year, despite the drug's potential to prolong life in the girl. "In my mind, I wasn't going to put that kid through a bunch of misery so she could live another six months. I would rather have her live two good months than have her live six bad months," explained Lindsey's father.[19] Anecdotal evidence presented to doctors suggested that a growing minority of AIDS patients were choosing similarly.

In the decade ending in 1995, scientists and clinicians produced a number of compounds that initially showed promise, but none proved substantially more effective than AZT. National Institutes of Health researcher Ira Pastan, for example, experimented with the Pseudomonas exotoxin in hope that it could selectively attach itself to HIV-infected CD4 cells and kill them, and University of Texas scientist Jonathan Uhr attempted similar tasks with ricin. But both teams ran into the barrier of the immune system itself, which tended to surround and defuse the toxins before they could effectively wipe out the AIDS-infected cells.[20] Meanwhile, French scientist Daniel Zagury reported promising results with a new immunotherapy treatment, but was then forced to cease his work when several patients died from viral infections related to the therapy.[21] And while NIAID director Anthony Fauci reported continued progress with ddI through the early 1990s, as of 1993 the drug had not yet been approved for mass distribution.[22]

Two promising advances had been made by 1994, however. The first was the medical treatment not of AIDS itself, but of some of its most toxic opportunistic infections. *Pneumocystis carinii* pneumonia, for example, one of the two most fatal infections associated with AIDS, retreated so markedly in the face of a combined regimen of AZT, aerosolized pentamidine, and Bactrim, that one AIDS physician concluded that AIDS was "a different disease than it was last year."[23] The second was the increasing use of combinations of drugs with AZT in an effort to bolster the primary drug's effect while circumventing the virus's ability to mutate to an AZT-tolerant form. AZT was combined with heparin, Dilantin, acyclovir, and Bactrim in various combinations in an effort to ward off seizures, fight infections, and generally strengthen the antiviral action of the central drug. While no combination proved to be a panacea, various combinations did seem to work marginally better than AZT alone for some patients, and for a few patients the improvement was substantial. "It was as if somebody had pressed a switch," commented one patient who began such a regimen after fighting AIDS for two years.[24]

This early success with drug combinations seemed auspicious. While no single drug seemed to circumvent all of HIV's defenses, a number of drugs in development in the early 1990s posed the potential of negating some of the virus's many weapons. Drug companies Merck, American Cyanamid, IAF Biochem International, Hoffmann-La Roche, Abbott, and Bristol-Myers Squibb all had drugs at varying stages of development and testing by 1991, which fell into the general categories of nucleoside inhibitors and nonnucleoside inhibitors (both of which inhibited the production and functioning of reverse transcriptase), protease inhibitors (which worked on viral particle formation), and myristoylation inhibitors (which blocked viral integration). No one drug appeared to offer a miraculous cure, but a number working together might do the trick.[25]

COMBINATION THERAPY

In the winter of 1993, Boston medical student Yung-Kang Chow announced that by using three drugs together—AZT, ddI, and one of either pyridinone or neverapine—he could both disable HIV and prevent it from mutating. Within a few months, senior scientists in the same lab discredited Chow's findings—calling it an "unfortunate error"—but the three-drug combination did work better than other combinations of drugs in controlling the HIV's growth.[26]

Just three years later, a variation on Chow's regimen seemed to promise miracles. A combination of AZT, ddI, and one of several new powerful protease inhibitors could apparently stop the growth of the virus in humans almost entirely. In various clinical trials performed on tens of thousands of AIDS patients, the drug "cocktail" reduced viral

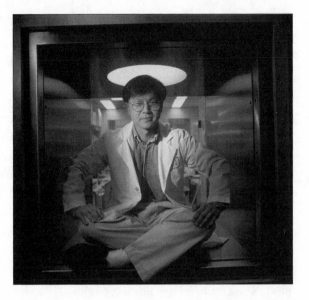

David Ho, in his "Man of the Year" spread in *Time*. (Ted Thai/TimeLife Pictures/Getty Images)

loads to undetectable levels in nearly 60 percent of all patients, with most of the remaining patients posting significant reductions.[27] And despite investigators' fears of rapid viral mutation to accommodate the cocktails, the antiviral effects lasted at least a year. "The data is true, and it's unbelievable," exalted Emory University scientists Raymond Schinazi. "There's no toxicity. It's a home run!"[28]

In the early months of the triple-therapy miracle, skeptics abounded. Researchers who had toyed with various pharmacological interventions for a decade or more could not believe that the solution was at hand. But as AIDS researchers presented their results, gleaned from tens of thousands of patients enrolled in clinical trials lasting multiple years, the skeptics, and then the general public, were won over. "If you had asked me in January 1996, 'Can you eradicate HIV infection,' I would have laughed in your face," remarked Julio Montaner of the University of British Columbia. "But now we've been able to demonstrate that we can effectively suppress viral production. And that is leading to a dramatic change in how we think of this disease."[29]

Although combination therapy was a result of hundreds of researchers toiling in university and corporate labs throughout the world, the individual most responsible for the breakthroughs was David Ho, a noted infectious-disease investigator who served as director of the Aaron Diamond AIDS Research Center in New York City. Ho had been drawn into AIDS research in the early 1980s while completing his infectious-disease training at Cedars-Sinai Hospital in Los Angeles. In diagnosing the many critical patients admitted to the hospital, Ho noted the unusual preponderance of young gay men suffering from immune disorders, and postulated the existence of a new infectious agent. Recalling the time later, he admitted that the prospect of a new infectious agent to which he could turn his investigative acumen excited him both professionally and intellectually.[30]

Ho's brilliance was amplified by his recruitment to direct the newly created Aaron Diamond AIDS Research Center, a brainchild of New York philanthropist Irene Diamond, whose husband had left her $200 million upon his death in 1984. Irene Diamond had made her career in Hollywood, where she notably sighted a script entitled "Rick's Bar" and had the foresight to produce from it the movie *Casablanca*. Sensitized to issues of homophobia by her Hollywood experience, she was drawn to the AIDS epidemic both for its medical challenges and its civil rights connotations. Speaking later about her perceptions of AIDS in the mid-1980s, when no dedicated AIDS research centers yet existed, she remarked, "I just had a gut feeling back then that this was going to be horrendous."[31]

Matching a city gift of $3.5 million with $8.5 million of her foundation's money, Diamond established the center in 1988 on the Upper East Side of Manhattan, and affiliated it initially with New York University. Recruiting the 37-year-old Ho as director, Diamond and partner Edward Kilbourne envisioned a young, iconoclastic group of scientists working exclusively on AIDS, unfettered by the traditional thinking of grant-review panels and federal overseers. "I detest bureaucrats," Diamond was known to remark.[32] Ho, in turn, hired 35-year-old researcher Richard Koup, who in turn helped recruit a cadre of energetic scientists. By 1996, Ho and Koup were the only two scientists at the center over 40. Recalled Koup years later, "Here every one of us was recruited as young people, we instantly had our own large laboratories, and all the labs exploded with terrific research."[33]

Ho's great breakthrough was his insight into the rate of reproduction of the virus. While most researchers had assumed that the virus gestated initially in a quasi-dormant state (thus explaining the long lag between infection and display of symptoms for most HIV victims), Ho found that in reality the virus began reproducing furiously immediately upon entry to the body. Working closely with various coworkers, Ho described viral loads and viral growth rates 10,000 times greater than those generally supposed. Such rates of reproduction, with concomitant high mutation rates, explained the virus's extraordinary ability to quickly mutate itself into drug-resistant forms, rendering traditional antiviral regimens useless. The discovery also convinced Ho that a combination approach to treatment was the most promising solution; stopping such an elusive adversary required attacking it at multiple points of vulnerability, denying it the opportunity to morph into a new form. In a sense, Ho understood that an injured AIDS virus was almost more dangerous than one not injured at all, for the injury gave the virus the information it needed to mutate itself into a new form. The only solution, he realized, was to kill the virus outright.[34]

The understated Ho was quick to share credit with colleagues at both the Diamond Center and at labs around the country. Whether collaborating with Diamond colleague John Moore, Alabama scientist George Shaw, or Diamond Center scientist Ned Landau (who discovered the cc-CKR5 "doorway" through which HIV invaded human cells), Ho was quick to emphasize the collaborative nature of scientific research in general, and of his work in particular. And although he antagonized some colleagues by refuting some of their earlier findings or hypotheses, in general he believed in a team model of science, particularly when dealing with so wily an adversary as HIV. For his brilliance, organizational acumen, and moral leadership, *Time* magazine designated him its "Man of the Year" for 1996, acknowledging the oddness of the man's anonymity. "Some people make headlines while others make history," the magazine's editors wrote. "And when the history of this era is written, it is likely that the men and women who turned the tide on AIDS will be seen as true heroes of the age."[35]

The great pharmacological breakthrough that had allowed for the development of combination therapy was the invention of protease inhibitor drugs simultaneously by three firms: Merck (which made Crixivan), Abbot (Norvir), and Hoffman-LaRoche (Invirase). These drugs attacked and neutralized the protease enzyme that was central to the virus's "packaging" capabilities, and in doing so decreased the viral load in most cells some 10,000-fold.[36] And although the prototype for the drugs was discovered as early as 1988, the companies required nearly eight years to create palatable, effective, and adequately safe versions of the drugs that could pass FDA approval.

The protease inhibitors on their own could temporarily halt the growth of AIDS, but so adaptable was the virus, and so quickly did it mutate that in the presence of Crixivan alone (or a Crixivan proxy) the virus would adapt before it could be decimated. By adding AZT (or AZT clones ddI, ddC, or 3TC) to the mix, as well as the nonnucleoside reverse transcriptase inhibitor neviripine (made by German company Boehringer Ingelheim), doctors were also able to attack the cell replication mechanism of the virus so that it could not duplicate its own genetic material. Any one of those drugs could alone reduce viral loads, but it took the combined force of the three to fully neutralize the virus.

Combination therapy could be compared to the variety of tools with which a fireman puts out a fire. Although water alone can do much of the job (similar to Crixivan), without ladders, axes, and foams the vestiges of the fire may continue to simmer, and may in fact reignite themselves after a bit of delay. To achieve real safety, the firemen can't leave until the fire is absolutely out—no smoldering embers, no isolated burning tinder, no heat-filled rooms that could gestate the fire anew. Similarly, for AIDS it was not adequate to extinguish 95 percent of the virus, even if that temporarily alleviated the patient's symptoms; to be safe, you needed to aim for 100 percent removal, or as close to it as possible.

One of the reasons that an effective antiviral therapy proved so elusive was the basic similarity of HIV's components to those of a human cell. The challenge for all infectious-disease researchers was to figure out how to kill a pathogen without killing a human host. Something as simple as common bleach, for example, could kill the AIDS virus, but it would also kill the patient. In the ongoing fight against bacteria, by contrast, scientists could take advantage of the ubiquitous cell wall specific to plant and bacteria cells. Because mammalian cells possessed no cell wall, any compound that exclusively attacked cell walls would be nontoxic to human cells.

Viruses, unfortunately, had no cell wall, nor much of anything beyond a piece of RNA and a protein coat. Thus, to attack the virus effectively, researchers needed to find a chemical or enzymatic process unique to the virus that could be halted or interrupted without disrupting processes in human cells. Scientists who worked on AIDS ultimately focused on two interesting components of the virus—the reverse transcriptase enzyme (which allowed RNA to replicate itself, a trick not performed by human cells), and the protease enzyme, which was instrumental in the virus's manufacturing of a new protein coat. Ultimately, scientists attacked both enzymes in an effort to thwart HIV's survivalist contortions as it attempted to modify its own protein coat and enzymatic structures to resist the new medications.

Combination therapy was a miracle—a true cure for what had been a 100 percent incurable and fatal disease. It was not, however, flawless. For one thing, the regimen was daunting—requiring some 30 different pills per day, taken at specific times, before and after specific meals, on either a full or empty stomach, with and without milk. Physicians worried that none but the highest-functioning and assiduous patients would be able to conform to the regimen's dictates over the long run. Indeed, as early evidence of combination therapy failure came to light (nearly 40 percent of all patients on combination therapy failed to achieve nondetectable viral loads), physician-investigators suspected noncompliance as a major source of failure. One early study of compliance and efficacy suggested that any patient missing over 20 percent of doses over a three-day period had a high likelihood of AIDS resurgence.[37]

Second, a sizable number of patients—perhaps 60 percent—began to show some viral recovery after a year. That is, although the viral load remained very low, it was no longer undetectable a year after combination therapy had been started. This suggested that effective as the three-punch treatment was, there was still a minuscule amount of virus that could tolerate the drugs and reproduce. Scientists were not overly concerned with this phenomenon—they suspected the effective antiviral therapies would require a continual stream of new drugs to offset the effects of ever-mutating drug-resistant viruses (similar to antibiotics and bacteria). However, the evidence suggested that the fight against AIDS would be chronic, and would not be won in any one round.

Third, the medications produced a host of unpleasant side effects, from diarrhea, to kidney stones, nausea, anemia, and partial paralysis. The drugs interacted with a host of common substances such as caffeine, Valium, and Xanax, meaning that patients would need to carefully monitor their intake of those substances while on combination therapy. Many patients ultimately resorted to antinausea medications, testosterone injections, and over-the-counter pain relievers to alleviate some of the worst symptoms of the therapy.

And last, the regimen was expensive: hugely so. Crixivan alone cost $5,000 per year, with Norvir running at $8,000 and Invirase at $7,500. AZT was still priced at some $6,000 per year, and Saquanivir was nearly $6,000 as well. When one added in the cost of the necessary blood assays (to measure viral loads and calculate doses), the cost for a typical AIDS patient could easily exceed $20,000 per year. While this was substantially cheaper than the cost of multiple hospitalizations for untreated opportunistic infections, and obviously preferable to death, it did mean that the miraculous treatment would remain an option solely for either rich individuals or denizens of rich countries. With average per capita medical expenditures in sub-Saharan Africa hovering at $5 per year, the drugs were simply not a viable treatment option for over half the world's AIDS victims. Noting the multiple drawbacks to the combination regimen, one University of California, at San Diego, researcher pronounced, "You can have a home run and still lose the ballgame."[38]

REACTIONS

Combination theory was a miracle, comparable with antibiotics, anesthesia, and the polio vaccine in the annals of the history of medicine. Sage scientists determined it a "quantum leap."[39] Within a week of its announcement at the 1996 Vancouver AIDS conference, over 75,000 AIDS patients in North America had already been placed on the regimen, and those patients routinely displayed tripled T cell counts within a month, and plummeting viral loads. Patients withdrew from antibiotics, chemotherapy, and the host of other interventions to which they had been clinging in an effort to thwart opportunistic infections. Described one physician: "Some of my patients are really coming back from the dead. I had a patient who came into my office just last week . . . I didn't recognize him, he looked so different after a month on Crixivan."[40] And recalled AIDS patient and writer Andrew Sullivan: "I was at a meeting of activists in New York, where David Ho described how people who'd had millions of copies of HIV in their blood now had zero. I just remember thinking, 'This period of complete helplessness is over.' "[41]

The miracle was not without complications, however. The side effects were very unpleasant, with patients complaining of skin sensitivity, dizziness, intense nausea, and uncontrollable diarrhea. "It would be unexpected and without warning—you'd have these colonic purges. I got to know every bathroom in every restaurant within about six blocks of my house and would often be running in to them and it was humiliating."[42] Others complained about the "sludge" that formed in their overworked kidneys, likening it to "carrying a bowling ball in there," and others experienced violent outbreaks of herpes.[43] "One Sunday afternoon I couldn't move, and I wanted to scream every time my skin was touched," recalled a patient on protease inhibitors.[44] So bad were the side effects that patients sometimes admitted preferring death to suffering them; and the attrition rate from ritonavir (seemingly the most toxic of the drugs) was estimated to be as high as 50 percent.[45]

The high cost of the drugs presented a mixed set of challenges.[46] Ironically, the poorest and most disenfranchised of AIDS sufferers were shielded from the cost by generous state Medicaid prescription drug programs, which usually reimbursed 100 percent of the drugs' cost. Individuals with private insurance were also mostly protected from financial liability, save for modest calendar-year deductibles or negligible copayments. But AIDS victims who had lost their jobs, and with them their private health insurance policies, were in a tricky fix. While eligible to continue purchasing their private plans for 18 months after dismissal (as required by federal COBRA regulations), these patients would almost certainly be denied coverage after their eligibility ran out, yet often were ineligible for Medicaid. For such men (and they were usually men) the drug bills could quickly drive them to penury. Some states established special funds to help reimburse for AIDS drugs, but these funds often reimbursed only a portion of the cost.

On the other hand, the high cost of the drugs, and likelihood of their continued use for long intervals, was the primary inducement for drug companies to develop the new molecules at all. On a worldwide scale,

AIDS was still relatively small—affecting fewer than 1.5 million people in the industrialized world. A limited disease such as this could be attractive to pharmaceutical companies only if it promised long-term payoffs as gleaned from chronic care, rather than one-time interventions. Science reporters David Dunlap and Lawrence Fisher noted: "The drug industry . . . is likely to stay the course. For one thing, now that these patients can live far longer, they can buy these expensive drugs for a long time."[47]

Compliance was the larger issue. The combination therapy regimen was complex and exacting. Some of the drugs needed to be refrigerated, while others had a short shelf life. And virtually all virologists and infectious-disease specialists were terrified that incomplete compliance would quickly breed a class of "superbugs" resistant to the drugs altogether. David Ho, for one, believed at the outset that the regimen was too taxing to be a viable long-term therapy. "Because of the toxicity issue and patients' noncompliance, we want to get a clue as to how long we have to take drugs. If it's ten years, it's not doable. If it's one year, like for tuberculosis, it's great," he reasoned.[48] Data already available by 1996 showed that protease or reverse transcriptase inhibitors taken in isolation quickly promoted resistance, and within a year of wide-scale adoption of combination therapy resistant strains of HIV were being observed in nearly 50 percent of patients.[49]

Unfortunately, the greatest increase in AIDS was in exactly that portion of the population least likely to be capable of complying with the exacting regimen—impoverished, poorly educated, frequently unemployed drug users. Such patients posed a quandary for physicians and public health-care workers, who worried that by treating them with the combination therapy they would be abetting the development of drug-resistant HIV. One director of an AIDS residential center related how an increased patient discharge rate was causing concern, as the patients often left the premises to return to IV drug use, unsafe sex, and even prostitution.[50] Alternatively, some treated patients attempting to return to their kin and communities encountered hostility and rejection. "Willie went home to his old New York neighborhood," related the residential center director, "and his father said, 'Come outside.' He gathered the men of the neighborhood and said, 'This is my son, Willie. He was a drug addict and now he has AIDS. I want him out of my life.' "[51] The prognosis for such castoffs was poor indeed.

Less problematic, but still unnerving, was the so-called Lazarus effect experienced by many patients on combination therapy. Individuals who had been presumed to have only a few years to live now found themselves with years, if not decades, of life ahead of them, and had to comport their lives to this new reality. Men who had withdrawn from employment were now compelled to seek work, while others had to face substantial consumer debt and second mortgages that they had assumed they would never live to pay off. New York City's Division of AIDS Services found its job placement service overwhelmed, while ex-employers faced requests from their discharged employees to find room in the workforce.[52] Efforts at retirement saving, which had largely been abandoned, became important again, as AIDS patients pondered the idea of growing old in poverty.

Patients' partners had to accommodate the new reality as well. Related one patient: "There was a time a year ago when a lot of little things that couples might argue about became incredibly unimportant in context. And now it's back to, 'You didn't wipe off the ketchup bottle.' "[53] Others patients suddenly had to refocus on the many banal life concerns that had largely been abandoned as they had battled AIDS—dental care, social engagements, skills training, and even decorating. Related one man of his previous laxity: "I got a card for my annual dental checkup and I didn't go—I didn't think I had to worry about my teeth, and then, after a year . . . they're getting pretty scuzzy and I went and got my teeth cleaned."[54] The patients welcomed their new life, of course, but found themselves puzzled, as pedestrian concerns assumed renewed importance. The effect was confusing, and largely unprecedented.

VACCINE RESEARCH IN THE 1990S

Even as miracles were being wrought in pharmaceutical interventions, vaccine research had continued through the early 1990s, albeit with few successes. By 1994, over a dozen experimental vaccines were in some stage of clinical trials, yet none seemed particularly promising. Part of the problem lay in the multiple forms of HIV—at least eight of which were known—which could possibly require multiple forms of vaccine.[55] But the bigger issue lay in the extraordinary adaptability of the virus to almost any antibody, owing to its high rate of mutation.

A few beacons glimmered. In one strange case, an Australian blood donor found to be HIV-positive turned out to possess a rare mutation of the virus that replicated extremely slowly and failed to progress to either ARC or AIDS. Blood recipients who accidentally received the virus displayed a similar absence of symptoms. Could this compromised virus provide the template for a live vaccine? While some scientists expressed cautious optimism, others feared that given HIV's high rate of mutation, the benign viral form, when injected into millions of people through an inoculation program, might change to a more typically virulent one.[56]

In another possible breakthrough, scientists in 1996 published findings of a newly discovered protein, which appeared necessary for HIV to attach to the CD4 proteins on cell membranes. The new molecule, fusin (CXCR4), was a co-receptor for HIV, without which infection was thwarted, or at least temporarily slowed. The newly enlarged understanding of the infection process seemed, at least to some researchers, to open a possible new opportunity in thwarting AIDS infection, although actually capitalizing on the opportunity proved elusive.[57]

Another possible point of attack was the creation of a new class of therapeutic vaccines—substances that would not prevent infection, but upon injection might slow the progress of HIV infection toward full-blown AIDS. As early as 1988, several drug companies had produced such vaccines in experimental form, which usually contained clones of the gp120 and gp160 proteins found on the HIV shell.[58] NIH director Bernadine Healy expressed cautious support for these developments, but the approach offered no hope of actually stopping new HIV infection.[59]

Most promising of all, however, was the 1992 discovery of a successful vaccine for the closely related simian immunodeficiency virus (SIV), from which HIV had mutated in the 1930s. Primate researchers reported that year that live crippled vaccine had been used to inoculate a group of monkeys against SIV, by removing the nef gene from the virus, thus thwarting its ability to reproduce. Calling the discovery "the most impressive . . . we have seen in any of our vaccine experiments," team leader Ronald Desrosiers suggested that the experiment could lead to an effective live-attenuated virus vaccine for humans.[60] But other scientists were more skeptical. Again, the aggressive mutation abilities of the virus made the placement of any live vaccine, however attenuated, into a human extremely dangerous, and the differences between SIV and HIV might be substantial enough to render any analogies useless. Even Desrosiers admitted that it could take "ten or fifteen years of safety testing before we can be comfortable putting this into thousands of people."[61]

A different line of inquiry focused on the handful of individuals who seemed naturally immune to HIV. Five percent of all HIV-infected individuals never progressed to full-blown AIDS, even without medication, while a handful—perhaps a total of 70 in the United States by 1993—never displayed any symptoms at all, even after living with the virus for years. Most of these hardy individuals displayed the usual drop in CD4 cells immediately after infection. For unknown reasons, however, the CD4 count leveled off after a few months, and then began to gradually rise. Researchers were unsure if these individuals had perhaps previously been exposed to a weakened mutation of the virus (thus receiving a natural vaccination), or if they had simply been born with naturally more adaptive immune systems, having been given the gift of a "genetically charmed life," in the words of one AIDS writer.[62]

By 1996, researchers believed that they had the answer to the genetic mystery. Individuals with dual copies of a defective CCR5 gene (constituting 1 percent of the white U.S. population) were almost wholly resistant to HIV, while those with a single copy of the defective gene (about 20 percent of the population) were somewhat resistant. The gene seemed available only to whites of European descent, and the discovery did not seem to hold particular therapeutic promise. People who possessed the normal CCR5 gene could not suddenly rid themselves of the protein within, while the potential for genetically engineering a class of people without CCR5 seemed remote. At best, the discovery seemed only to reveal an anomalous curiosity, of greater interest to medical historians than to clinical researchers. One such CCR5-deficient individual, Steve Crohn, was billed "The Man Who Can't Catch AIDS," by the *London Independent,* but the distinction was reserved for a lucky few.[63]

One important barrier to developing an AIDS vaccine was economic. Despite the visible horrors of AIDS, it in fact threatened only a narrow slice of the population of wealthy nations relative to other innoculable infectious diseases. While virtually every child in the developed world was routinely inoculated for smallpox, polio, pertussis, and diphtheria by 1990, few would be inoculated against HIV, even if an effective vaccine ever became available. The remote possibility of AIDS infection from live-attenuated vaccine meant that the numbers of people who would accidentally catch AIDS versus the number of prevented AIDS cases would be quite high—too high for most families to risk having their children undergo inoculation. At the same time, denizens of central and southern Africa, who were at high risk of HIV infection, were too poor to pay for an inoculation. Thus the potential market for an eventual vaccine was quite small.

The limits of potential profits mainly dissuaded large pharmaceutical companies from investing heavily in an AIDS vaccine, leaving the work to boutique biotechnology firms and small start-up drug companies. But even those firms seemed ambivalent about the goal. One of the leaders in the effort to develop a vaccine, Massachusetts-based Repligen Corporation, abruptly ceased its efforts in 1994 citing a "lack of available funding."[64] In fact, the available investor capital for AIDS vaccine research by that year was probably under $25 million—a relative pittance compared with the sums invested in drugs for anxiety, erectile malfunction, high cholesterol, and hypertension. If a vaccine was to be developed, it would need to be funded largely by nations and nongovernmental organizations, and none save the United States seemed willing to invest substantial sums in the task.

By 1997, the AIDS profile in industrialized nations had changed markedly. AIDS deaths dropped by 12 percent from mid-1995 to mid-1996, and promised to drop even more in the next year.[65] (In New York City deaths dropped over 30 percent, although this was not representative of the country.) The Clinton administration promised to raise funding for AIDS drug treatment by 35 percent (to $385 million) while the NIH began to overhaul its AIDS funding apparatus in an effort to redirect funding streams to the most promising areas of development.[66] A cautious optimism, so markedly absent from all connected with AIDS over its first decade and a half, was now present.

The nonindustrialized world was nonplussed, however. The costs of the drugs, coupled with the required refrigeration conditions and meticulous timings of dosages, rendered the breakthroughs irrelevant. Moreover, a time of moral uncertainty had begun, as Western nations pondered their obligations to the suffering millions of central and southern Africa, as well as to the burgeoning patient populations of Southeast Asia. Should the West direct its efforts to finding ways to fund the combination therapy in the developing world, or should it persevere in its effort at vaccination? And what about prophylaxis? Didn't the governments of the African nations have a responsibility to exhaust their own preventive efforts before the United States and other wealthy nations invested billions in subsidized medications? A miracle had been wrought, but like most miracles its effects were more complicated and troublesome than had been initially foreseen.

CHAPTER 12

ASIA

FOREIGNERS

AIDS in Asia was met with a blunt xenophobic response. In Thailand, China, Japan, and Burma, where the first dozen AIDS deaths were documented by 1987, governments assured their citizens that they need avoid only foreign travelers, sex clients, and blood donors to remain AIDS-free. Bangkok massage parlors frowned on Western clients (or barred them entirely), Chinese health officials blamed foreign blood donations in an effort to dismiss accusations of miscegenation between Chinese and Westerners, and the Japanese foreign ministry considered reclassifying visas of resident aliens based on AIDS status.[1] As late as 1987, a senior Chinese government official declared that his primary task was to "prevent AIDS from coming into China," suggesting that no indigenous epidemic yet existed.[2] Canadian officials repaid the favor by warning their own citizens to avoid acupuncture treatment in China lest they be exposed to contaminated needles.[3]

The Soviet Union, by contrast, followed Cuba's policies on AIDS control, with mandatory testing of suspected AIDS carriers, prison sentences for individuals who knowingly spread the virus, and expanded policing powers granted to public health officials. Although the Moscow government suggested that testing and arrest would be most likely reserved for those at highest risk—IV drug users and sex workers—the policy implied totalitarian force. At the same time, Soviet health officials began condom education efforts and urged "chaste behavior" for all citizens.[4]

Japan, always leery of foreigners, initially tagged virtually all AIDS cases as foreign impositions. Despite the tens of thousands of Japanese men traveling annually to Thailand for "sex tours," the Japanese media preferred to focus on infected blood products (of which Japan was the world's largest importer) and alien prostitutes as the primary cause of HIV infection in Japan. The effort reached its apogee when a Filipino prostitute working in Matsumoto was identified with AIDS in 1986 and quickly deported.[5] Within a year, however, neither the Japanese government nor the media could deny the presence of dozens of ethnic Japanese prostitutes infected with AIDS. In response, the Japanese government commenced an AIDS-prevention campaign, while the nation's media outlets strengthened their reporting of the disease.[6]

Although virtually all Asian countries, as well as the Soviet Union, claimed to harbor only minuscule epidemics in 1987, by 1989 statistics told otherwise. In August of that year, World Health Organization AIDS chief Jonathan Mann reported that nearly a third of IV drug users in Bangkok tested positive for HIV, and by October the rate exceeded 40 percent.[7] Asian AIDS scholar Chris Beyrer noted that 5 percent of Thai drug users were seroconverting each month—"an unprecedented rate of increase."[8] Despite earnest government protestations to the contrary, the Asian epidemic was self-sustaining, independent, and robust. "Disaster seems written in each new batch of statistics," noted the *Economist*.[9] In 1992, Mann predicted that the Asian epidemic would supercede the African one imminently, and he predicted that the continent would account for 42 percent of worldwide AIDS cases by 2000.[10]

HEROIN

Initially the problem in Asia was heroin.[11] Long the dominant intoxicant in Thailand and Burma, heroin use in Asia facilitated the epidemic's spread into the area's urban male population. Thailand's 15,000

AIDS-infected addicts of 1988 turned into 40,000 a year later, which morphed into over a half million in Thailand and India combined by 1991.[12] By decade's end, injection drug use accounted for 80 percent of AIDS in Kazakhstan, 75 percent in Malaysia and Vietnam, and possibly 50 percent in China.[13]

In Thailand, though, heroin was only the jumping-off point for a commercial-sex-charged epidemic, which flowed out of the brothels of Bangkok and Chiang Mai and into the country's northern provinces from whence a disproportionate number of the nation's millions of prostitutes emanated, and where many eventually returned. Similarly, in Japan, the virus moved into the urban sex trade where it simmered throughout the 1990s, controlled but undiminished. In China, meanwhile, the epidemic exploded into western villages and towns, where it gestated in contaminated rural medical clinics, spread through unsterilized needles, combined plasma donations, and shared medicine bottles. By 1995, WHO estimated that the Asian AIDS epidemic would top 3 million.[14]

Intravenous drug use in Asia carried with it all of the accumulated dangers of such drug use in the United States, with the added burden of users drawing their potion from a communal drug pot into which contaminated needles were repeatedly dipped and drawn. As in America, poor addicts sought out shooting galleries (*lo chich* in Vietnam), but unique to several Asian countries was the existence of dealer-injectors who both sold the product and injected it from the drug pot, leaving little latitude for concerned users to sterilize the communal needles or even use their own. One study found that a large pot might provide product to as many as 50 customers, all serviced with the same needle dipped repeatedly into the potion, with no regard for hygiene or contamination.[15] Further, Western-style drug treatment clinics were practically unknown in many nations of the region, although by decade's end Nepal, Thailand, and Vietnam reported nascent methadone programs.[16]

In Burma, the general IV drug epidemic was exacerbated by a growing national heroin addiction, a direct result of the nation's enlarged role in heroin production. By 1988, the country was the single largest producer of heroin in the world (estimates of its share of the world market ranged from 40 to 60 percent), and the drug was suffusing the countryside.[17] By 1988, a United Nations study of Myanmar found drug abuse prevalence in small towns to range from 2 to 25 percent, with over three-fourths of all users favoring heroin as their drug of choice.[18] The users, nearly all male, were broadly distributed in age, ethnicity, marital status, occupation, and education. The problem was pervasive.

Extreme poverty in Burma transformed a narcotics problem into one of AIDS, as virtually all of the addicts made use of communal injection equipment. The injector-dealers would repeatedly use and resharpen needles, while some rural purveyors whittled needles from bamboo or plastic. The repressive government seemed disinclined to rein in the practice, allowing dealers to sell their wares unimpeded by police or health officials. By 1994, United Nations observers in Burma reported the highest HIV rates ever found in addict groups: 74 percent in Rangoon, and over 90 percent in rural Myitkyina.[19] One exiled activist reflected bitterly that while meeting to discuss human rights could earn a participant a 15-year jail term, "you can sell heroin in the college dormitory and nobody will bother you."[20]

THE SEX TRADE

For Thailand, and later Vietnam, Cambodia, and Burma, IV drug use was merely the point of departure for an epidemic transmitted largely through the nation's commercial sex industry. Long famous around the world for their youth, beauty, compliance, and sheer physical adeptness, Thailand's prostitutes served not only the local population, but hundreds of thousands of international tourists who traveled to that country intentionally seeking unique experiences and thrills. Sex shows in Bangkok featured performers copulating onstage in every possible position and combination; young boys masturbating en masse; public displays of homosexuality, bestiality, and pederasty; and the famed Thai specialty of young women propelling Ping-Pong balls out of their vaginas at assorted targets. "It's about as exploitative a scene as anyone could want, and all the staff are for hire," noted Thai observer Chris Beyrer.[21]

Tourists venturing out of Bangkok could have their golf games caddied by prostitutes, their billiard balls racked by prostitutes, their drinks served by prostitutes, and their meal orders taken by prostitutes. On specially packaged sex tours, men from Japan, Germany, Switzerland, and other more staid nations could find succor and satiation in boys and girls of all ages, types, and appearances. Brochures showing Thai women in various states of undress invited foreign tourists to "sample the wares" and "pick the local flowers," while one glossy shot of a young topless Thai girl prominently displayed on Lauda Air flights was simply captioned, "From Thailand with Love."[22] Only when children's rights activists protested was the ad pulled, or at least repositioned in a less visible media outlet.

Thailand's sex workers were drawn disproportionately from the northern region surrounding Chiang Mai where social acquiescence (and frequently encouragement) spurred girls and boys to sign on with sex recruiters as young as age 13, shortly after finishing mandated schooling. These young workers were able to send home substantial amounts of money from their labors, leading to increased living standards in the province, and could return after several years facing little stigma. Sociologists struggled to understand the unusual absence of social taint attached to the returning women, and settled only on the embedded tradition of young women (rather than young men) supporting their aging parents, and a general societywide permissive attitude toward extramarital sex and prostitution. One observer of the Thai scene even suggested that the returning prostitutes were lauded by local men as "successful and worldly," having accrued stature by "contributing to the local community."[23]

The size of the Thai sex industry was vast. Estimates varied, but one count reported 2 million adult and 800,000 child prostitutes in the nation, out of a population of 61 million. Overall, 15 percent of all Thai women had engaged in, or would engage in, prostitution at some point during their lives, and in certain northern villages the rate approached 70 percent.[24]

A permissive culture not only condoned prostitution, but use of prostitution. Thai men frequented brothels more so than did American and other Western men, and began using the brothels at a younger age. Reliable data was elusive, but one study of several regions in the country showed that about half the nation's men admitted to using prostitutes at some point in their lives, while in the north the rate of prostitution usage was estimated to be as high as 85 percent. Teenagers were frequently introduced to sex through a brothel visit, while brothel-shopping in Bangkok and Chiang Mai was a common activity for young men out in a group.

As in Africa, wealthier men, of generally higher social status, were more likely to patronize prostitutes or engage in extramarital affairs than were poorer men. Wealthier men had the discretionary cash with which to purchase sex services, and were more attractive to potential paramours and second wives. Further, as in virtually all third-world cities, single men who had migrated to cities for work were the most likely to seek out prostitutes, and the most likely to possess the spare cash necessary for the transaction. The poorer men, who had remained on farms and in villages, had neither cash, opportunity, nor the social autonomy to exercise their prerogative.

By 1991, AIDS in the Thai sex industry was rampant. Official government estimates placed the infection rate at 14 percent of all prostitutes, but reporters and health workers suspected the true rate was much higher.[25] One staff member from the Save the Children Fund observed that of the 18 teenage "waitresses" at one village teahouse, every one of them was HIV-positive. Infected prostitutes returned home to spread the disease to boyfriends and husbands, who thereupon spread it to a larger network of contacts. In one six-month stretch of 1989, the national AIDS rate actually doubled, and by 1991 the country had a half million cases, which could possibly double over the following year.

AIDS in Thailand was not evenly distributed. Unlike in Africa, where AIDS followed the trucking routes, in Thailand it followed the lives of prostitutes. Infected northern women, returning to their homes after multiyear sojourns in Bangkok and Chiang Mai, fostered a rural epidemic that was seven to eight times worse than that in the rest of the nation. The HIV infection rate in Thai army recruits in 1991 was just under 2 percent, but in the north it hovered at 15 percent.[26] And while the government would begin a large (and ultimately effective) anti-AIDS campaign that year, the epidemic was already poised to seep into China, Burma, and Vietnam.

PREVENTION AND TREATMENT

Asian nations responded inconsistently. Politically liberal Thailand, armed with a relatively free press and an honest acknowledgment of its prostitution problem, was best prepared to meet the epidemic with a Western-style safe-sex education program. In the late 1980s, Senator Mechai Viravaidya inaugurated a highly visible condom education and distribution program, in which he personally went through the nation's bordello districts handing out condoms, teaching Thais about condom usage, and generally demystifying the role of condoms in AIDS prevention. At the same time, Prime Minister Anand Panyarachun instigated an aggressive condom distribution program in brothels and sex shops, and threatened to close institutions that did not comply. To reinforce the message, radio stations were required to run AIDS-education ads at least once per hour.[27]

Thai authorities made liberal use of billboards, bus station ads, and pamphlets to spread the message. Glossy photos showed AIDS patients riddled with skin lesions, and emaciated sex workers expressing regret at their decisions. Shots of beautiful young women were embellished with captions suggesting that AIDS was often invisible and unknowable. Other ads targeted injection drug use, with addicts offering testimonials as to how they got AIDS, mothers crying over their dead children, and in one shocking image, a policeman examining the hanging body of an obvious suicide with a caption reading, "Of course, she has AIDS so she killed herself."[28]

The Thai program worked initially, and by some estimates may have saved as many as 350,000 lives over its first five years. Nevertheless, by 1996 its effects seemed to be diminishing. The nation's sex industry seemed only partially receptive to the safe-sex message, and large numbers of young people, both male and female, admitted to eschewing condoms.[29] One 1993 Thai study found that few women asked men to wear condoms, and, more perniciously, exposed the prevailing assumption by both sexes that by limiting their sexual liaisons to neat and well-educated partners they could avoid AIDS.[30] True, fewer Thai men admitted using prostitutes, and more prostitutes were using condoms (possibly 60 percent by 1994), but Thais seemed simply to invest more heavily in illicit nonpaying sexual relations to compensate. WHO estimated that 2 percent of the Thai population was infected by 1994, and that barring a miraculous therapeutic breakthrough, life expectancy could drop to 40 by 2010.[31]

Imperfect as the Thai prevention campaign was, however, it was substantially more successful than those in other Asian countries. Burma's military government seemed to willfully ignore the burgeoning epidemic, despite its ferocious rate of spread (all of the Asian epidemics were rooted in the unusual subtype E of the virus, which appeared to spread more efficiently through heterosexual contact than other HIV strains), and the nation's ubiquitous heroin problem. "The whole country is in denial" noted one Rangoon-based health official.[32] By 1997, the government had not even acknowledged that an epidemic existed, claiming an official caseload of 14,000 people. Unofficially, the government tabulated over a half-million AIDS cases by that time, and most outside AIDS experts suspected that the real number might be half again as large.[33] One observer of the Burmese epidemic noted wryly, "The generals who rule Burma have chosen a different strategy to fight the disease: they lie about it."[34]

Governments of the Catholic Philippines, and of the Muslim nations of the region such as Indonesia and Malaysia, faced the opprobrium of fundamentalist religious leaders as they attempted to educate the public about condoms. In the Philippines, Manila archbishop James Cardinal Sin tagged the government's AIDS program as "intrinsically evil," while leading antigovernment demonstrations that included burning boxes of condoms.[35] In Indonesia, Muslim clerics denounced condom campaigns as attempts to foster promiscuity and demanded that they be limited to married couples, while in Malaysia the government responded to religious pressure by simply postponing its education implementation plans. "I think there's a fear of having to deal with some sticky issues," noted Marina Mahathir, president of the Malaysian AIDS Council. "You have to talk about sex, and all the conservative elements of this society don't want to talk about it."[36]

Medical conditions mirrored those in Africa, with Western medicine available to only small portions of the populations of Thailand, Burma,

Cambodia, and Vietnam. Hospitals were grossly inadequate, medications were in short supply, and combination therapy was wholly beyond the means of all but the smallest portion of the population. In Burma, the poorest of the region's nations, medical shortages were so extreme as to immobilize the system. Chris Beyrer described the situation thus:

> Surgical equipment is re-used until it is useless. Disposable gloves are rewashed until they're in shreds. Rubbing alcohol, a common disinfectant, was in such short supply in 1994 that nurses were diluting it ten to one with water; it would smell like disinfectant to patients but it would not be of much use. The NAP admits that only 65 percent of blood is screened before transfusion—and even this low rate applies only to Rangoon. There are at least two states (out of 14) that have never done an HIV test, and where all transfusions are with unscreened blood products.[37]

Throughout Southeast Asia, AIDS essentially bypassed the medical system. Unable to provide patients sterile surroundings, antibiotics, aerosolized pentamidine, AZT, or combination therapy, hospitals instead dispensed Tylenol, blankets, and food when available, and nothing at other times. AIDS patients returned home, when relatives would have them, or else died in squatters shacks and makeshift shelters. Even international aid programs could promise only limited succor, as the medical infrastructures of the afflicted nations were inadequate to absorb substantial amounts of equipment and drugs.

Despite the poor medical care and imperfect education campaigns, by the end of the decade the continent was fairing far better than the worst parts of Africa. While in central and southern Africa several nations were reporting HIV infection rates of 20 percent or higher, in Asia no country's rate exceeded 5 percent. And while certain subpopulations—sex workers, heroin addicts, sexually active gay men—posted rates substantially higher, these miniepidemics did not seem to be generally moving into the larger population. The education campaigns had worked to some degree, or else distinct social mores had somehow thwarted an accelerating tragedy. But the looming pandemic of Africa cast a pall over Southeast Asia, and impelled health officials and educators to focus their efforts at containing an epidemic that was still manageable. "There's a huge window of opportunity because HIV levels are very low in the general population," noted United Nations epidemiologist Bernhard Schwartlander.[38]

INTERNATIONAL HELP

The United Nations took the lead in organizing international aid to the stricken countries of Southeast Asia, mostly in the form of coordinating the efforts of several large nongovernmental organizations. Funds from the United Kingdom's Department for International Development, the Swedish International Development Cooperation Agency, the Asian Development Bank, US AID, and the United Nations' own Development Program (UNDP) were funneled through the UN to fund education and treatment efforts.[39] The sum of all such philanthropy, however, was modest next to the size of the region's own internal efforts. Thailand, for example, the most aggressive of the region's nations in addressing the epidemic, was funding over 70 percent of its AIDS programs out of general tax revenues as early as 1991, and over 90 percent by 1993.

Ironically, the United Nations was at least partially responsible for Cambodia's spreading epidemic. UNTAC troops sent there in the aftermath of the Khmer Rouge genocide drove up demand for prostitution, and appeared to accelerate the epidemic's spread. Unattached and wealthy (by local standards), United Nations troops spread their income throughout the cash-strapped economy, which responded by opening brothels, luring new women into the sex trades, and recruiting women from Vietnam.[40]

Increased prostitution meant an increased spread of AIDS, particularly when the primary clients were young and largely uneducated troops. Soldiers who had served in Cambodia posted unusually high infection rates of HIV subtype E, found almost exclusively in Southeast Asia. According to one report, 15 percent of Indian soldiers who had served in Cambodia came home infected with HIV. And while official protestations that prostitution was nonexistent in Cambodian society before the presence of UN troops were largely prevaricated, the troops did impel expansion of the sex trade in a culture that had previously been fairly intolerant of it. Moreover, unlike in Thailand, most prostitutes would have little chance to reintegrate themselves into the mainstream of society. By Cambodian standards, they had been tainted beyond redemption.

CHAPTER 13

BACKSLIDING

AIDS declined in America in the half decade after the introduction of combination therapy. By 1998, AIDS was killing only 5.9 Americans out of every 100,000 per year (from a high of 15.6), and ranked no higher than 14th on the nation's roster of leading causes of death (down from 8th).[1] In New York City, still the center of the nation's epidemic, new AIDS cases among IV drug users had dropped from 6,340 in 1993 to 2,109, while in New York State AIDS-related deaths in prisons declined from 181 in 1996 to 60.[2] Across the nation, quarterly AIDS deaths had dropped from 12,000 to 4,000, while reported new AIDS cases had dropped from 20,000 to 10,000. Further, new epidemiological estimates published in *Science* in 1996 suggested that the epidemic at its apogee may have been less widespread than had been assumed—perhaps only 900,000 Americans had been infected in 1993 rather than the previously assumed 1.2 million.[3] All together, the AIDS threat in the United States seemed to be diminishing.

However, the *rate* of decrease was declining by 1998. The epidemic seemed to be approaching a plateau of incidence, in which the epidemic would neither expand into the general population nor fade away in the manner of smallpox and pertussis. The CDC reported in September of

1999 that among the most vulnerable groups—minorities and young gay men—the rate of infection seemed to be falling hardly at all, and that new prevention programs seemed incapable of reaching the targeted populations.[4] Moreover, even in more responsive groups, adherence to safe-sex guidelines seemed to be waning. "In this era of better therapies, it is clear that people are becoming complacent about prevention," noted Helene Gayle, AIDS program director at the CDC.[5]

In fact, a complex set of facts was emerging. On the one hand, in those communities that were most vulnerable to AIDS, incidence was hardly falling at all. Among both gay men and IV drug users, approximately 2 percent were becoming infected each year. This was better than the 10 percent infection rate of the late 1980s, but substantial enough to perpetuate a continued significant epidemic.[6] The continued epidemic in the IV-drug-using population was particularly troubling, for all evidence suggested that members of this group were so compromised in life skills and decision-making processes that they would remain insensitive to essentially all public health measures. "Life is regressive," noted columnist George Will. "People with problems have a high probability of acquiring more problems."[7]

At the same time, large numbers of AIDS patients were living with the disease for much longer periods of time, thanks to the newly discovered combination therapies. That is to say, while AIDS was still spreading, it was no longer killing people. By December 2000, almost 325,000 Americans were living with AIDS: the highest number ever reported.[8] Median survival time had increased from 11 months to 46 months, and was growing constantly longer. Of the people diagnosed in 1996, three-quarters were alive two years later, and two-thirds were alive the year after that.[9]

Gay men, in particular, were living longer. Although they constituted a shrinking portion of the total epidemic, in 1999 they were still over 40 percent of all domestic AIDS cases, and their extended life-spans meant that they would continue to be a significant portion of the epidemic regardless of declining infection rates. The Gay Men's Health Crisis reported that it was turning its efforts away from helping patients with wills, and toward helping patients with employer discrimination suits and housing issues, as the focus of their clients' concerns turned from dying to living. "And we're offering seminars now on reentering the workplace," noted a GMHC spokesman.[10]

The picture that emerged was mixed. People were living much longer, but at the same time were continuing with myopically destructive behavior. And in some ways the new medications were actually exacerbating irresponsible choices, as gay men (in particular) relaxed their guards upon recognizing that AIDS no longer constituted a death sentence. For IV drug users, on the other hand, the impact of the new drugs was less profound. Capable of neither raising nor lowering their level of vigilance, they continued with their lives, affected by neither therapeutics nor prevention.

BAREBACKING

Undermining the declining mortality rates was a return to unsafe gay sex practices. Starting in the early 1990s, and accelerating in the years after the introduction of combination therapy, many gay men dismissed the need for condoms and monogamy. From 1994 to 2000, the percentage of gay men who reported using a condom "every time" dropped from 69.6 to 49.7 while the percentage of men reporting unsafe practices with multiple partners rose from 23.4 to 48.8.[11] Nearly half of gay men in their 20s reported regularly having sex without condoms, and percentages among black and Hispanic gay men appeared higher still.[12]

The practice, known as "barebacking," was particularly appealing to young men who had lost few friends and lovers to AIDS in the late 1980s. Coming of age in the postcocktail era, the men perceived AIDS to be simply a treatable disease—unpleasant, but not fatal. In addition, young men were increasingly using sex-enhancing drugs such as ketamine ("K"), gamma hydroxybutyric acid ("GHB"), and ecstasy ("X"), further blurring their judgment and increasing their feelings of invulnerability. "Sometimes I can let my hair down and I decided that this was going to be one of those nights," admitted one clubgoer. "It [ketamine] definitely relaxes me."[13]

Barebackers created a separate AIDS subculture in major American cities in the late 1990s. Communicating through advertisements in gay newspapers and magazines, and increasingly on dedicated Web sites, aficionados held barebacking parties where condoms were barred and HIV-positive status was assumed.[14] Participants in the subculture viewed themselves as more liberated and more genuinely gay than the aging generation who had lived through the initial AIDS onslaught, and they were reluctant to conform themselves to what they perceived to be overly repressive norms. "It's not my experience to lose half my friends and feel the debilitating effects of the virus," one sexually active HIV-infected man admitted. "I can't help but feel that the idea of either getting HIV or transmitting HIV is not that horrible."[15]

The practice was particularly notable in the youngest sexually active men—college students or recent graduates, just going public with their sexual orientation and exploring gay bars, clubs, and other gay gathering places. One telling statistic was that new gonorrhea infections, which had declined with the safe-sex practices of the 1980s, were returning. New infections rose by 13 percent from 1997 to 1999, with more than half of all such infections occurring in men between 15 and 24. In one survey, 20 percent of gay male college students admitted to having had more than one sexual partner over the preceding month (the comparable statistic for straight male college students was 9 percent), and only 36 percent reported always using condoms.[16] One college student explained the phenomenon: "I know a lot of guys my age just coming out, and [they] are having too much fun to worry about AIDS."[17]

AIDS rates in the population climbed concomitantly. By the year 2000, 4.5 percent of gay men in their 20s were becoming infected each year, while the figure for young gay black men was nearly 15 percent.[18] Over the five years from 1995 to 2000 the rate of new HIV infections among young gay men in San Francisco tripled, and elsewhere in the country the growth was nearly as great. At the same time, the incidence of AIDS in the gay community as a whole was increasing, with infection rates among walk-in patients at San Francisco clinics rising from 1.3 percent in 1997 to 3.7 percent in 1999.[19] Health experts reiterated their constant message concerning safe sex, condoms, monogamy, and committed relationships, but increasingly the message was ignored. Explained the spokesman for San Francisco's Stop AIDS Project: "Fifteen years ago, you would see skeletons walking down the street—it was easy to identify who had AIDS. The fact that most everyone you see looks healthy—people don't equate that with an epidemic."[20]

Gay men rationalized their behavior in different ways. Some pleaded hardship: it was simply unrealistic to expect a sexually active young man to don condoms for the remainder of his life, argued some. One man expressed disbelief that such an arrangement was even viable. "I can't see trying to hang around for a long life sucking on rubbers," he said. "I can't see how other guys do that. Do they do that?"[21] Many men echoed the sentiment, some suggesting that the aggregate sacrifice of sexual pleasure was simply not worth the added utility to be gained by remaining HIV-negative. "The prospect of going through the rest of your life having to cover yourself up every time you want to get intimate with someone is an awful one," admitted one man.[22] Stated another more succinctly, "It feels good, because there's no rubber."[23]

Other men admitted relief when finally testing positive for HIV, claiming that they had felt marginalized in an AIDS culture. Having lived with the fear of contracting AIDS for years, and sporadically taken precautions, a diagnosis of HIV infection brought for these men a certain measure of peace, as if knowing their true risk allowed them now to take definite action toward safeguarding their health. Counterintuitive as this sentiment sounded to nongays, many gay men admitted to it. "Now I've got HIV and I don't have to worry about getting it," explained one man. "I was tired of having to be careful, of this constant diligence that has to be paid to intimacy."[24] Another man, still HIV negative, expressed almost a longing to become infected. "There have been times when I thought there'd be a certain freedom if I seroconverted," he explained. "It would be done with. The biggest life adjustment would be that I'd have to take care of myself more: eat right, quit smoking, get enough sleep."[25] And yet another admitted that at least with AIDS he would not have to "live through 50 years of burying dead people."[26]

More bizarre were the sporadic gay men who actively sought HIV infection. These "bug chasers" seemed to enjoy the thrill of courting danger, or conflated HIV infection with a perverse sort of intimacy. But these men were marginalized, even in heavily infected social circles. Eschewing a condom in the heat of passion might be an acceptable foible, but consciously seeking illness bordered on insanity. Commented one man living with AIDS: "I can't imagine someone being HIV negative and taking risks with this disease. This morning my back is out again, I have sciatica. I have a herpes shingle going right up my back. I'm just now finishing all my drugs. Yesterday I had to take injections to make my bone marrow grow, and my life is no fun. Sometimes I wish I were dead."[27]

The majority of HIV-negative barebackers were simply ignorant of the true risks they were courting. Having come to sexual maturity in an era of treatable AIDS, they lacked the fear or respect for the virus exhibited by their older compatriots who had watched so many of their friends die. "There's a generation gap," explained AIDS Action Committee director Larry Kessler. "Younger people now coming of age, some of whom weren't born when the epidemic started, think, 'Oh, that's an old '80s thing. It won't affect me.' "[28] Or if they understood the risk of infection, they often did not fully appreciate the onerousness of complying with combination therapy. Too many viewed the disease as the gay man's diabetes—somewhat unpleasant, but eminently treatable and largely inconsequential.

The resurgence of unsafe sex produced a renewed demand for gay bathhouses, which had been closed in most cities since the mid-1980s. In San Francisco, where the demands grew quite vociferous by 1999, gay men had enjoyed the presence of gay "sex clubs" over the preceding decade, but not baths. The sex clubs were entirely open, affording participants no opportunity for privacy from monitoring eyes, which watched incessantly for condom use and general safe-sex practices. Advocates for reopening the bathhouses argued that such a move might, in fact, facilitate *safer* sex, as gay men could more easily discuss matters of HIV status in the privacy of a locked cubicle. Opponents dismissed the argument, claiming that the frenzied rate of sexual activity in the cubicles largely precluded conversation. Former New York City health commissioner Stephen Joseph had fought against reopening bathhouses for years, calling such plans the "height of bureaucratic folly," and the "dereliction of public health responsibility."[29]

Proposals to reopen the baths did not meet with widespread disapproval. Many people felt that unsafe-sex practices were common in the absence of the baths, and that reopening them would be inconsequential. Moreover, at least a few agreed with bathhouse proponents' arguments regarding the safety inherent in privacy, or at least felt that bathhouses could become venues for the dissemination of safe-sex facts and pamphlets. Readers surveyed by the *San Francisco Chronicle* opined, "There's nothing wrong with reopening them as long as the patrons practice safe sex," and, "Banning the baths in 1984 was the right decision for that time, when less was known about AIDS and AIDS prevention. Now people are better informed."[30] But police and public health officials thought otherwise. "Believe me, this place will never open," stated one policy commissioner during a 1994 debate over opening a new San Francisco bathhouse.[31]

RATIONALIZATION

The return to unsafe sex prompted a spate of theorizing and rationalizing from gay observers, theorists, and apologists that mixed the insightful with the pathetic. Most frequent was the conjecture that a life of sex that was 100 percent safe was too hard. "I'm a human being. I'm not a god. I try my best not to share this with anyone. . . . That's all I can do," one participant in San Francisco's Stop AIDS Project explained.[32] Many others agreed, suggesting that living the safe-sex life was so onerous that death might actually be preferably. Another participant in the Stop AIDS Project admitted, "I did not value my life enough to prevent myself from getting totally blasted and ending up as a receptacle for somebody else."[33] Andrew Sullivan, the columnist and editor, wrote that, try as he might, he could not avoid all sexual slips in his quest for safety, lest he so squelch his libido that he would deny his own humanity. Such slips, he suggested, might even be heroic:

> I simply refused to take cover completely, to end any sexual adventurism, to abolish all risk. Like those inhabitants of Sarajevo who after months of siege and the constant threat of snipers, began once again to walk down the streets slowly and upright and in full view, I rebelled against the logic and plague and judgment. There was foolishness in this, of course. But also an unrepentant assertion of freedom, an assertion that the deepest personal struggles do not end in the mid-

dle of a crisis. Indeed in the middle of a crisis, a refusal to end them is a mark of the ultimate resistance.[34]

Some gay men suggested that the relapse was a reasonable response to a standard that was homophobic in effect, if not in intent. In his 1997 book *Sexual Ecology,* Gabriel Rotello decried those community leaders who had refused to condemn the "brotherhood of promiscuity" that developed in the early 1970s, and who continued to apologize for gay sexual excesses in the 1990s by suggesting that safe sex was simply unattainable, for anybody.[35] One reviewer of the book chastised these community leaders, who had dismissed demands that "gay men could or should accomplish a degree of behavioral change that no self-respecting heterosexual man would ever think of imposing on himself."[36]

Some gay men admitted that sex without condoms was simply too much fun to give up, and that the constant vigilance was exhausting. "I have to constantly be on guard and watch and think, and I can't ever relax," one man explained. Another man described the euphoria of unprotected sex: "Anal sex is a complete giving of yourself to that person, where you're totally exposed. . . . It's like a spiritual dimension, like Catholicism."[37] Reinforcing this point was the disturbing finding from a 1997 poll that found that over half of surveyed gay men admitted that they would rather have a great sex life than live to 75.[38]

A growing consort of gay voices responded to these rationalizations by urging gay men to become more responsible adults, and to accept the restraints that accompanied adulthood. These exhortations came from gay physicians, public health professionals, social workers, and politicians, who all sought to draw gay men from the culture of sexual indulgence that had been central to the gay revolution in the 1970s, toward a more mature gay sexuality that would more closely mirror heterosexual culture. Rotello urged his peers in an article in the *Nation* in 1997 to trade the gay nightclub for the gay community center, and to express spirituality not in orgiastic excess but in gay synagogues, churches, and meditation centers.[39] Ronald Bayer, professor of public health at Columbia University who had been studying the epidemic from its onset wrote in 1995, "I am even more aware of and concerned about personal and moral responsibility,"[40] while one gay man in Manhattan summed up the sentiment tersely, "Don't just use a condom, use your conscience."[41]

Responsibility within certain gay circles became the new mantra of enlightenment. Disgusted with their community's failure to rise to its greatest challenge, these leaders and critics demanded that gay men discard an archaic and flawed philosophy, and respond to the scourge with strength and mettle. Harvey Fierstein, a popular Broadway actor, wrote in an admonishing column in the *New York Times:* "HIV is an almost completely avoidable infection. You need to be compliant in some very specific behaviors to be at risk. In fact, if every person now infected vowed that the disease ended with him, we could wipe out the ballooning number of new infections."[42] Andrew Sullivan described the movement in his book *Love Undetectable:* "[W]ith AIDS, responsibility became a central involuntary feature of homosexual life. . . . In some ways, even the seemingly irresponsible outrages of ACT UP were the ultimate act of responsibility. They came from a conviction that someone had to lead to connect the ghetto to the center of the country."[43]

The tension between the radical gay liberationists who argued that sex in its most raw form was emblematic of gay dignity and autonomy, and those who argued to the contrary that unity must grow from restraint and responsibility, exemplified the tremendous ambivalence that existed among gays, and sometimes within individuals. When Randy Shilts, a celebrated gay reporter for the *San Francisco Chronicle,* died in 1994, he was mourned nearly universally by gays, yet during his life he had been vilified and mocked as a "gay Uncle Tom" for urging bathhouse closings.[44] And Andrew Sullivan, who had established himself as the nation's foremost conservative gay writer, and who had advocated gay marriage over "a life of meaningless promiscuity followed by eternal damnation," was exposed in a gay newspaper for having sought "barebacking" partners on a Web site dedicated to that activity using the screen name RawMuscleGlutes.[45] In a sense, Sullivan had done nothing wrong. He was candid about his HIV status, and had explicitly sought partners who were themselves HIV-positive. Nonetheless, the incident proved embarrassing for Sullivan, and further highlighted the allure of unprotected sex for even mature and informed gay men.

FIGHTING OVER NEEDLE
EXCHANGES

A decade after their inception, needle exchanges continued to provoke spirited debate. By 1995, 75 needle exchange programs existed in 55 American cities. In 14 states, the programs were explicitly legal, while in another dozen states police failed to enforce needle laws as a matter of policy. And the number kept expanding. In 1992, Connecticut rescinded a ban on nonprescription sales of syringes; in 1994, Richard Riordan, the mayor of Los Angeles, declared the city to be in a state of emergency, thus allowing it to flout the state's prohibition of needle exchanges; Maine passed a law in 1997 allowing all residents to possess up to 10 hypodermic needles; and in 2000 the Illinois legislature passed a law almost identical to Maine's.[46]

The legislative developments were misleading, however. Many, if not most, elected officials around the country—governors, state representatives, and county freeholders—rejected needle exchange proposals, and expressed doubt as to whether such programs were consistent with the goals of the state. In New Jersey, where the electorate had historically supported moderate candidates from both parties, the Governor's Advisory Council on AIDS recommended in 1996 that the state implement a needle exchange program, given the growing needle-transmitted AIDS epidemics in Newark, Jersey City, Paterson, and Camden. David Troast, the chairman of the council, deemed a needle exchange to be "the single most important strategy not now being practiced in New Jersey," and claimed that such a program would reassure drug users that "we [the state] care about you," and that "we want to keep you alive and get you into rehabilitation."[47]

But Christine Todd Whitman, the state's moderately conservative Republican governor, rejected the argument. Having visited with some of the state's many crack-addicted babies in pediatric wards while campaigning, Whitman was impressed at the tremendous and permanent psychic damage wrought through drug use, and suspected that such emotional scars could be actually more destructive to a community than the deaths brought by AIDS. "When you have a newborn infant who is unable to bond, because it's constantly crying, it's in withdrawal, it's addicted to drugs, the psychological and emotional damage can be just devastating," the governor explained. While Whitman acknowledged the dangers of unchecked AIDS infection, she reminded the state's citizens that AIDS could be arrested, to some degree, with drugs, while the affects of infantile drug addiction were essentially permanent. "The child born addicted never really has a chance," she stated.[48]

Despite the proliferation of needle exchange programs across the country, it was Whitman's view that better reflected the beliefs of the electorate. President Clinton refused to lift a federal funding ban on needle exchanges, and Donna Shalala, the secretary of Health and Human Services, did not confront him on the issue.[49] Most Americans, lacking familiarity with either epidemiology or infectious-disease medicine, recoiled from the idea of facilitating IV drug use, regardless of the motivation, and politicians responded accordingly. "If someone comes into my pharmacy, I'm not going to sell them needles if they are going to use them for drugs," stated Ron Stephens, New York State legislator and pharmacist. "I believe allowing an addict to have access to needles is just enabling them to further their addiction they suffer from."[50] And Gary Bauer, president of the conservative-leaning Family Research Council, explained: "It strikes the average voter in the gut as being against common sense. . . . I don't see how this administration could do anything on this that wouldn't blow up in their face."[51]

Scientific studies of the early needle exchanges generally failed to support the claims of the exchanges' proponents, although results were inconsistent. A study of the Amsterdam needle exchange, the world's oldest, failed to demonstrate that the exchange had protected participants from HIV infection.[52] A study of the Vancouver exchange similarly discerned no difference in HIV incidence between heavy and light users of the needles, suggesting that the exchange did little to actually reduce rates of AIDS transmittal. And in a Seattle study, the exchange appeared to play no role in the reduction of other blood-borne diseases, such as hepatitis B or C.[53] On the other hand, a study of the New Haven, Connecticut, exchange found that the rate of HIV infection in the returned needles had declined by a third over several years, while a study of the Tacoma, Washington, exchange indicated an eightfold drop in hepatitis infection.[54]

No study supported the widely held conjecture that needle exchanges prompted the uninitiated to use injection drugs, or even to exacerbate a preexisting drug addiction.[55] Although many people assumed that needles provided by the government would make drug use appear more legitimate, if not altogether more attractive, data indicated otherwise. In Amsterdam, at least, the mean age of drug users actually rose during the years of its needle exchanges, and one public health physician who investigated its effect found that injection drug use among the young connoted being a "loser."[56] Nonetheless, the issue remained essentially untouchable for national politicians in the United States, as did AIDS in general. "Remember when Clinton's HIV-positive aide, Bob Hattoy, told the Democratic National Convention that America needed a President who wouldn't be afraid to say the word 'condom'? Clinton still hasn't said the word," wrote Doug Ireland, a columnist for the *Village Voice*, in 1998.[57]

CONSERVATIVE RESPONSE

HIV's migration from gays to IV drug users in the late 1990s proved immaterial for conservatives' perception of the disease, which remained rooted in visions of moral obloquy and divine justice. Conservatives continued to understand AIDS as primarily a failure of moral rectitude, secondarily of abnegation of personal responsibility, and only last as a human tragedy, with those few examples of victims outside of the known risk groups falling into the last category. Reports of high levels of adultery in Africa, commercial sex in Asia, and injection drug use around the globe, further reinforced this perception.

Renewed unsafe-sex practices among American gays outraged conservatives, whose generally contemptuous attitudes were now tinged with disbelief. Conservative leaders, politicians, and columnists pointed to the destructive behavior as evidence of extreme moral dissolution. "Is it, then, willful suicide, or hubris, or the former posing as the latter, that has lately been leading so many young homosexuals knowingly to engage in the kind of unprotected sex that is most calculated to leave them with AIDS?" Midge Decter queried in the *National Review*.[58] One angry letter-writer rebuked Ronald Johnson, of the Gay Men's Health Crisis, for comparing AIDS to the bubonic plague in the 14th century. "Mr. Johnson and his colleagues consistently promote AIDS as a mainstream disease with little more purpose than to gather compassion and support from people from all walks of life, while simultaneously rejecting responsibility and accountability for those most at risk," went the missive.[59] Another writer caustically dismissed pleas for his sympathy: "I am monogamous, not a drug-user and not gay. Considering that approximately 98 percent of the people who get AIDS fall into one or more of those categories, I personally could not care one iota about researching a cure for the disease."[60]

Anti-AIDS sentiment on the Right combined with general antigay sentiment in the mid 1990s, as gays advocated for legalized gay marriage, gay spousal benefits, and rescinding the many sodomy laws still technically in force around the country. Gay marriage, in particular, proved provocative to the coalition, as Christian fundamentalists allied themselves with mainstream social conservatives to block legislation in several states that would allow gays to legally wed. In Congress, Robert Dole in the Senate and Robert Barr in the House of Representatives sponsored the Defense of Marriage Act, which President Clinton promised to sign. Frank Riggs, Republican of California, sponsored legislation in the House to deny federal housing grants to cities and counties that required contractors to provide spousal benefits to gay partners. Even the generally liberal columnist Jack Germond recoiled from the idea, promising to "move to Canada" if courts upheld gay marriage.[61] And in the nation's midwestern heartland, the movement met with near total condemnation. "Boycott Hawaii!" an announcement in a Topeka, Kansas, church bulletin ran, after a Hawaii judge endorsed gay marriage. The announcement continued:

On December 3, 1996, a judge in Hawaii ordered that same-sex couples be allowed to marry. Henceforth, Hawaii is a moral leper colony, where none but the dregs of humanity will voluntarily go. Henceforth, Hawaii is fit only for fags, perfectly suited to be a sanatorium for the compulsory quarantine of all guilty, homosexual AIDS carriers. There they can eat, sleep, and copulate, and the whole of Hawaii will be their toilet. Hawaii, the Islands of the Damned. Anteroom to Hell. Sperm Bank of Satan.[62]

Antigay sentiment at times seemed to evolve into general antisex sentiment, as social conservatives tarred long-established sex education curricula and publications as culprits in the AIDS epidemic. While conservatives had long worked to block sex education courses in public schools in southern and midwestern states, now even liberal New England and California harbored antisex activists. A survey conducted in Massachusetts by the conservative-leaning *Massachusetts News* revealed that nearly half of Massachusetts residents felt that gay pride clubs in high schools encouraged teenagers to declare their homosexuality at too young an age, while 40 percent thought that homosexuals had chosen their sexuality rather than having had it biologically dictated. In the same study, 85 percent of respondents disagreed that teenagers ought to be able to exercise sexual freedom without parental consent.[63] Robert Dornan, seeking the Republican presidential nomination for 1996, attacked AIDS education for federal workers as evidence that the Clinton administration "promotes homosexuality or bisexuality as just another healthy lifestyle choice."[64] And everywhere, Americans who generally sympathized with privacy considerations, expressed reservation about the moral neutrality of homosexuality. One Rhode Island writer, who described himself as generally compassionate, explained his intolerance of homosexuality: "One need not be a rocket scientist to recognize that when men attempt sexual relations with men, or women [attempt sexual relations] with women, something has gone wrong. It is indeed abnormal, 'aberrant' and, to many faiths, such behavior is immoral."[65]

The conservative ethos spilled onto the ongoing debates regarding testing and reporting of AIDS cases. By 1997, only 26 states required reporting by name of individuals who tested positive for HIV, and virtually none of the states most heavily affected by the epidemic—New York, New Jersey, California—did. Only 12 states classified AIDS as sexually transmitted, and only 16 classified it as communicable at all. Moreover, only 4 states—Arkansas, North Carolina, South Carolina, and Oregon—required partner or spousal notification by authorities, meaning that in 46 states a man could test positive and continue sleeping with his ignorant wife without violating a law.

This sort of "AIDS exceptionalism" flouted virtually all public health precedents, whose efficacy in the past had relied heavily on careful record keeping, quarantine, isolation, and dissemination of information.[66] Public health professionals faced civil libertarians and gay activists over the issue, with the sanitarians arguing for the primacy of health protection, while their adversaries argued for privacy protection. But as the debate progressed, all but the most strident defenders of privacy began to turn. AIDS was simply too lethal, and notification too important to the public's health, to continue to compromise safety in the name of privacy. In late 1998, the Centers for Disease Control recommended that health-care providers be required to submit names of patients testing positive for HIV to a central record-keeping authority, and even left-leaning public health professionals registered agreement. "I was not always a supporter of named reporting and, in fact, gave testimony on behalf of the American Civil Liberties Union when named reporting was first considered in Colorado in the mid-1980s," wrote Lawrence Gostin, a professor of public health at Johns Hopkins University. "Yet, named reporting is sufficiently important to the health of persons with HIV infection and to the public good to justify it."[67]

Contrary to arguments made by privacy advocates, named reporting did not seem to dissuade people from getting tested, and there was no evidence from those states that had been requiring reporting that names had been released to the general public, or indeed to anybody except partners for the purpose of partner notification.[68] One of the strongest arguments against reporting, that a diagnosis of AIDS was tantamount to public disclosure of homosexuality, was simply specious. Only 40 percent of AIDS cases were among gay men by 1997, and reporting cases of rectal gonorrhea, a far more accurate marker of homosexuality, had been required for decades. Moreover, the availability of effective drug cocktails made testing and reporting, for the first time, of benefit to the patient as well as to the public's health.

Conservative advocates of testing drew strength and support from the case of Nushawn Williams, an HIV-positive man who infected at least 11 teenage girls (the youngest of them 13 years old) in and around Chautauqua County in western New York State in 1996 and 1997. Although Williams had infected at least six women after having tested positive for HIV, he had broken no law, nor had state regulations required that his test be reported. Nettie Mayersohn, state assemblywoman from Queens, responded with outrage: "The laws in New York

State border on insanity. If a person walks into a doctor's office and tests positive for HIV, no one has to be notified. The guy can walk out and he's free to transmit the disease."[69] Area residents responded with anger, with one writing that "the intentional spread of a deadly virus, for which there is no cure, sounds like nothing short of murder to me," and even liberal state legislators agreed that the laws concerning testing and reporting needed to be reexamined.[70]

Despite the shift of AIDS from gays to IV drug users, from the first world to the third world, and from incurable disease to treatable long-term ailment, the political alignment of AIDS foes and advocates in the United States had scarcely shifted by 1997. Social and political conservatives continued to view the disease as derived from immoral, if not depraved, behavior, and demanding of stringent condemnation and policing, while gay advocates, civil libertarians, and social and political liberals continued to view the disease as representing a challenge to civil rights and privacy protections. Neither side had adequately accommodated the changing demographics of the epidemic, nor did either recognize that improved medical treatment could possibly change the terms of the debate.

BLACKS

The resurgence of HIV transmission in the gay community in the late 1990s was most apparent in the black community. Black Americans had made up a disproportionate share of HIV's victims since the late 1980s, and the disparity between black and white infection rates had only grown over the decade. By 1999, blacks, who made up 12 percent of the nation's population, constituted 45 percent of new AIDS cases. In some states, the disparity was even more pronounced. In Massachusetts, for example, where blacks made up only 5 percent of the population, they accounted for 37 percent of new AIDS cases in 1998, meaning that they were overrepresented in that state's epidemic by 750 percent. In the Deep South, by contrast, their infection rates were hardly worse than those of their white peers.[71]

But concentrated as the epidemic was in America's blacks, it was even more so in black gay men. In large cities, a fourth of all young black gay men were HIV-positive by 1999, compared with 15 percent of young gay Hispanic men, and 3 percent of young gay white men.[72] *New York Times* columnist Bob Herbert called the rates "stunning," and compared them with the worst centers of the African epidemic.[73] Nearly half of all gay men surveyed nationwide admitted to having had unprotected anal sex over the preceding six months, but black men seemed particularly cavalier about condom use, and posted AIDS rates double that of all gay men.[74]

Black women also posted substantially higher infection rates than their white counterparts, but here the etiology of infection appeared to be different. While black gay men's high infection rate resulted from inadequate condom use, black women's infection rates resulted from IV drug use, and from unprotected heterosexual intercourse with infected black men. In some areas, particularly in the Deep South, black women dominated the epidemic, constituting, in 2000, nearly 30 percent of all AIDS cases in Mississippi, 31 percent in Alabama, and 27 percent in North Carolina. The ratio of black to white female HIV infection was 15 to 1 in 1995, and was predicted to climb to 20 to 1 by 2005. The epidemic was caused almost entirely by high rates of drug use in the community, with some 65 percent of all black IV drug users infected with HIV by 1998, and concomitantly high rates among women. A group of social workers attempting to educate blacks about the disease tried to dispel the common knowledge of the day: "Myth," they wrote. "AIDS is an 'equal opportunity disease.' "[75]

Homophobia in the black community was partly responsible. While homophobia, or at least discomfort with gays, was widespread in America, among blacks it was ubiquitous, having enjoyed a "long, pernicious tradition," in the words of Henry Louis Gates Jr., a professor of African American studies at Harvard.[76] In the highly masculinized culture of urban black America, homosexuality was viewed as a taint on the entire community, a "white man's perversion," in the words of Benoit Denizet-Lewis, a Boston-based writer.[77] Gay black men remained disproportionately closeted, even among educated peers who might have been expected to espouse greater tolerance toward alternative lifestyles, and adopted a life approach of "Down Low." Whether the homophobia grew from the social distortions of systematized racism, or whether it was an organic outgrowth of northern black culture, it embodied black discomfort with the "sensitive man" icon of the late 20th century. "In a vain attempt to recapture their denied masculinity, many black men mirrored America's traditional fear and hatred of homosexuality," wrote Earl Ofari Hutchinson, a black writer, in 2000.[78] Rued one gay black man living in Atlanta: "If you're white, you can come out as an openly gay skier or actor or whatever. It might hurt you some, but it's not like if you're black and gay, because then it's like you've let down the whole black community, black women, black history, black pride. You don't hear black people say, 'Oh yeah, he's gay, but he's still a real man, and he still takes care of all his responsibilities. What you hear is, 'Look at the sissy faggot.' "[79]

Accusations of black homophobia were generally rejected by black leaders. For a group that had been the target of the worst and most prolonged bigotry in the nation's history, return accusations of bigotry seemed misplaced. When a handful of black leaders, among them Jesse Jackson and Coretta Scott King, suggested that the accelerated spread of black AIDS resulted at least in part from homophobia in the community and an unwillingness to confront unpleasant truths, they were generally dismissed. Moreover, when Magic Johnson publicized his own HIV status while repeatedly denying any participation in homosexual liaisons (which was statistically unlikely to be true), few black leaders stepped forward to condemn his lack of candor. Carl Bean, a black Los Angeles minister and director of that city's Minority AIDS Project, only exacerbated the problem when he pronounced on the Johnson case, "Whatever Magic says about his life, the message is what you do isn't what matters, it's the way you do it."[80] A half decade later, this type of mass denial of homosexuality would be one of the primary causes of accelerated AIDS transmission among gay black men.

Black churches embodied the community's discomfort with identifying and acknowledging black homosexuality. A black gay AIDS epidemic undermined the community's image of itself, and invited denial if not outright derision. Black homosexuality was the "pink elephant that nobody wants to talk about," admitted Kwabena Rainey Cheeks, a pastor in Washington, D.C.[81] Few black ministers acknowledged the largely homosexual nature of AIDS among black men, and fewer still extended themselves to openly gay parishioners. David Satcher, the U.S. surgeon general, who had grown up attending black churches, admitted that it had been difficult to find ministers who were "even willing to talk about it in their pulpits," and Alton Pollard III, director of black-church studies at Emory University, stated, "The black church can't even talk about sex itself, and you can't get to sexuality until you get to sex."[82] Illustrating the situation perfectly was the pronouncement of outspoken Pittsburgh minister Johnnie Monroe, who confronted his congregation with the direness of the black AIDS epidemic, only to offer the bromide, "One of the things that we are facing is the fact that AIDS does not only hit homosexuals, does not only hit those who abuse drugs."[83]

But of course, the truth was almost precisely the opposite. For American blacks, AIDS was a disease born almost exclusively of either homosexuality or drug use. In attempting to universalize the disease among his black congregants, Monroe grasped for the same political tool as had gay organizers a decade before—a depiction of an epidemic worthy of attention and sympathy because it was ultimately a disease of everybody. To reserve the disease for black gays and drug users was to marginalize it and place it beyond the bounds of black Christian charity. "It's all right if it's the gay population that dies," bitterly pronounced Irene Monroe, an openly gay minister. "It's a travesty to them if their heterosexual population begins to die. You can salvage their souls, but you cannot salvage the souls of black queers."[84]

Not all black churches and leaders denied the scope of the problem. In the mid-1990s several iconoclastic ministers and community organizers spoke about the growing plague and spurred congregants to take note of the threat it posed. In Manhattan, Balm of Gilead, an organization working to promote AIDS awareness within black churches, claimed 5,000 congregations among its associates.[85] Various black mayors, governors, and municipal politicians formed the National Black Leadership Commission on AIDS to raise public understanding and lobby for funds. In Washington, D.C., congressional black leaders such as Ronald Dellums of California and Donna Christian-Christiansen of the Virgin Islands focused the attention of the Congressional Black Caucus on the issue, and worked to raise awareness among all legislators. "The face of AIDS has changed, and it is now ours," declared Christian-Christiansen.[86] And in Philadelphia (and elsewhere to a lesser degree), blacks moved into leadership positions within the local ACT

UP organization to replace the declining numbers of gay activists for whom, in the wake of combination therapy, the disease seemed no longer quite as compelling.[87]

At the same time, Eugene Rivers, a Boston-based minister, worked to raise awareness among black Americans of the scope of the African epidemic, which he viewed as appropriately a concern of the African-American community. In 1999, he wrote an open letter to African-Americans urging them to focus efforts and resources on the situation in sub-Saharan Africa, asking them, "What verdict will our descendants render upon their ancestors who stood silently by as a generation of African children was reduced to a biological underclass by this sexual holocaust?"[88] Calling particularly on black churches to focus their resources on the "needs and interests of millions of orphans in Africa," he outlined a plan of international aid, education, and lobbying.[89] Dellums of California echoed the call after visiting several of the most afflicted nations. "Look folks, 12 million Africans have already died. You should stand up with moral outrage," he declared on a nationwide speaking tour, delivered predominantly in black churches.[90]

One barrier to effective intervention in the black community was black leaders' reluctance to discuss black promiscuity, either in the United States or in Africa. Although Rivers referred to sexual promiscuity in Africa as "violence against women," few black ministers would openly broach the topic. Julian Bond, chairman of the NAACP, questioned whether it was appropriate for pro-black lobbying groups to advocate abstinence. "We're not a birth control organization," he claimed of his group. "That's not our mission."[91] But Rivers insisted on promoting "ancient African chastity," and suggested that others do likewise. Noted Eva Thorne, a Rivers acolyte: "People don't want to talk about when black is ugly. They only want to hear about 'black is beautiful.'"[92]

Public health officials identified the high rate of HIV transmission among blacks, but were unsure of how to respond. Great efforts had been extended to educate blacks on the dangers of drug use and unprotected sex, yet the community seemed unreceptive to the message. Many social workers and health educators suspected that the problem lay in the medium, rather than the message. Blacks would respond to AIDS education programs, they argued, provided that those programs were culturally sensitive to black audiences. "Generic" messages, in the opinion of Buffalo minister Heshimu Sparks, would not reach black audiences, nor would generic pamphlets that had simply been reprinted with photos of blacks.[93] Rather, a new education effort, designed by and for blacks, was required, "a new and intense and creative effort—led by black Americans," in the words of Bob Herbert. Joey Pressley, executive director of the New York AIDS Coalition, assented. "The prevention message for black people . . . must take into account community norms, social networks, cultural issues and history," he wrote. "The message can no longer be 'use a condom every time.' "[94]

Education efforts had been stymied by continued black skepticism about the very nature of the epidemic, among other reasons. As late as 1999, blacks still expressed heightened suspicions that AIDS had been maliciously created by white scientists—government or private—with the explicit intention of infecting, and ultimately killing, large numbers of blacks. Nearly half of all black Americans expressed belief in the "reports" that AIDS had been produced in a germ-warfare laboratory, while 43 percent believed that the government was hiding the full truth about the disease.[95] Various black celebrities, including Spike Lee and Moe Dee, expressed concern that AIDS existed to exterminate blacks, and Will Smith, a popular movie star, stated in an interview that "possibly AIDS was created as a result of biological-warfare testing."[96] The speculations were absurd, but the distrust was real, and any health educator would need to dispel the conspiracies before she could actually begin to teach.

PROBLEMS WITH COMBINATION THERAPY

The effects of rising rates of new infections among both gays and blacks in the late 1990s were to some extent ameliorated by the ubiquitous combination therapies available in the United States. Even as the affected populations engaged in riskier behaviors, death rates declined, owing almost entirely to the effect of the drugs. Moreover, the mere existence of the drugs facilitated unsafe behavior, as gay men, particularly, rationalized their unsafe behaviors with the knowledge that any contracted disease was treatable.

Such thinking belied the inconvenience, cost, and limited efficacy of the medication. Despite advancing to a second generation of drugs by 1999, combination therapy remained supremely unpleasant, inconvenient, and expensive. It was still composed of between 32 and 40 pills daily, each requiring specific directions and conditions for optimum efficacy. Some patients on the therapy reached out to young people engaged in unsafe behavior in an effort to inform them of the burden of the treatment. "When I talk to young people, I tell them about when I was taking 32 pills a day. I say, 'Thirty-two pills versus HIV. Thirty-two pills. HIV . . .' over and over," explained one Brooklyn woman.[97] Others tried to warn about the extraordinary cost of the medications that could quickly bankrupt an uninsured individual before driving him or her into the local Medicaid program. The fact that sales of the drugs were plateauing by 1999 in the United States, despite continued growth of the epidemic, suggested that many of the newly infected were incapable of tolerating the regimen, either because of lifestyle or insurance status. Dean Mitchell, vice president at Glaxo Wellcome, noted: "Some of the people who are now testing positive for HIV are at the lowest level of resources. They are not as assertive as gay men. They have to work their way around the system."[98]

The high cost of the drugs, and the reluctance of private insurers to pay for them, drove increasing numbers of AIDS patients to Medicaid in the late 1990s. By 1998, health statisticians discovered that only 32 percent of all AIDS patients had private health insurance, and that Medicaid was the primary insurer for 55 percent of all adult AIDS patients and for 90 percent of pediatric ones. Medicaid AIDS drug expenditures had doubled in three years from $606 million to $1.3 billion, and 19 states had placed caps on their emergency drug assistance plans in an effort to place more of the burden on the federal government.[99] One AIDS patient explained the terrible burden of paying for his drugs and the need to enroll in Medicaid. "I've always thought of going on Medicaid as a failure of financial planning for middle-class people, and this really caught me off guard."[100]

Further undermining the drugs' curative potential was growing evidence of drug-resistant strains of HIV. Pharmaceutical researchers had strongly suspected from the early days of anti-HIV development that the virus would prove adept at mutating toward resistant forms. Its high mutation rate and long gestation period promised to make the virus stubbornly successful at rapidly evolving new strains, and this promise had impelled physicians and public health officials to limit combination therapy to those patients who were most likely to fully comply with the complicated regimens. Incomplete compliance, leading to incompletely killed viruses, would greatly facilitate the organism's evolution.

Despite these prophylactic efforts, resistant strains were appearing by the late 1990s. By 1999, 14 percent of patients appeared to be infected with resistant strains—up from 4 percent in 1996—and 6 percent of patients were infected with strains that were resistant to two or more drugs.[101] By 2001, the portion was above half, with 42 percent resistant to all protease inhibitors and 70 percent resistant to at least one transcriptase inhibitor. NIAID director Anthony Fauci warned about the "genetic plasticity" of the virus, and various studies found the rates of resistant strains increasing exponentially.[102] "We could be right back where we were in 1984, when the virus was unstoppable," warned Larry Kessler of the Boston-based AIDS Action Committee.[103]

Drawbacks aside, however, the impact of combination therapy continued to be profound, and its price relatively low compared with the potential cost of hospitalization for all infected patients. By 1999, as many as 300,000 Americans were being treated with combination therapy, with 91 percent boasting CD4 cell counts below 500 per cubic millimeter. Total cost for all care of these patients, including outpatient visits, drugs, and periodic hospitalization, was $7 billion, which was just under 1 percent of the nation's health-care expenditures. Considering that the prevalence of the disease in the population had failed to drop, and that as late as 1995 health planners were warning that AIDS could bankrupt the United States health-care system, the total cost was modest. The drugs had indeed delivered a therapeutic and financial miracle, even if they were not the therapeutic panacea or vaccine of which most health planners dreamed.[104]

CHAPTER 14

PANDEMIC

By the year 2000, 21.8 million people had died of AIDS, and 50 million people had been infected with HIV. Over 2.5 million people were dying yearly, and 5.6 million people were becoming newly infected.[1] While over 90 percent of all new infections were in Africa and Asia, even the healthy and wealthy United States had suffered; its 440,000 AIDS deaths over the previous two decades totaled more than all United States military fatalities in World Wars I and II combined.[2]

Africa continued to be worst hit. Over half of all AIDS fatalities had been among the 400 million people living in the southern half of that continent, cutting 20 years from life expectancy in some countries. Africa experts noted that AIDS was killing 10 times the number of sub-Saharan Africans killed each year in all of the region's wars combined, and that the future promised worse, not better.[3] "AIDS is hitting Africa so fiercely that it now compares to the great epidemics of history—the Black Death of the Middle Ages . . . and the influenza pandemic of 1918–1919," wrote Lawrence Altman, a medical reporter for the *New York Times*.[4] Other observers resorted to similar hyperbole, calling it an "epidemic of Biblical proportions."[5]

Moreover, Africa was desperately short of cash. The region's extreme poverty relegated its people to spending less than $10 a year on health care. "Most people in Africa can't even afford to take a bus to get care at a free clinic," Michael Specter, a reporter for the *New Yorker,* wrote in 2003.[6] In such an environment, combination pharmaceutical therapies costing between $10,000 and $15,000 annually were beyond reach. Even the cheapest drug, AZT, which used alone could do little but thwart perinatal transmission of the virus, was too expensive for most Africans. Only a radical change in societal sexual norms offered hope, and thus far most Africans resisted this.

Next worse, in rates of infection and transmission, was the Caribbean. Echoing Africa, many of the region's isles harbored cultures of promiscuity that facilitated transmission while undermining the hygienic sanctity of marriage. At the same time, poverty nearly as crushing as that of sub-Saharan Africa forced growing numbers of women into prostitution, or to the status of "girlfriend for hire," while social mores dictated that both girls and boys would begin sex early, and engage in it frequently. One study of school-aged children in several English-speaking islands found 42 percent had had sex by age 10, and 62 percent by age 12.[7]

Data for the Caribbean was notoriously unreliable. Haiti, for example, which most public health experts ranked as the most heavily infected nation in the region, claimed only 5,000 AIDS cases in 1998, whereas United Nations officials believed the correct number to be 330,000.[8] A number of countries maintained no statistics at all, while others recorded only cases of full-blown AIDS rather than all HIV infections. The most highly infected countries—Haiti, Bahamas, Barbados, Guyana, and the Dominican Republic—probably had a prevalence of infection ranging from 3 to 5 percent, but nobody was exactly sure.[9] The island nations, heavily reliant on tourism, were reluctant to publicize the problem, and outside public health practitioners and reporters were often rebuffed.

Despite the muddied data, public health experts did know that the Caribbean epidemic was heavily heterosexual, perhaps 60 percent so. As in Africa, the preponderance of infected individuals were heterosexual adults between 18 and 40, while gay transmission for most countries was responsible for as little as 10 percent of all infections.[10] The numbers could not quite be reconciled, as use of injection drugs in the region was very low, and there was little reason to believe that the region harbored a unique vector. More probably, instances of homosexuality and bisexuality were being underreported, and according to one researcher perhaps redefined. Fernando Zacharias, a physician with the Pan American Health Organization, estimated that possibly 17 percent of all men on some islands had had sex with another man, but most would not describe themselves as homosexual unless they had been receptive anal partners.[11]

The epidemic in Russia and other former republics of the Soviet Union was expanding. Over half of all intravenous drug users in some areas were testing positive for HIV, and the total reported number of AIDS cases was growing exponentially—from 10,000 in 1999 to 70,000 in 2000.[12] And as in the Caribbean, the infections were almost certainly being substantially underreported. Injection drug use was escalating rapidly, particularly among the young: the number of IV drug users 14 and younger in Saint Petersburg, for example, increased 2,000 percent between 1997 and 1999.[13] At the same time, rising alcoholism, falling employment, and extremely high rates of violent crime were testament to societies in distress. AIDS tended to thrive in such circumstances, and the Russian epidemic appeared to be robust.

But without question the future of AIDS belonged to Asia. China and India, between them harboring nearly half of the world's people, had come late to AIDS but were now catching up. By 2000, over 1 percent of India's 1 billion people, 10 million, were probably infected, but nobody really knew. In Miraj, the worst-hit city, 1 in 20 was infected. Prostitutes professed general ignorance of the disease, and condom use was rare. At the same time, the nation's public health agencies had been reluctant to work too aggressively at testing, marking, educating, or even informing patients who tested positive for HIV. One doctor claimed he never shared information with HIV-positive prostitutes lest they "become too depressed and commit suicide."[14] China claimed only a half-million cases by 2000, but again the figure was unreliable. If only 2 percent of the 1.3 billion Chinese ultimately became infected, not an unlikely scenario, the world would have another 26 million AIDS cases. Writing in 1999, David Ho speculated that the Asian epidemic could ultimately infect between 100 million and 1 billion people if no workable vaccine emerged.[15]

The epidemic had failed to meet the most pessimistic of predictions. Eight years earlier, WHO had speculated that possibly 100 million people worldwide would be infected by 2000, yet the true count was somewhat less than half of that.[16] On the other hand, in the worst-off nations life expectancy had declined precipitously, and would most likely continue to do so. To emphasize the magnitude of the disaster, statisticians presenting at the World AIDS Conference at Barcelona in 2002 estimated probable life expectancy in the year 2010 for several countries with and without AIDS. For most Western countries, including the United States, the difference was trivial. But in South Africa, life expectancy would drop from 68 years to 37, in Zimbabwe from 71 to 35, and in Botswana from 74 to 27. [17] Such stunning declines exceeded anything in history, and their effect on the economic, civic, and cultural lives of the affected countries would be profound and unpredictable.

Furthermore, coepidemics of tuberculosis, including new antibiotic-resistant strains, were developing alongside AIDS in much of the nonindustrialized world. Long prevalent as a low-grade infection (public health experts estimated that up to one-third of the world's population carried the bacillus), tuberculosis was overwhelming weakened immune systems, obsolete antibiotics, and poorly fed and hydrated young bodies to kill more people each year than AIDS and malaria combined.[18] Over half of all AIDS patients in Africa and Asia had tuberculosis, creating a new form of hyperopportunistic infection that failed to respond to what few drugs and what little medical treatment were available. In fact, tuberculosis was probably killing over a third of all AIDS patients, and infectious-disease specialists estimated that people with HIV infections were 30 to 50 times more likely to develop active tuberculosis from a latent infection than were those without HIV.[19] Arata Kochi, manager of WHO's tuberculosis program, observed, "TB and HIV are feeding off each other at an alarming rate. When they're together, they multiply each other's impact."[20]

AFRICA

The epidemic in sub-Saharan Africa raged unabated in 2000, and had actually increased in force despite a decade of international efforts to educate, control, and assuage. In central and southeast Africa, eight countries posted double-digit infection rates for adults between 15 and 49, and Botswana, Zimbabwe, Zambia, Swaziland, and Namibia all exceeded 20 percent.[21] Reporters describing the epidemic reached for new comparisons in an effort to transmit the unimaginable scope of the tragedy: four out of five deaths of people between 25 and 35 were AIDS-related; half of people reaching voting age would die before retirement; new babies were being born with life expectancies of 40 years rather than the previous 70.[22] One particularly discursive correspondent for *Time* magazine wrote: "Corpses stack up in morgues until those on top crush the identity from the faces underneath. Raw earth mounds scar the landscape, grave after grave without name or number. Bereft children grieve for parents lost in their prime, for siblings scattered to the winds."[23]

By 2000, 2 million Africans were dying of AIDS each year. By comparison, the total number of all Americans who had died of AIDS since the epidemic's beginning was just over 440,000. And the epidemic continued to spread. In west Africa, Sierra Leone faced a growing epidemic, even as it struggled to rebuild following a 10-year civil war. Epidemiologists estimated that 10 percent of the country was infected (despite official claims of under 3 percent) and over 20 percent of army recruits were testing positive for HIV infection. Infected soldiers spread the disease to the hordes of prostitutes who materialized around their bases, who in turn spread it to their civilian partners and spouses. And this was in a part of the continent that had hitherto appeared to be largely beyond the reach of the epidemic.[24]

While Africa's epidemic was largely a case of the same as elsewhere, but more so, aspects were unique. Low rates of circumcision appeared to correlate well with AIDS transmission in southern Africa, despite the fact that this was not true in (largely uncircumcised) Europe.[25] Certain studies suggested that African women appeared to progress more slowly from infection to full-blown AIDS (and ultimately to death) than did their Western counterparts, leaving them infectious for longer periods of time.[26] Higher rates of tuberculosis throughout the continent, coupled with limited access to antibiotics, meant that Africans generally had weaker respiratory systems. Also, southern Africa's epidemic was largely caused by type C of the HIV virus (as opposed to type B in North America and type A in east and west Africa) which was possibly more virulent.

Some researchers surmised that Africans had generally weaker immune systems than did Europeans and Americans, or immune systems that were specifically susceptible to HIV. The theory posited that because of high levels of untreated bacterial and viral infections throughout the continent, many Africans were living with highly "activated" immune systems with higher CD4 cell counts. These extra CD4 cells provided a broader target for HIV, meaning that a smaller initial infection could cause AIDS or ARC than was true in Europe and the United States. The theory was contentious, but even highly regarded AIDS researchers refused to dismiss it.[27]

Large numbers of African babies appeared to be catching the disease while breastfeeding in a pattern of epidemic spread rare in the West. While data were sketchy, one study found infection rates almost a third higher among infected African women who were breast-feeding than among their Western counterparts. Possibly the African women simply carried higher viral loads, or the babies themselves were weaker and more susceptible to infection. One researcher suggested that ancillary infections of the breast tissue might be playing a role, but nobody knew for sure. What the United Nations was quite sure of, though, was that of the 500,000 new pediatric infections per year worldwide, 90 percent were taking place in Africa.[28]

Where Africa clearly differed from the West was in cleaving to a variety of political and cultural norms that facilitated the spread of infections. For two decades, for example, large parts of the continent had been rent by wars that were accompanied by large standing armies, roving tribal forces, and the general presence of soldiers intermixed with civilian populations. (Congo, at its worst, had been occupied by troops from seven different armies *concurrently*.) The soldiers copulated with prostitutes, girlfriends, hangers-on, and sometimes forcibly with local civilians. (Toward the end of the 1990s, South Africa posted the highest rate of rape in the world.) HIV infection rates among the troops were extraordinary. Many armies harbored infection rates of over 50 percent, and one study of Zimbabwean troops placed the rate at nearly 80 percent.[29]

Many African governments contributed to the rate of spread by failing to invest heavily in AIDS education, or by opposing it outright. For some African leaders, it was simply a point of nationalistic pride. High AIDS rates called into question their administrative efficacy (or even political legitimacy), and contributed to the perception that theirs were not legitimate nations with functioning governments. For others, the impetus was more economic. In tourist-dependent countries, such as Kenya, Tanzania, and Zimbabwe, high AIDS rates, if publicized, would frighten away tourists and diminish revenues. President Daniel arap Moi of Kenya had been particularly reluctant to admit the scope of his nation's AIDS epidemic; even as 60 percent of Nairobi prostitutes were testing positive for HIV, the president continued to insist that the country had only a modest problem.[30]

In either case, governments of most sub-Saharan countries were late in admitting the scope of the problem, late in designing education and intervention schemes, and late in implementing those schemes. Through the late 1990s, physicians in many of the afflicted countries continued to routinely hide AIDS diagnoses and falsify causes of death on official documents. "I write TB or meningitis or diarrhea but never AIDS," remarked one physician in South Africa.[31] Other doctors admitted to succumbing to pressure regarding reporting blood tests, or even in writing AIDS diagnoses in their own (confidential) medical files. The continent, it seemed, had adopted a "Don't ask, don't tell" attitude, to the detriment of the public's health.

In some areas, notably Muslim sections of west Africa and heavily Christian areas of east Africa, religious leaders resisted spreading safe-sex messages. As in the United States, condom education conflicted with articulated norms regarding monogamy and contraception, regardless of the reality of the population's behavior, and thus could not officially be tolerated. One telling figure was the 80 million condoms sold in Nigeria in 2000 for a population of 110 million: a total of 2 condoms for each adult male in the country for the entire year.[32] Given the high rates of extramarital and premarital sex in the country, not to mention sex within the confines of marriage, the low number indicated a near total disregard of prophylaxis. Safe-sex education was not reaching its targeted audiences, if indeed it was being touted at all.

And of course there was the promiscuity. After a decade and a half of ever-increasing incidence of AIDS across virtually all countries in the region, sub-Saharan Africa refrained from extramarital sex hardly at all. Sex with wives, girlfriends, secondary and tertiary wives, prostitutes, on-the-road girlfriends, young acolytes, and students was pervasive. In several countries in central Africa, schoolteachers were among the most infected of all of the nations' professional groups, and they in turn spread the virus to the multitudes of students with whom they slept. Older men in several countries clung to the belief that sex with a virgin, or at least a young woman, could cure them of their ills—including AIDS. Young women engaged in sex with older married men to win cash, or favors, or protection, or simply social status. Christine Varga, a researcher based in Durban, South Africa, reflected, "For young people, sex is a must to be taken seriously by their peers."[33] A paper presented at the 1999 international AIDS conference in Zambia revealed that 80 percent of all men in that country maintained multiple sex partners.[34]

The outrageous death tolls wreaked havoc on social structures in the affected countries. Across Africa, by 2000 there were nearly 11 million orphaned children.[35] Bereft of the meager support available to them while their parents lived, they now became wards of overburdened state agencies, or of their grandparents who now found themselves raising another generation in the years when they had expected to be cared for by their grown children. Orphans in Africa faced a bleak future. Many lost social and cultural attachments to become homeless runaways: easy prey for recruitment into criminal gangs and warring minority factions. As they aged, these unsocialized individuals promised to become more socially disruptive, rather than less so. Fearing the societal affect of these aging vagabonds, the South African presidential spokesman Parks Mankahlana publicly stated his reservation about rearing these children to adulthood: "We don't want a generation of orphans," he said.[36]

In the worst-affected countries, AIDS brought normal population growth to a halt, and in certain cases led to population decline. In Botswana, Lesotho, Namibia, South Africa, Swaziland, Zambia, and Zimbabwe, AIDS rates of 20 percent or more were harbingers of rural depopulation and stagnant economies. UNAIDS data suggested that AIDS-afflicted households in these countries consumed 41 percent less food and produced 67 percent less income than did non-AIDS-afflicted households. AIDS-afflicted households did consume more health care—400 percent more by some estimates—even as their incomes declined. In countries that were deeply impoverished before AIDS, the crisis threatened to paralyze the health systems. One United Nations economist estimated that by 2005 Zimbabwe, among others, would spend 65 percent of its national health-care budget on AIDS.[37]

Despite substantial declines in agricultural production, however, the economies of the worst-affected countries were not expected to shrink substantially, if at all.[38] Alan Whiteside, an economist at the University of Natal, estimated total AIDS-related declines for most sub-Saharan economies at .5 percent per year.[39] In nations with huge supplies of cheap unskilled labor, even massive death tolls would do little to slow economic growth, and wage premiums for the survivors might actually strengthen the economic landscape.

Nobody could really predict the ultimate effects of the epidemic. Many historians and economists studied the consequences of the medieval Black Death, and agreed that while it had forestalled economic development for a century, it ultimately enabled Europe's rise to technological supremacy. Labor shortages in the wake of the epidemic had led to greater investments in technology and capital improvements, while freeing up arable land and other natural resources.[40] Whether Africa would follow this model, or disintegrate further into warring chaos and ensconced corruption, could not be predicted.[41]

SOUTH AFRICA

The South African epidemic stood out in 2000 for its sheer size and for the scope of its potential economic cost. Although the epidemic was about a decade behind that of central Africa, 20 percent of the population was now infected with HIV, and this number promised to increase to nearly 30 percent over the following decade. Moreover, the epidemic was proving to be particularly devastating to working adults, with 25 percent of sexually active women testing positive for HIV nationwide, and over 35 percent of sexually active women testing positive in the most highly infected rural precincts.[42] In the Khutsong mining area, where single men toiled in isolation from families and communities, nearly 45 percent of men in their early 30s tested positive for HIV, as did nearly 60 percent of women in their mid-20s.[43] Noting the extreme size of the South African epidemic, Abt Associates, a consulting group, called it the "greatest catastrophe South Africa has ever confronted" in a report issued in 2000, and projected a national infection rate of 27 percent by 2010 that would produce nearly 2 million orphans.[44]

The causes of the epidemic mirrored those elsewhere in Africa, albeit with certain unique attributes. As elsewhere, the low status of women precluded them from being able to negotiate terms in sexual relations, and placed them at the financial mercy of their husbands and boyfriends. Through the traditional practice of *lobola,* men purchased younger wives with mixed dowries of livestock and cash, allowing them the community status accorded to husbands and fathers coupled with the prerogative to philander with impunity.[45] At the same time, a rash of postapartheid violent rapes accelerated the spread of AIDS, while at the same time further undermining the ability of women to negotiate sexual parameters. By 2000, South Africa had the highest rate of rape in the world, with a woman being raped every 26 seconds and the police and courts seemingly uninterested in aggressively policing the crime. In one notorious example of judicial indifference, a Bloemfontein judge granted leniency toward a 23-year-old rapist who had abducted and raped two 10-year-old girls, explaining that the act was simply a product of the man's virility.[46]

As elsewhere in Africa, prostitution—formalized or not—increased the epidemic's reach, although here again South Africa added its own unique twist. Whereas in most African countries prostitutes followed truckers, in South Africa they followed the miners who patronized them at unprecedented levels. Although under apartheid South Africa had maintained a not-undeserved reputation as being somewhat prudish (as bespoke its Calvinist past), in the years following apartheid prostitution, pornography, and the sex industry rushed in to fill the historical void.[47] In mining towns and precincts, rates of infection for local women were the highest in the world, reaching 66 percent in Carleton-ville in 2000.[48] Desperate prostitutes would offer sex for as little as the equivalent of four U.S. dollars, placing their services well within the reach of virtually any man with even menial employment. And with many of the mines employing between 5,000 and 10,000 men, most unaccompanied and all in their years of peak sexual activity, the problem seemed unsolvable. "You've got men living in single-sex hostels without their wives. What do you think they're going to do, play backgammon?" one AIDS researcher from the University of Pretoria remarked.[49]

Prostitution was hardly confined to the mining towns. In the wake of apartheid's dissolution, South Africa welcomed prostitutes from many lands, while wealthier urban clientele eagerly sought the services of the new transplants. One enterprising reporter hired a high-priced "elite" prostitute to guide him through that city's sexual attractions and discovered the sorts of outrageous sex shows and novel sexual experiences hitherto associated primarily with Bangkok. Prostitutes from both east Asia and east Europe were sought after by clients seeking the next exotic thrill, and police willingly ignored most of the activity, which was still technically illegal. The reporter wrote of the Johannesburg sex trade, "It's not unusual these days to find your 'escort' has olive skin and almond eyes, or her name is Svetlana and her preferred drink is vodka."[50]

But while its problems with sex, prostitution, and misogynistic violence were hardly unique, South Africa's extraordinary indifference to the epidemic was. The country's president, Thabo Mbeki, for several years refused to acknowledge that the country had an AIDS problem, then refused to acknowledge that HIV was the cause, and then refused to admit that combination antiretroviral therapy was the most appropriate and promising remedy.[51] Mbeki postulated that Western scientists at best knew nothing, and at worst were themselves promulgators of a new genocidal agent. Vowing to seek a homegrown African remedy to the threat, and calling pro-pharmaceutical protesters "paid marketing agents for toxic AIDS drugs from America," Mbeki authorized his subordinates to use "native" African approaches in responding.[52] While his minister of health prescribed garlic to treat the disease, other government functionaries expressed skepticism over the validity of scientific inquiry at all. "Western scientists once said to us the earth was flat. Now we know it's round. I bet one day we look at AIDS the same way," one official of the governing African National Congress reflected.[53]

The obliviousness was even more insidious because South Africa was one of the few countries on the African continent that was wealthy enough to actually be able to afford to purchase combination therapy drugs for a substantial number of infected citizens. South Africans earned over $3,000 per capita in 2000 and maintained a Western-style health system. And although the system had disintegrated somewhat in the years since apartheid's end, and better served whites than blacks, it still delivered the best medicine in sub-Saharan Africa to nearly all who called upon it. Archbishop Desmond Tutu, the nation's winner of the Nobel Peace Prize, expressed his frustration at the government's intransigence, even as he himself had previously espoused certain Afrocentric dogma. "What is distressing is that we really are fiddling while our Rome is burning . . . people are dying, but unpleasant truths we tend to deny," Tutu said in 2001.[54]

But even in relatively wealthy South Africa, AIDS and AIDS-related tuberculosis were overwhelming the health-care system. Tuberculosis had climbed to a quarter million cases per annum by 2001—15 times the United States caseload of 16,000 for a nation with one-seventh the population—and now comprised over 10 percent of hospital admissions. At the same time, non-TB AIDS cases comprised over 5 percent of all hospitalizations, versus .2 percent a decade earlier.[55] Furthermore, the sexual nature of the dual epidemics undermined the usual efficacy of the predominantly female South African nursing corps, which confronted cultural barriers regarding discussions of sexuality between unrelated men and women, or even between whites and blacks. Neil Jorgensen, a white Afrikaner physician attempting to limit AIDS infections among Zulu tribes in the Hlabisa area, could not use local nurses to educate tribesman about sex and condoms, and was forced to do much of the educating himself. Even then he faced charges of cultural insensitivity. One reporter described a confrontation: "One worker stood up and shouted at him [Jorgensen] that white men had no business telling Zulu men how to sleep with their wives and girlfriends, and that condoms were a white plot to keep blacks from multiplying."[56]

The threat to the nation's economy was immense. Already over a fifth of all miners and construction workers were infected, and possibly a fourth of the nation's teachers.[57] Health insurance premiums, still largely borne by private employers, promised to triple by 2010, which would force the population to divert funds from savings and investment.[58] The United Nations estimated that the epidemic was slowing economic growth by .4 percent per year, which would lead to a GDP 17 percent smaller than expected by 2010 in the absence of a breakthrough in treatment.[59] While the wealthiest and most highly trained professionals in the workforce—physicians, attorneys, scientists, and bankers—were not particularly hard hit by the epidemic (in contrast to other sub-Saharan African nations)—teachers were. By 2000, teachers were dying at irreplaceable rates, which in turn undermined the nation's ability to replace infected health-care workers and government bureaucrats who were also dying quickly. By at least one estimate, over half the South African workforce would die in the succeeding decade.[60]

A few individuals scored victories. Abdurrazack Achmat, an energetic and enterprising gay South African, founded the Treatment Action Campaign to protest government policies on HIV-drug distribution as well as high drug prices being charged by pharmaceutical companies.[61] Justice Showalala founded the Inkanyezi project to care for AIDS victims, bringing meals to the disabled and rudimentary nursing care to those suffering from opportunistic infections.[62] And the ANC lobbied, and ultimately prevailed, against a law prohibiting the manufacture of off-patent drugs for use in combination therapy.[63] By 2003, the average price of a year's supply of antiretroviral drugs had fallen from $10,000 to $2,000 owing to the efforts of these individuals and organizations.[64] At that price, the drugs were still beyond the means of most of the population, but at least a few more people could now afford them.

SAFE SEX

Most public health professionals' initial instinct was to promote safe sex throughout the developing world. Given the financial and environmental barriers to implementing combination therapy in these countries, as well as the unavailability of a vaccine, widespread adoption of

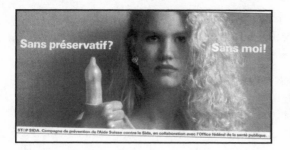

Safe sex educational efforts took a variety of forms in different countries, such as a poster campaign in Switzerland, or a public health class in Kampala, Uganda. The Swiss poster reads, "No Condom, No Sex." (Swiss Federal Office of Public Health and Corbis)

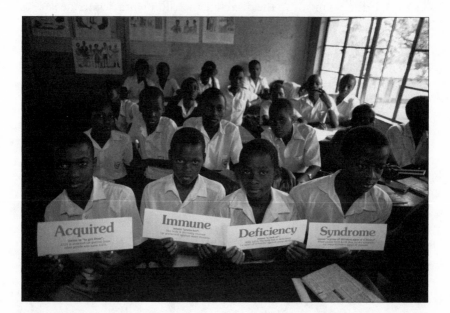

condoms seemed the most promising approach to stemming the epidemic. Condoms were cheap, effective, and easy to transport. Moreover, new condomlike technologies such as female condoms and vaginal gels were being developed that could further the array of safe-sex choices for residents of third-world countries.[65]

Money was not a barrier. International organizations had increased funding drastically over the previous decade, to the extent that by 2000 over $1.8 billion was being committed annually for AIDS-related work in the developing world. (The United Nations and its co-sponsors alone were spending $700 million.)[66] The sum was inadequate to fund combination drug treatment, but it was more than adequate to finance the purchase and distribution of adequate numbers of condoms.

But condom campaigns were largely ineffective. In some cases, governments resisted acknowledging an AIDS epidemic at all, while in others governments refused to divert adequate amounts of foreign aid to condom distribution, or funneled funds through corrupt contractors who provided faulty condoms.[67] But the greater barrier was men's unwillingness to wear the condoms, and women's lack of autonomy in controlling their own sexual behavior.

AIDS in the third world underscored the essentially powerless position of many women throughout the world. Whether deprived of economic independence, legal protections, or cultural autonomy, millions of women simply lacked the ability to assert with whom, where, when, and how they would have sexual relations. Multiple surveys indicated the unwillingness of many men throughout the developing world to wear condoms—77 percent of Brazilian men, for example, claimed to never use condoms, as did 80 to 90 percent of men throughout central and southern Africa—and women risked violence and rape in demanding that they do so.[68] Women claimed to risk accusations of infidelity for even suggesting that their husbands wear condoms, and in many countries courts routinely dismissed charges of domestic violence and rape.[69] Prostitutes, particularly children pressed into prostitution, had even less ability to control the environment of their sexual liaisons. One study of girls living on the street in São Paulo found that nearly half had been raped, and a similar study of street children in Rio de Janeiro indicated that over a quarter had been forced into anal intercourse.[70] Almost none regularly used condoms.[71]

The problem was profound and seemingly without solution. Changing women's sexual autonomy would require wholly restructuring many traditional societies, including granting women access to property, civil rights, privacy rights, and most of all education. As late as 2000, the majority of women in heavily AIDS-afflicted countries were ignorant about the mechanism of HIV infection, the need for condom use, or even knowledge of their own fertility cycles. Traditional societies were loathe to openly broach these topics with men or women, and retreated to a sanctioned modesty regarding AIDS and sex education. One editorial writer said that of all the basic steps that needed to be taken to fight AIDS, the most important was to "stop being squeamish about sex."[72]

A few countries succeeded in stemming the infection. Thailand, for one, implemented an aggressive safe-sex education and condom distribution campaign in the late 1980s that succeeded in getting significant numbers of Thai prostitutes to insist on condom use by their patrons, and in getting the patrons to comply. Largely the brainchild of Senator Mechai Viravaidya, the Thai campaign succeeded, in part, because Thais never had been particularly squeamish about sex. Mechai was known to hand out condoms on the street and ultimately earned the sobriquet "Mr. Condom." And although a million Thais had caught AIDS by 2000, public health planners suggested that the number would have been 40 percent higher in the absence of Mechai's effort.[73]

But the two other countries that had most visibly succeeded in lowering the AIDS transmission rate by 2000 had not relied on condoms. Cuba, as previously discussed, had resorted to aggressively testing its population, maintaining records of testing results, and quarantining infected individuals.[74] Uganda, by contrast, had managed to contain AIDS by actually transforming the country's sexual practices. Cleaving to the "ABC" program ("Abstain, Be faithful, wear a Condom"), the country had promoted the values of monogamy, deferred sexual activity, and "zero grazing." By 2000, the percentage of Ugandan women reporting multiple partners over the previous year had fallen from 8.4 to 2.5, and the HIV infection rate among adult women had fallen from 21.2 percent to 6.2.[75]

The large-scale rejection of condom usage in the nonindustrialized world, even in the midst of catastrophic infection and death rates, suggested that the cost of condom usage was actually much higher than most health planners wished to admit. Whether symbolically emasculating men, or simply robbing both partners of substantial levels of sexual pleasure, condoms were deceptively abhorrent to much of the world.[76] The fact that two of the three nations most successful in reducing AIDS transmission had done so without relying on increased condom usage indicated to public health professionals that condoms should be discarded as the preferred method of fighting AIDS. Increasing state policing powers, or redefining the terms of acceptable sexual engagement, had actually proven easier than getting men to wear condoms. The condom, it seemed, was not the answer.

INTELLECTUAL PROPERTY

In January 2001, Tina Rosenberg, an investigative journalist who had won a MacArthur "genius" grant for her reporting on revolutionary movements in Latin America, wrote a lengthy article for the *New York Times Magazine* urging Western governments to cease defending patent rights for production of antiretroviral drugs so that the millions of infected people living in third-world countries could have some chance of purchasing the drugs. Citing the example of Brazil, which had successfully lowered its AIDS death rate by manufacturing generic versions of the drugs, Rosenberg urged the world to violate patent protections, facilitate the manufacture of off-brand drugs, and fund the distribution of these drugs to all poor nations afflicted with substantial AIDS epidemics. In powerful language she condemned resistance to this idea as fundamentally immoral:

> Brazil is showing that no one who dies of AIDS dies of natural causes. Those who die have been failed—by feckless leaders who see weapons as more alluring purchases than medicines, by wealthy countries (notably the United States) that have threatened the livelihood of poor nations who seek to manufacture cheap medicine, and by the multinational drug companies who have kept the price of antiretroviral drugs needlessly out of reach of the vast majority of the world's population.[77]

By 2001, Brazil was manufacturing a year's supply of triple therapy for $3,000, and hoped to reduce the price by two-thirds within a few years' time. In Senegal, wealthy individuals could purchase a year's supply for $1,000, and India was working toward producing a year's supply for $700. But by standards of international intellectual property law, virtually all of these drugs were illegal.

Pharmaceuticals developed by Western drug companies were protected by patents of 20 years, at which point they were available to the general public to be copied by whomever wished to do so. In an effort to amortize the cost of researching and developing a new drug, as well as the hundreds of drugs that failed to pass FDA testing, drug companies priced the drugs far above the cost of manufacturing—sometimes several thousand percent over. Since the market share of the branded drug could decrease by 90 percent once patent protection ended, the companies worked to maximize profit during this 20-year window, through aggressive marketing and high pricing.

Drug companies priced drugs differently depending on their targeted markets. Drugs sold in the United States, where competing private insurance plans were willing and able to pay exorbitant prices, were priced at one level. Those sold in Canada, Western Europe, and Japan—wealthy countries with national health insurance systems—were priced at a middle level in deference to the market pressure exerted by the national payers. And those sold in nonindustrialized countries were sold for even less.

Drug companies, not surprisingly, fought the effort to circumvent their patents. Convinced that breaches in intellectual property protection in certain countries might lead to widespread flouting of patent conventions, pharmaceutical executives tried to undermine the piracy movement by repricing their drugs, agreeing in Geneva in 2000 to reduce the wholesale price of HIV drugs by 70 percent.[78] Under such a plan, a year's supply of combination therapy might drop from the current $18,000 per year in the United States to as little as $1,000 per year for central and southern Africa.[79] Further, drug companies argued that nearly 80 percent of AIDS-drug-related patents were not even registered in Africa, as the companies that owned the patents had simply not found the effort to register the molecules worth their while.

But the lowest prices for combination therapy were still well beyond the reach of most poor Africans, even aided with levels of foreign hand-outs. By one estimate, if combination therapy for Africa was priced at $1,000 per patient per year, the total annual bill for the continent would be $3 billion—10 times the total annual public drug budget of South Africa, the region's dominant economic power.[80] While Rosenberg argued against the preservation of intellectual property rights in a time of international crisis, the property rights were not the greatest barriers to drug distribution. Rather, the region's poverty was so extreme as to negate even magnanimous actions by corporate pharmaceutical makers and eleemosynary efforts by international aid agencies.

It was in India, rather, where incomes and the national budget were adequate to exploit inexpensive generic AIDS drugs, but not so ample as to be able to pay Western prices for the branded ones, that the debate became more consequential. One large generic Indian drug maker, Cipla, claimed that it could produce an annual course of combination therapy for as little as $600. In response (and at the urging of the World Health Organization), the five largest AIDS drugs makers—GlaxoSmithKline, Merck, Hoffman-La Roche, Boehringer, and Bristol-Myers Squibb—agreed to offer their drugs to African nations for little more than cost. Glaxo, for example, agreed to sell a day's dose of Combivir in Africa for $2 (versus $17 in the United States).[81]

The ethical issues involved were deceptively complex. Although to some observers the choice seemed stark and clear—wealthy shareholders enriching themselves at the expense of millions of people dying unnecessarily—this was hardly the case.[82] People would invest neither their time nor resources into creating anew if they were not confident of ultimate ownership of their creations. The mass migration of highly trained and gifted engineers and scientists from third- to first-world nations exemplified the desire of most people to capitalize on their creative powers, rather than simply donate them to the common good. A society that failed to reasonably guarantee property rights would quickly lose investment capital—both financial and intellectual.[83]

Pharmaceutical companies exploited the profits from successful drugs to fund their research operations. As only very few experimental molecules ultimately became marketable drugs—as few as 1 in a 1,000—drug companies were compelled to maximize revenues on those drugs that ultimately proved profitable. Of the generic producers, Andrew Sullivan wrote derisively, "They're the Napsters of the world—only worse, because they charge for what they steal rather than give it away for free."[84] For the mainline companies the calculus was simple: the world needed to guarantee patent protection or cease benefiting from any new drugs coming from applied pharmaceutical research. The *Wall Street Journal* opined dryly, "Needless to say, the prospect of widespread intellectual property seizure will not encourage further research on the fast-mutating HIV virus."[85]

Few nations heeded Rosenberg's call to disregard patents already registered, but the message succeeded in drawing attention to the scarcity of drugs throughout the developing world. Whereas prior to 2001 most donor nations had concentrated their efforts on education and condom awareness, in the aftermath several governments and nonprofits committed themselves to trying to fund the drugs themselves. Doctors Without Borders began treating Africans with combination therapy for free in 2001, and several large mining concerns at the same time agreed to provide combination therapy to infected employees. At the same time, the Bill and Melinda Gates Foundation pledged $100 million to fighting AIDS in Africa, much of which would go to purchasing medicine. These efforts, coupled with international governmental funds totaling nearly $1 billion that year, purchased substantial amounts of the drug therapy, particularly at the reduced prices now being charged by pharmaceutical companies for their products in Africa and Southeast Asia. By 2003, double the number of Africans were on combination therapy as had been two years before, and the trend was accelerating.[86] By that time, too, Brazil claimed that every AIDS patient in the country who was deemed medically appropriate was being treated with combination therapy.[87]

Even infinite amounts of money would not completely solve the problem, however. The drugs remained highly toxic, commonly causing diarrhea, nausea, liver failure, and pancreatic damage. As many as 20 percent of patients who began the drug treatment found that they could not tolerate it. Compliance with the treatment plan was probably no higher than 80 percent, and that was in wealthy developed nations where patients could easily refrigerate the drugs and take them on schedule with appropriate doses of food and drink. New resistant strains of the virus were constantly evolving, and the expected lower compliance rates in Africa would only accelerate this process. And distribution in a continent that measured its paved roads by the hundreds of miles, rather than by the thousands, in which railroads, modern highways, private automobiles, and electric power were all scarce or nonexistent, and in which cultural and linguistic norms were inconsistent with modern medicine, was sure to be difficult.[88]

INTERNATIONAL AID

The cost of combination therapy dropped precipitously in poorer countries between 2000 and 2003, from $18,000 to as low as $700 in certain African countries where the major drug companies had begun to distribute drugs at cost, or even at a loss. Some international health planners speculated that the cost of the drugs in central Africa might drop to as low as $350 per person per year. But even at these prices, the total cost of treating all affected individuals was immense, and far beyond the budgetary resources of the worst-afflicted countries. In 2001, the United Nations produced an extremely rough estimate for the cost of treating all AIDS patients worldwide who were presently beyond the reach of Western medicine—between $7 billion and $10 billion—a number so vast that it dwarfed the current foreign aid commitments of the industrialized nations.[89]

At the time, foreign aid commitments varied broadly. The United States had committed $330 million, the United Kingdom $200 million, and minuscule Norway and Canada had pledged $110 million and $73 million, respectively.[90] From there national commitments declined quickly. Sweden had committed $60 million, Nigeria $10 million, and other countries far less.[91] By 2001, the total annual foreign aid coming into Africa, to choose one heavily infected region, was approximately $250 million to treat some 4 million new AIDS cases annually. By contrast, at that time the United States was spending nearly $1 billion per year in government funds on AIDS at home to treat one-tenth the number of new cases annually.[92]

Proponents of greater U.S. funding pointed out that the United States' annual commitment to fighting AIDS in the third world amounted to about one one-thousandth of the annual Pentagon budget, and that on a per capita basis the United States trailed the largesse of most European countries, including even Portugal.[93] Solomon Benatar, a professor at the University of Cape Town, in South Africa, implored Western nations to donate more, lest they miss the opportunity to thwart an evil on a par with the slave trade and apartheid. He wrote in February 2000, "If there are any lessons to be learned from the past, the incredible lightness of moral blindness is surely one."[94] One savvy reporter pointed out that South Africa's budget for fighting AIDS was only $13 million, when its annual budget for military acquisitions was $6.5 billion, "including three German submarines for a navy that faces no threat."[95] And Robert Borosage, founder of the Campaign for America's Future, wrote with disgust: "If there were a way to strafe or bomb AIDS, we'd be there. But we don't do plagues."[96]

By 2002, the world was beginning to respond. Professor Jeffrey Sachs, director of Columbia University's Earth Institute, and one of the most visible and widely recognized economists anywhere, had begun to campaign aggressively for substantial increases in donations from Western to poor countries, whether to alleviate poverty, fund investment, or help in treating AIDS. Mainstream foreign policy analysts, often skeptical of the value of foreign aid to third-world development, began to appreciate that AIDS was a problem that countries could not be held accountable for, and that required massive handouts and donations, pure and simple. "It's simply the right thing to do," insisted the editorial staff of London's politically moderate *Economist* newsmagazine. "A colossal number of lives could be saved, and immeasurable suffering relieved, for about $25 per rich-country citizen each year."[97] Sachs argued for deploying "weapons of mass salvation," a jab at the United States's search for weapons of mass destruction in Iraq.[98]

Money began to flow the following year. President George W. Bush pledged $15 billion to fighting global AIDS over 10 years, while Bill Gates pledged $100 million from his foundation to fighting AIDS in India, with more to come for Africa and beyond.[99] Money was promised from Nelson Mandela's Children's Fund, the Diana, Princess of Wales Memorial Fund, and from MTV, which pledged all proceeds from its AIDS Awareness Concert heard by possibly 2 billion people.[100] Commitments came from Levi Strauss, the Paul Allen Charitable Foundation, Youth AIDS, and Doctors Without Borders. Bill Clinton had agreed to chair the International AIDS Trust with Nelson Mandela, after donations had fallen off in the wake of the terrorist attacks of September 11, 2001. "We cannot call a cease-fire when the killing continues," he remarked about the continuing need to fight AIDS, even in the midst of the War on Terror.[101]

The Gates Foundation led all other foundations by a wide margin. Endowed with over $25 billion, the foundation had already pledged $25 million to Harvard for public health research on AIDS, $50 million to Botswana, and $100 million to India.[102] As the decade progressed, Bill Gates himself elevated AIDS relief, along with third-world medical care in general, to a privileged place in his foundation's work, and worked to inform himself on the challenges facing prophylaxis, treatment programs, vaccine development, and third-world development in general. Given a personal fortune exceeding the entire annual Indian government budget, his potential to spur change was immense.

NEW HORIZONS

AIDS was spreading. India, the world's second largest nation in population had the world's second largest AIDS epidemic by 2001, after central Africa. Over half of the sex workers in Bombay were infected, as were a third of people with sexually transmitted diseases, and 2.5 percent of women in prenatal clinics.[103] Of the 4 million infected, nearly 70 percent were women, leading public health workers to suspect a similar transmission pattern as that found in Africa. Married men from rural areas were patronizing prostitutes in the nation's cities and bringing home the virus to their unsuspecting wives. And as in Africa, the women dared not complain or even report their concerns for fear of stigma and ostracism. "If you want to stay in your village, don't tell anybody," counseled one infected woman from a small village near Chennai.[104]

China had a surging epidemic. After years of official denial, the government admitted in 2001 that at least 600,000 Chinese were infected with HIV, and that the country could have 10 million AIDS cases by 2010 if the virus's spread was not stymied.[105] Described by one medical writer as a "rumbling volcano," the Chinese epidemic differed markedly from the African and Southeast Asian epidemics in that it did not seem to be spread primarily through sexual contact.[106] Rather, IV drug use appeared to be the primary culprit, accounting for up to 70 percent of all cases, with prostitutes appearing to be only a secondary nexus of the disease. In the major cities, if public health records were to be believed, fewer than 10 percent of prostitutes were testing positive by 2002, as compared with 70 to 90 percent in major cities of other heavily affected nonindustrial countries.[107]

Although China admitted to a few sexually transmitted cases of AIDS in the mid-1980s, the epidemic's spread into the country accelerated in the late 1980s as IV drug users in the provinces abutting Myanmar, Laos, and Vietnam began to test positive. Yunan Province, in particular, appeared to be the jumping-off point for the disease, much as Bangkok had been in Thailand and Port-au-Prince had been in North America. While the Communist government had been able to substantially reduce prostitution in China in the 1950s, it had been unable, or unwilling, to stem heroin use, and the behavior had been quasi-sanctioned for decades. Now it proved to be the entry point for the disease that China had theretofore been able to avoid. By 2001, 70 percent of IV users in the province were infected with HIV, and users in other provinces were close behind.[108]

The Chinese accelerated the spread of their epidemic through the practice of collective blood donations, in which dozens, or even hundreds, of people in a town or village donated blood, and were then reinjected with the collective plasma after the corpuscles and leukocytes had been filtered out. The practice allowed one donor to infect an entire village—in one incident 400 people became infected in an afternoon.[109] And even when blood pooling was not practiced, blood donors contracted the disease when unsterilized equipment was used to draw blood. Given the widespread practice of selling blood (the *Economist* described it as "something of an industry," and commercial blood-buyers were a common feature of rural villages), the infection could spread through both city and village with scarcely a sexual vector present.[110]

But most ominous was the growing epidemic in the former Soviet Union. Numbers were wholly inaccurate. As late as 1994, Russia reported only 136 AIDS cases, and the Ukraine only 27.[111] But by 2000, Russia reported 80,000 registered cases of HIV infection, and most public health experts suspected that the true number was at least 10 times higher.[112] A United Nations team estimated 75,000 new HIV infections in Russia in 2001 alone, which represented a 1,500 percent increase over 3 years. Ukraine reported 1 percent of its population to be infected, which theoretically made it the most heavily infected of the ex-Soviet republics. In truth, virtually no one knew the real numbers.[113]

The ex-Soviet epidemic was closely tied both to the disintegration of social order in the wake of the breakup of the Soviet Union and to the general anarchy and lawlessness that had descended upon Afghanistan following withdrawal of Soviet troops from that country in the late 1980s. To finance their continuing campaigns, warring tribal leaders in Afghanistan had turned to the sale of heroin, which had been distributed through Russia and eastern Europe en route to its final destination in Amsterdam and other Western European cities. Along the way, the drug found demand amid the chaos and unemployment of ex-Soviet states.[114] By 2000, inflation in Russia exceeded 20 percent annually, unemployment approached 10 percent, and the percentage of the population living below poverty approached 40 percent. The combined stresses on the population pushed Russians from their traditional drug—vodka—to the newly available highly refined heroin being produced nearby.[115]

Initially the Russian epidemic appeared to be almost exclusively spread through IV drug use—"There could be no AIDS because Russian people had no sex," one observer quipped.[116] By 2001, for example, only 1 percent of sexually active Russian adults were infected with HIV according to the best estimates available, compared with 20–30 percent in the worst-hit African countries. By contrast, IV drug users throughout the country tested positive for HIV at extremely high rates: in Moscow, Saint Petersburg, Irkutsk, and even Temirtau in central Kazakhstan, between 50 and 80 percent of tested IV drug users were infected.[117] All statistics pointed to 90 percent of the Russian and Soviet satellite epidemics being spread through needle use.

But general social disintegration and rising prostitution rates promised to expand the epidemic into the non-drug-using population as well. By 2001, public health indicators pointed to a society in crisis on multiple fronts: healthwise, economically, morally, and socially. Hepatitis

A, B, and C were spreading rapidly through the population by contaminated water and food supplies, sex, and needles. "Hepatitis is really everywhere. It's like the common cold," Evgeny Bocharov, an infectious-disease specialist noted.[118] Only 60 percent of Russian children were vaccinated against polio by age 2.[119] Masha Gessen, a Moscow-based writer, urged the nation to admit that it had a "third-world style crisis," and to "swallow its pride" and learn from African nations.[120] The health-care system had been deeply weakened by progressive budget cuts (most Russian doctors' incomes barely surpassed the poverty line). Alcoholism rates approached 30 percent, life expectancy had declined by 15 years from a decade earlier, birth rates were the lowest in the world, and the population was shrinking rapidly. By 2050, the country would be only half the size that it had been at the time of the breakup of the Soviet Union, and this was assuming that AIDS did not make continued inroads into the population.

Russians used a variety of drugs, but the newest insidious substance was hymka, an inexpensive injectable liquid opiate that was quickly gaining adherents across the country. At the same time, prostitution was increasing in the wake of widespread economic dislocation, and AIDS was beginning to spread into the sex industry. Traditional Russian bathhouses were doubling as brothels in many cities, and condom awareness was years behind the West. In Kalingrad, illegal commerce, organized crime, rampant prostitution, and drug transit combined to create the densest concentration of HIV infection in the world.[121] One Russian medical researcher described the situation: "It's as if we're standing on the beach watching a giant wave coming right at us. We know it, we see it, and we can do almost nothing about it. We're just going to get swept away."[122]

Other countries were not far behind. In Nepal, Iran, Indonesia, Myanmar, and Cambodia, tests of IV drugs users, or sex workers, or prisoners registered infection rates of 10 to 50 percent.[123] Indian truck drivers, similar to their African counterparts, engaged in extramarital sex at high rates with the ubiquitous prostitutes along their routes.[124] In Cambodia, to the consternation of officials, outside public health experts estimated the adult infection rate at 14 percent. Brazil, a country that had moved to aggressively treat AIDS patients with inexpensive generic antiretroviral drugs, hosted 100,000 cases of either AIDS or

HIV infection by 2001 and continued to record new infections at the rate of 14 per 100,000 annually.[125] And in Romania, Nicolai Ceauşescu's horrific legacy of despotism and savagery lived on in the epidemic of AIDS among the nation's orphans. Consigned to orphanages because of poverty or legal strictures on reproduction, the children, mostly girls, had been routinely given micro–blood transfusions in an effort to strengthen them. The procedures, performed with unsterilized equipment, had infected as many as a third of all babies in some of the orphanages. Now they were dying, and the impoverished medical system could do little.[126]

VACCINE

All along, scientists had engaged in efforts to produce a consistently workable vaccine. For most infectious diseases, among them polio, smallpox, rubella, pertussis, and measles, vaccines had proven to be the ultimate form of treatment. A successful vaccine was cheap, reliable, long-lasting, and relatively devoid of side effects. A good one could permanently rid the world of an infectious scourge, end the need for expensive medical or hospital-based interventions, and save the world countless billions of dollars in treatment costs and lost productivity. A vaccine was the holy grail for AIDS researchers, and drew $350 million of United States government support annually by 2002.[127]

Work toward developing an AIDS vaccine was hampered, however, by the general unwillingness of large pharmaceutical companies to direct their research labs at the problem. This was the result of the strange economics of AIDS; vaccines were not a particularly attractive project for for-profit firms because the countries with the greatest need for the vaccines were those least able to afford them. By contrast, no Western country hosted a high enough HIV infection rate to justify mass vaccination of the population. Moreover, combination therapy for AIDS patients in Western nations had proven to be lucrative to drug companies, providing a strong disincentive to develop a vaccine. Generally, "Big Pharm" refused to invest heavily in the vaccine effort.[128]

A few smaller companies did direct resources at vaccine development. A small genetic engineering firm, Tanox, was testing a potential vaccine in FDA phase II trials by 2002, and a half-dozen others were in phase I trials with experimental molecules.[129] Most promising was AIDSVax, at the time in phase I trials.[130] The drug replicated the gp120 protein on the T cells, and could potentially stimulate the immune systems to create antibodies that would bind to the proteins, thus blocking HIV from binding in place.[131] Although far from perfect, and diverging from the preferred vaccine model of a live-attenuated virus, AIDSVax appeared to be effective in 40 percent of patients.[132]

Forty percent efficacy was low for a vaccine, but seemed the most researchers could realistically hope for, given the hyperadaptive capabilities of HIV and the multiple forms in which it existed. But a vaccine effective less than half the time it was used against a disease nearly 100 percent fatal raised troubling ethical questions. For one, should it be used at all? AIDS, after all, was in theory a highly preventable disease. Researchers who favored mass education and shifts in cultural attitudes toward promiscuity and unprotected sex feared that widespread use of a semieffective vaccine might actually accelerate the epidemic's spread. Vaccinated individuals, thinking themselves safe from infection, might engage in dangerous practices placing themselves at higher risk for exposure. Newer, more virulent forms of AIDS further imperiled an only partially protected populace.[133] Observing these barriers to vaccine development, physician and writer Charles Krauthammer had asked in 1997, "Why embark on a huge national venture to create a vaccine for a disease that is already extraordinarily preventable?"[134]

Moreover, how did you ethically recruit the necessary controls to trials of AIDS vaccines? If you recruited 1,000 individuals and placed them on placebos, would you fool them into thinking that they were inoculated against the virus, and thus encourage them to engage in risky behavior? Scientists and physicians who oversaw clinical trials took pains to warn their subjects that they might be receiving a placebo, and that even if they were receiving a vaccine it might be ineffective, yet they worried nonetheless. Past data on research methodology suggested that people involved in studies disproportionately believed themselves to be on the drug, rather than on the placebo, and the return to risky behavior by gay men in the United States in the late 1990s suggested that safe-sex practices were adhered to in direct proportion to the level of jeopardy that people felt themselves to be in.

Moreover, what was the role of combination therapy within the process of clinical testing for vaccines? Clearly you could not demand that an HIV-infected individual refrain from using combination therapy, yet without doing so the trials were useless. Facing this odd ethical conundrum, drug companies were forced to turn to Africa (and to a lesser extent, Asia) for research subjects, which raised troubling questions regarding appropriate use of economically vulnerable populations to such ends. For some ethicists and policy analysts, such testing recalled the infamous Tuskegee experiment in which rural black syphilis patients in the American South were left untreated by public health physicians for decades after the development of effective antibiotics.[135] Other ethicists considered the alternatives—a total cessation of vaccine developments—and decided that compromises in the protocols were morally justified.

In the end, however, most experts on health in developing nations understood that a vaccine was the only potential long-term solution. Despite the development of new antiretroviral drugs, combination therapy remained too expensive for nonindustrialized nations, even when made available in generic form at cost. Logistical barriers such as poor roads, lack of electricity, poorly developed distribution networks, cultural aversion to Western medicine, and illiteracy all suggested that combination therapy would never be able to reach more than a small fraction of infected people in the third world. Rather, a simple, reliable, long-acting, robust vaccination, available in injectable or oral form, was the only possible solution to the international AIDS pandemic. With 50 million people infected worldwide by 2003, and potentially enormous epidemics just beginning in Russia, India, Pakistan, and China, the best that Western medicine had to offer was simply not good enough. Seth Berkley, director of the International AIDS Vaccine Initiative, stated in 2003: "You have to ask yourself what on earth the people on this planet are doing. If you stand back and think about what the world will look like a hundred years from now, and you look at even the most conservative numbers, you will see that in the end only a vaccine will matter. Nothing else."[136]

EPILOGUE

Like most natural disasters, AIDS teaches no obvious lessons and lends itself to no glaring moral pronouncements. Arising from chance genetic mutation, a virus came into being that was uniquely adapted to evade the myriad defenses created by the world's medical scientists. That it did, and continues to do so, has had tragic consequences. That we humans, the target of the virus, may have mishandled certain aspects of countering the disease, compels us to reflect.

A disease as ferocious as AIDS feels intentional; a fair and just world does not simply visit a lethal scourge on millions of innocent victims without an accompanying message. From the epidemic's beginning, many observers of the disease have sought that message, finding clues in biblical prophecy, moral paradigm, natural law, and common decency. Gays brought it upon themselves through their own obscene behavior; drug users invited death by mocking life; Africans refused to conform to the norms of Western monogamy; the world turned a silent ear to the suffering, the marginal, the weak, the black, the gay, the poor, the "other." AIDS demonstrates our own fundamental inhumanity; AIDS defines a world in which we refuse to take essential responsibility for our fellow human beings; AIDS is what happens when people refuse to care—about themselves, their lovers, their friends, their compatriots, their fellow denizens of the earth. AIDS is God's revenge.

Such sweeping condemnations are unhelpful. AIDS results from a simple virus—a strand of RNA inside a crystalline protein coat. The virus, one of millions that have evolved since life began on this earth, is without consciousness, intentionality, or meaning. It simply is, as are we. That our biological niches overlap and clash has no moral meaning, any more than does Dutch elm disease, or maggots feasting on a carcass, or red tide blooming in the ocean. Nature is vast and complex, forming and shaping new species and continuously redefining the biological space in which life flourishes. AIDS has hardly threatened us; there are nearly a billion more people alive today than there were when AIDS first presented itself a quarter century ago. If this is the Noahide flood that will be our ultimate undoing, we've survived handsomely.

But if AIDS is not moral, it is certainly political. From its onset, the disease has invited abuse and exploitation for political gain, whether from conservatives who labored to portray it as divine intervention, or from liberals who used it to illustrate the necessary primacy of civil rights. It is important to note that much of the politicization came to naught. For all the opprobrium wrought by conservatives, conservative-minded governments repeatedly enacted generous research budgets, aggressive public health measures, and daringly candid information campaigns. Likewise, for all the fears articulated by liberals regarding sanctity of privacy, abrogation of civil rights, and general demonization of AIDS victims, the rights and privileges of AIDS patients have rarely been violated. In the United States, at least, people have left most AIDS victims blessedly alone, to suffer or heal in privacy. That they may seek to avoid the afflicted is not unexpected.

But in a few areas, both domestic and abroad, AIDS politics have seriously hindered efforts to fight the disease, or have accelerated its spread, or have made more miserable the lives (and deaths) of its victims. In the United States, for example, gay opposition to bathhouse closures in the early 1980s delayed health agencies from taking this significant step toward limiting the epidemic's spread. While interested men could have found alternate locations for anonymous sex, maintaining the bathhouses facilitated the liaisons, and thus forestalled efforts at containing the epidemic. On the other hand, once gay organizers recognized the extent of the tragedy in their midst, they created highly effective community organizations targeting AIDS education, fund-raising, and treatment. Gays, in many ways, were both their own best friends and worst enemies.

Liberal public health officers and medical professionals similarly po-liticized the epidemic in insisting from the mid-1980s on that this was a disease of all, and that the nation as a whole needed to change its ways. In fact, readily available statistics always showed unambiguously that this was a highly contained epidemic of a few—gay men and IV drug users and their partners. Furthermore, from an early point in the epi-demic, Nancy Padian's research demonstrated that the virus simply did not transmit effectively in heterosexual intercourse between healthy adults, particularly from women to men. Portraying the disease as a threat to all Americans was a highly politicized exercise in wishful thinking, done in part to spur congressional generosity in research funds, in part to win the sympathy of Americans, in part to protect gays from stigma, and in part to get Americans to take seriously whatever modest threat might actually confront them. Ultimately, however, the policy may have backfired, as monogamous and generally law-abiding Americans resented the conflation of themselves with the drug using and the promiscuous. Michael Fumento's prolonged philippic on the "myth of heterosexual AIDS" was more than anything a protest against having marginal and extreme practices projected onto himself and most other Americans.

Conservative moralizers who attacked AIDS victims as deserving their ignoble end in payment for immoral lives were odious. In sub-scribing to their point of view, they bound themselves to a history of theologians, preachers, and prophets who viewed disease as God's re-venge, whether Miriam's leprosy or King George's madness. On the other hand, their message was received in part because they correctly apportioned some of the blame for contracting AIDS to the victims themselves. People who slept with hundreds of lovers may not have been special targets of a vindictive God, but they were engaging in just the sort of recklessness that tended to bring misfortune. Even before AIDS, promiscuous gay men contracted sexually transmitted diseases and bowel ailments at high rates. While some took such ailments as warn-ing signs of excess, most ignored them and continued in their solipsistic ways. Similarly, injecting narcotics is simply one of the most self-destructive actions a body can partake in. Those who did so may not necessarily have *deserved* their premature deaths (in a moral sense), but they were certainly flouting sensible and safe conventions in total disregard of prudence, health, and self-preservation. People who placed such little value on their own health and well-being were hardly being punished by AIDS, but perhaps they were experiencing the fruits of lives poorly lived.

The disease was less politicized abroad, yet was far worse. With the exception of a bizarrely recalcitrant South African government, most governments accepted the words and advice of well-meaning international health advisers and public health experts while doing little. At times they denied the extent of the epidemic in their midst, but generally these lies did little to worsen the sickness or accelerate transmission. (An important exception was the Chinese government's continued endorsement of mixing of blood products while denying the existence of an AIDS outbreak in its rural western villages, needlessly killing tens of thousands of people.) The epidemic in the third world, rather, was one born largely of misogyny and archaic social norms.

In both Africa and the Far East AIDS was a disease of the sex trade. In both places the main vector of transmission was prostitution, although in both places the epidemic could not have thrived without a helpful push from either narcotics use (in Asia) or preexisting genital sores (in Africa). Moreover, in both areas the role of promiscuity, polygamy, and what Westerners called adultery, was so ingrained in society that even the most well-intentioned governments could do little to stem the epidemic. Indeed, in all of the third world, only Thailand and Uganda could really claim substantial success in fighting AIDS by 2002, and Thailand achieved the success through condom use. Uganda alone proved itself capable at lowering promiscuity, and even there the monogamy campaign reduced AIDS deaths by no more than one-third from initial projections.

Many AIDS experts have declared a vaccine the only answer. In the decade since combination therapy became available in the West, it has not been greatly improved on, nor has it shown itself to be a promising intervention for any but the richest countries (although Brazil and India have demonstrated the efficacy of concerted campaigns with counterfeited or generic drugs). In the absence of social change, virtually all of central and south Africa, much of central and eastern Asia, and Russia and Ukraine will remain mired in the epidemic's grip. While the epidemic may level out (it seems to have finally slowed its growth in central Africa, and in no country has it infected more than 35 percent of the population), it will remain a huge scourge on humanity long into the future, robbing families of their loved ones, communities of valued citizens, and the land of possibly a third of its populace.

But if a vaccine is one answer, women's education is the second. Throughout the third world, promiscuity and adultery are coupled with female illiteracy, and in fact are tolerated mostly by women who have no choice in the matter. Women who are educated are better able to care for their health, better able to provide for themselves, and better able to resist the malignant actions of those who claim to love them. In both the United States and abroad, women who contract AIDS are most often one step removed from the initial foray into irresponsibility—they are the partners of the drug users in the United States, the wives of the sexual dalliers in Africa. The exceptions, of course, are the prostitutes themselves, but here again the infected women appear to be more agents of male malfeasance than active participants in their own demise. Whether northern Thai girls all but forced into teenage prostitution, or Russian prostitutes fleeing to Turkey and South Africa in an effort to escape poverty and starvation, women choose prostitution as the least horrible of a variety of bad choices. Social norms, themselves, are the culprit, coupled with illiteracy, ignorance, and subservience.

The West faces a conundrum. Having essentially solved its own AIDS problem, it now faces a humanitarian disaster produced largely by the countries in question. AIDS has become a uniquely third-world disaster, stemming from preindustrial social and sexual norms, in which marriage, monogamy, and sex education are deemphasized and sexual expression is valued. While the West can provide money and medicine, and perhaps some unwanted advice, it cannot change whole societies. These must change on their own, and all evidence points to the process being slow and attenuated. At best, the West can lead by example, demonstrating to the third world the advantages of gender equity, universal literacy, and mandatory education.

Outside of Africa, signs are more hopeful. The insidious Russian

AIDS epidemic is born of poverty rather than misogyny, and can thus be relieved by employment, investment, and growth. While the ex–Soviet Union is largely a mess of aging demographics, organized crime, corruption, and alcoholism, its economies are growing and several of its governments are progressing toward democracy. AIDS there is a result of aberrant social conditions, which may be relieved in the relatively near future. The West may have a role to play, but only upon first eliciting promises and covenants for government reform, fiscal prudence, and sound public health policies.

Asia, too, gives evidence of being able to solve its own problem. Growing literacy rates and general comfort with sexuality will facilitate condom education (as demonstrated by Thailand), testing of prostitutes, and measured attitudes toward adultery. Although data are not yet firm, it is quite possible that east Asia's epidemic will come to resemble that of the West, firmly enmeshed in the society's drug-using castoffs and impoverished streetwalkers, but largely absent elsewhere. Moreover, the region's economic growth portends widespread use of Western-style combination therapies, so that AIDS for Asia may become a manageable chronic disease while constantly killing relatively small numbers of the most marginal of its citizens.

The West can do little. AIDS is strangely preventable, yet stubbornly resistant to modern medical intervention. The virus has proven itself a formidable foe, evading vaccines and antidotes, while mocking our own imprudence, and self-indulgence. It has exposed much of what is worst in human nature, while giving us little opportunity to shine. It is a mirror that selectively reflects our ugliest warts and deepest weaknesses.

ABBREVIATIONS USED IN NOTES

Publications

AJPH   *American Journal of Pubic Health*
BG   *Boston Globe*
JAMA   *Journal of the American Medical Association*
LAT   *Los Angeles Times*
NEJM   *New England Journal of Medicine*
NYT   *New York Times*
PHR   *Public Health Reports*
TNR   *The New Republic*
WP   *Washington Post*

Manuscript Collections

AB   Ann Brock papers (Bush Library)
CA   Cliff Alderman papers (Bush Library)
CEA   Council on Economic Advisors files (Bush Library)
COS   Chief of Staff files (Bush Library)
DC   Daniel Casse papers (Bush Library)
DM   Donald MacDonald papers (Reagan Library)
DPC   Domestic Policy Council files (Bush Library)
GB   Gary Bauer papers (Reagan Library)
JB   Jean Becker papers (Bush Library)
JC   Julie Cooke papers (Bush Library)
JK   Johannes Kuttner papers (Bush Library)
JL   Jay Lefkowitz papers (Bush Library)
JR   James Renne papers (Bush Library)
JS   John Sununu papers (Bush Library)

JW	James Warner papers (Reagan Library)
KC	Kenneth Cribb papers (Reagan Library)
KS	Kathy Steffy papers (Bush Library)
NCAIDS	National Commission on AIDS files (Archives II, RG 220)
OCA	Office of Cabinet Affairs files (Bush Library)
OFL	Office of the First Lady (Bush Library)
OIA	Office of Intergovernmental Affairs files (Bush Library)
OLA	Office of Legislative Affairs files (Bush Library)
OPD	Office of Policy Development files (Bush Library)
PPI	National Commission on AIDS: Public Policy Issues (Archives II, RG 220)
RB	Richard Breeden papers (Bush Library)
RP	Robert Pastorino papers (Reagan Library)
RS	Robert Sweet papers (Reagan Library)
RS2	Richard Schmalensee papers (Bush Library)
RS-WGHPA	Papers of the Working Group on Health Policy: AIDS (Reagan Library)
SD	Stephanie Dunce papers (Bush Library)
T&S	Testimony and Statements files, NCAIDS papers (Archives II, RG 220)
WE	Will Eagle papers (Bush Library)

[NOTES]

Prologue

1. For general discussion of the simian roots of HIV, see Barry Schoub, *AIDS and HIV in Perspective: A Guide to Understanding the Virus and Its Consequences,* 2nd ed. (New York: Cambridge University Press, 1994), pp. 12–17, as well as Jared Diamond, "The Mysterious Origin of AIDS," *Natural History,* 9/92, pp. 25–29. Primary work in genetic tracing, which supports this hypothesis, has been presented in Feng Gao, et al., "Chimpanzees as Original Source for HIV," *JAMA,* 1/19/00, v. 283, p. 310; and Joan Stephenson, "HIV's Origins Traced to 1930s," *JAMA,* 3/8/00, v. 283, p. 1279. For reports on geneticist Beatrice Hahn's early dating work, see D. Christensen, "AIDS Virus Jumped from Chimps," *Science News,* 2/6/99, 155:6, p. 84; and Alice Park, "When Did AIDS Begin?" *Time Atlantic,* 2/21/00, 155:7, p. 60.

2. For an interesting discussion on the species leap from monkey to humans, see Diamond, "Mysterious Origin of AIDS," pp. 25–29.

3. In fact, viral transmission from monkey to man had probably occurred multiple times over the preceding several thousand years in several different mutations, but the epidemic didn't "take" until the 20th century. See the interview with Beatrice Hahn in Richard Kno, "HIV Origin Is Traced to Chimps: Researchers Track Virus to West African Subspecies," *BG,* 2/1/99, p. A3.

4. For a more detailed discussion, See Barry Schoub, *AIDS and HIV in Perspective* (New York: Cambridge University Press, 1994), pp. 12–17. Schoub considers the Hooper thesis regarding infected polio vaccine and ultimately dismisses it.

5. Simon Garfield, *The End of Innocence: Britain in the Time of AIDS* (London: Faber and Faber, 1994), pp. 3–7.

6. See Kno, "HIV Origin Is Traced to Chimps."

7. Gina Kolata, "Boy's 1969 Death Suggests AIDS Invaded U.S. Several Times," *NYT,* 10/28/87, p. A15.

8. I.C. Bygberg, "AIDS in a Danish Surgeon (Zaire, 1976)," *The Lancet,* 4/23/83, p. 925.

9. "Former Nun Got AIDS in Haiti, Doctors Find," *NYT,* 9/17/83, p. A7.

10. Robert Biggar, Philip Nasca, and William Burnett, "AIDS-Related Kaposi's Sarcoma in New York City in 1977," *NEJM,* 1/28/88, 318:4, p. 252; see also the case of Donald Lombardo, a gay New York man who probably contracted AIDS sometime before 1977, as described in Edward Hooper, *The River: A Journey to the Source of HIV and AIDS* (Boston: Little, Brown, and Company, 1999), pp. 58–59.

11. David Huminer, Joseph Rosenfeld, and Silvio Pitlik, "AIDS in the Pre-AIDS Era," *Review of Infectious Diseases,* 11–12/87, 9:6, pp. 1102–08.

12. Jane Getchell, Donald Hicks, et al., "Human Immunodeficiency Virus Isolated from a Serum Sample Collected in 1976 in Central Africa," *Journal of Infectious Diseases,* 11/87, 156:5, pp. 833–37; also W. Carl Saxinger, Paul Levine, et al., "Evidence for Exposure to HTLV-III in Uganda Before 1973," *Science,* 3/1/85, v. 227, pp. 1036–38.

13. Nathan Clumeck, Jean Sonnet, et al., "Acquired Immunodeficiency Syndrome in African Patients," *NEJM,* 2/23/84, 310:8, pp. 492–93.

14. Hooper, *The River,* chapter 1.

15. See "AIDS Wars," *The Economist,* 9/16/00, 356:8188, p. 87; also Jon Cohen, "Disputed AIDS Theory Dies Its Final Death," *Science,* 4/27/01, 292:5517, p. 615.

Chapter 1

1. CDC, *"Pneumosystis Pneumonia*—Los Angeles," *Morbidity and Mortality Weekly Report,* 6/5/81, 30:21, p. 1.

2. Eva Hoffman and Margot Slade, "Rare Cancer in Homosexuals," *NYT,* 7/5/81, p. D7.

3. AP, "2 Fatal Diseases Focus of Inquiry," *NYT,* 8/29/81, p. A9.

4. Walter Dowdle, "The Epidemiology of AIDS," *PHR,* 7–8/83, v. 98, pp. 308–12.

5. Larry Kramer, "A Personal Appeal," *New York Native,* 8/24–9/6/81, no. 19, reprinted in Kramer, *Reports from the Holocaust* (New York: St. Martin's Press, 1989).

6. "CDC Updates Trends in AIDS Epidemic," *American Family Physician,* 11/82, 265, p. 290.

7. Ibid.

8. Lawrence Altman, "New Homosexual Disorder Worries Health Officials," *NYT,* 5/11/82, p. C1.

9. Stephen Morin and Walter Batchelor, "Responding to the Psychological Crisis of AIDS," *PHR,* 1–2/84, v. 99, p. 4.

10. Arthur Felson, "A Multicolored Mosaic," in Len Nungesser, ed., *Epidemic of Courage: Facing AIDS in America* (New York: St. Martin's Press, 1986), p. 5.

11. David Black, "The Plague Years," *Rolling Stone,* 3/28/85.

12. Ibid.

13. Jean Seligmann, Mariana Gosnell, et al., "The AIDS Epidemic: The Search for a Cure," *Newsweek,* 4/18/83, p. 74.

14. Ibid.

15. See Diane Apuzzo-Berger, "A.I.D.S.: Could You Be at Risk?" *RN,* 2/83, pp. 67–70. See also Barry Vinocur, "Being Gay Is a Health Hazard," *The Saturday Evening Post,* 10/82, p. 26.

16. Altman, "New Homosexual Disorder Worries Health Officials;" Lewis Hassell, "Preventing the Acquired Immunodeficiency Syndrome," *NEJM,* 12/1/83, 309:22, p. 1395.

17. Quoted in Susan Lawrence, "AIDS—No Relief in Sight," *Science News,* v. 122, 9/25/82, p. 203.

18. Seligmann, Gosnell, et al., "The AIDS Epidemic: The Search for a Cure," p. 76.

19. See, among others, J. L. Marx, "New Disease Baffles Medical Community," *Science,* v. 217, 8/13/82, pp. 618–21.

20. For discussion of early speculation into Haitian causes of AIDS, see Donald Francis, James Curran, and Myron Essex, "Epidemic Acquired Immune Deficiency Syndrome: Epidemiologic Evidence for a Transmissible Agent," *Journal of the National Cancer Institute,* 7/83, v. 71, pp. 1–4; "Herpes Virus May Have Role in AIDS," *American Family Physician,* 4/83, 27:4, pp. 268–69; and Matt Clark, Mariana Gosnell, et al., "AIDS: A Lethal Mystery Story," *Newsweek,* 12/27/82, pp. 63–64.

21. Francis, Curran, and Essex, "Epidemic Acquired Immune Deficiency Syndrome," pp. 3–4;

22. Robert Bock, "Searching for the Cause of AIDS: Is HTLV the Culprit?" *Bioscience,* 11/83, 33:10, pp. 619–20.

23. Ibid., p. 620. Roche laboratories investigator Arthur Davis suspected an autoimmune etiology after noticing infected thymus glands of early AIDS victims.

24. Seligmann, Gosnell, et al., "The AIDS Epidemic," p. 77.

25. Ibid.

26. Bock, "Searching for the Cause of AIDS," p. 620.

27. Frances Fitzgerald, "The Castro—1," *The New Yorker,* 7/21/86, pp. 34–35.

28. Ibid., p. 51; John-Manuel Andriote, *Victory Deferred: How AIDS Changed Gay Life in America* (Chicago: University of Chicago Press, 1999), pp. 8–9.

29. Fitzgerald, "The Castro—1," p. 36.

30. See Richard Rodriguez, "Late Victorians: San Francisco, AIDS, and the Homosexual Stereotype," *Harpers,* 2/84, pp. 56–60; Fitzgerald, "The Castro—1," pp. 51–55; and Randy Shilts, *And the Band Played On: Politics, People, and the AIDS Epidemic* (New York: St. Martin's Press, 1987), p. 15.

31. Benjamin Heim Shepard, *White Nights and Ascending Shadows: An Oral History of the San Francisco AIDS Epidemic* (Washington, D.C.: Cassell, 1997), p. 31.

32. See Fitzgerald, "The Castro—1," p. 54–56.

33. Tom Morganthau, Vincent Coppola, et al., "Gay America in Transition," *Newsweek,* 8/8/83, p. 30.

34. Michael Norman, "Homosexuals Confronting a Time of Change," *NYT,* 6/16/83, p. A1.

35. Michael Daly, "AIDS Anxieties," *New York,* v. 16, 6/20/83, pp. 24–29.

36. Norman, "Homosexuals Confronting a Time of Change," p. A1.

37. Andrew Holleran, Introduction to Larry Kramer, *The Lonely Heart* (New York: New American Library, 1985), p. 25.

38. Edmund White, "The Artist and AIDS," *Harper's,* v. 274, 5/87, p. 22.

39. Morgenthau, Coppola, et al., "Gay America in Transition," p. 30.

40. Quoted in Andriote, *Victory Deferred,* p. 21.

41. Morgenthau, Coppola, et al., "Gay America in Transition," p. 30.

42. Andriote, *Victory Deferred,* p. 21.

43. Fitzgerald, "The Castro—1," p. 64.

44. As quoted in Andriote, *Victory Deferred,* p. 25.

45. Ibid., p. 26.

46. Fitzgerald, "The Castro—1," p. 63.

47. Ibid., p. 64.

48. Lindsy van Gelder, "Death in the Family," *Rolling Stone,* 2/3/83, pp. 18–20.

49. Philip Weiss, "Inside a Bathhouse," *The New Republic,* v. 193, 12/2/85, p. 14.

50. See Stephen Joseph, *Dragon Within the Gates* (New York: Carroll and Graf, 1992), pp. 102–5.

51. Frances Fitzgerald, "The Castro—II," *The New Yorker,* 7/28/86, pp. 49–50.

52. Lion McKusick, James Wiley, et al., "Reported Changes in the Sexual Behavior of Men at Risk for AIDS, San Francisco, 1982–84," *PHR,* 11–12/85, v. 100, p. 622.

53. CDC "Self-Reported Behavioral Changes Among Homosexual and Bisexual Men—San Francisco," *JAMA,* 254:18, 11/8/85, pp. 2537–38.

54. Barbara Kantrowitz, Vicki Quade, et al., "Fear of Sex: A Deadly Threat Is Changing the Rules of the Dating Game," *Newsweek,* 11/24/86, p. 40.

55. Ellen Goodman, "A Question of Life and Life Style," *WP,* 7/9/83, p. A21.

56. "Homosexuals Find a Need to Reassess," *NYT,* 5/29/83, section 11, p. 8.

57. Andrew Holleran, *Ground Zero* (New York: Penguin, 1989), pp. 123–24.

58. Douglas Feldman, " 'Totally Safe Sex' or AIDS," *AJPH*, 5/86, 76:5, p. 588.

59. Arthur Felson, "A Multicolored Mosaic," p. 7.

60. "Homosexuals Find a Need to Reassess," p. 8.

61. Leon McKusick, William Horstman, and Thomas Coates, "AIDS and Sexual Behavior Reported by Gay Men in San Francisco," *AJPH*, 5/85, 75:5, p. 495.

62. Ibid.

63. "Homosexuals Find a Need to Reassess," p. 11.

64. McKusick, Horstman, and Coates, "AIDS and Sexual Behavior Reported by Gay Men in San Francisco," pp. 493–94.

65. Ralph Blumenthal, "At Homosexual Establishments, A New Climate of Caution," *NYT*, 11/9/85, section 1, p. 29.

66. Joyce Purnick, "City Shuts a Bathhouse as Site of 'Unsafe Sex,' " *NYT*, 12/7/85, section 1, p. 31.

67. Fitzgerald, "The Castro—2," p. 52.

68. "And the Band Stopped Playing," *Newsweek*, 3/21/90.

69. "San Francisco Curb on Baths," *NYT*, 4/10/84, p. A14.

70. Shilts, *And the Band Played On*, p. 447.

71. Weiss, "Inside a Bathhouse," p. 15.

72. As quoted in "The Bathhouse War: San Francisco's Move to Fight AIDS Creates Rift Among Gays," *WP*, 4/19/84, p. D1.

73. Fitzgerald, "The Castro—2," p. 53.

74. Aric Press, Susan Agrest, and Daniel Pedersen, "AIDS and Civil Rights," *Newsweek*, 11/18/85, p. 86.

75. "The Bathhouse War: San Francisco's Move to Fight AIDS Creates Rift Among Gays," p. D1.

76. Mark Uehling, "AIDS and Civil Rights," *Newsweek*, 11/18/85, p. 86.

77. Larry Kramer, "1,112 and Counting," *New York Native*, 3/14–27/83, no. 59, reprinted in Kramer, *Reports from the Holocaust*, p. 34.

78. Quoted in Vincent Coppola, Richard West, and Janet Huck, "The Change in Gay Life-Style," *Newsweek*, v. 101, 4/18/83, p. 80.

79. As quoted in Dennis Altman, *AIDS in the Mind of America* (Garden City, N.Y.: Anchor Books, 1987), p. 49.

80. Felson, "A Multicolored Mosaic," p. 18.

81. Kramer, "1,112 and Counting," p. 39.

82. Ronald Kessler, "Weekend Vigils Are Set in 16 Cities to Call Attention to AIDS," *WP*, 10/7/83, p. B3.

83. Altman, *AIDS in the Mind of America*, p. 49.

84. Fritz Witti and Michael Goldberg, "The NIH and Research into the Acquired Immune Deficiency Syndrome," *PHR*, v. 98, 7–8/83, pp. 312–18; "Public Health Menace," *U.S. News and World Report*, 6/6/83, p. 56; also, "AIDS: Public Enemy No. 1," *Newsweek*, 6/6/83, p. 95.

85. Kramer, "1,112 and Counting," pp. 34–35.

86. Altman, *AIDS in the Mind of America*, p. 60.

Chapter 2

1. Joseph Carey, "Rx for AIDS: A Grim Race Against the Clock," *U.S. News*, 9/30/85, p. 48; Jerry Adler, Nikki Greenberg, et al., "The AIDS Conflict," *Newsweek*, 9/23/85, p. 19.

2. Abigail Trafford, Gordon Witkin, et al., "The Politics of AIDS—A Tale of Two States," *U.S. News and World Report*, 11/18/85, p. 70.

3. Mark Starr and David Gonzales, "The Panic over AIDS," *Newsweek*, 7/4/83, p. 20; "A Plague on All Their Houses?" *The Economist*, 11/2/85, p. 27.

4. Bob Levin, "Facing a Fatal Disease," *Maclean's*, 1/6/86, p. 48.

5. "AFRAIDS," *TNR*, 10/14/85, p. 7.

6. Mary Bruno, Connie Leslie, et al., "Campus Sex: New Fears," *Newsweek*, 10/20/85, p. 82.

7. "AFRAIDS," p. 7.

8. See Joseph Berger, "Rock Hudson, Screen Idol, Dies at 59," *NYT*, 10/3/85, p. D23.

9. Matt Clark, Marianna Gosnell, et al., "AIDS," *Newsweek*, 8/12/85, p. 23.

10. Steven Petrow, *Dancing Against the Darkness* (Lexington, Mass.: Lexington Books, 1990), p. 3.

11. Evan Thomas, Cathy Booth, and Michael Riley, "The New Untouchables," *Time*, 126:12, 9/23/85, pp. 24–27.

12. Ibid.

13. "Fear of AIDS Infects the Nation," *U.S. News and World Report*, 6/27/83, p. 13; E. R. Shipp, "Concern over Spread of AIDS Generates a Spate of New Laws Nationwide," *NYT*, 10/26/85, p. 30.

14. Selwyn, *Surviving the Fall*, p. 50.

15. See the complete analysis of the case in Mark Carl Rom, *Fatal Extraction* (San Francisco: Jossey-Boss, 1997), particularly chapters 1 and 4.

16. Christine Russell, "U.S. Issues New Policy on Transfusions to Avoid AIDS Disease," *WP*, 3/4/83, p. A3; Penny Chorlton, "Warning on AIDS: Blood Donors Sent Letters Not to Make Donations if They Are in High Risk Groups for Disease," *The Guardian*, 12/22/84.

17. Matt Clark and Pamela Abramson, "The Blood-Bank Scare," *Newsweek*, 1/28/85, p. 62.

18. "Blood Banks Turn Away 'Directed Donations,'" *Los Angeles Times*, 10/6/85, p. A3.

19. See Bradley Bender and Thomas Quinn, "Medical Response to AIDS Epidemic," *NEJM*, 310:6, 2/9/84, p. 389, for growth modeling of the early epidemic.

20. See James Mason, "Public Health Service Plan for the Prevention and Control of Acquired Immune Deficiency Syndrome," *PHR*, v. 100, 9/85, pp. 453–55.

21. "Sex Transmits AIDS," *The Economist*, 7/5/86, p. 14. By contrast, the U.S. Department of Health and Human Services estimated only 270,000 American cases by 1991. Reported in Jean Seligmann, Mary Hager, and Karen Springen, "Spreading Alarm About AIDS," *Newsweek*, 6/23/86, p. 68.

22. Tom Morganthau and Mary Hager, "AIDS: Grim Prospects," *Newsweek*, 11/10/86, p. 20.

23. J. Silberner, "AIDS: Disease, Research Efforts Advance," *Science News*, v. 127, 4/27/85, pp. 260–61.

24. Erik Eckholm, "Screening of Blood for AIDS Raises Civil Liberties Issues," *NYT*, 9/30/85, p. A1. Also, A. R. Moss, "Predicting Who Will Progress to AIDS," *British Medical Journal*, v. 297, 10/29/88, pp. 1067–68.

25. David Anderson, "AIDS: An Update on What We Know Now," *RN*, 3/86, pp. 49–50.

26. Gerald Clarke, "AIDS: The Growing Threat," *Time*, 126:6, 8/12/85, p. 42.

27. See "AIDS: Deadly but Hard to Catch," *Consumer Reports*, 11/86, p. 725.

28. See J. Silberner, "AIDS: Disease, Research Efforts Advance."

29. James Warner to Gary Bauer, 3/5/87, GB papers, OA 18329/AIDS: Memo to Bauer Re: Heterosexual Transmission.

30. Sam Roberts, "Medical Detectives Hunt Clues to AIDS Outbreak," *NYT*, 6/4/83, p. 25.

31. Merle Sande, "Transmission of AIDS: The Case Against Casual Contagion," *NEJM*, 314:6, 2/6/86, pp. 380–81.

32. "Is Nobody Safe from AIDS?" *The Economist,* 2/1/86, p. 79. See also Carol Harris, Catherine Butkus Small, et al., "Immunodeficiency in Female Sexual Partners of Men with the Acquired Immunodeficiency Syndrome," *NEJM,* 308:20, 5/19/83, pp. 1181–84.

33. "The New Plague, in Perspective," *NYT,* 9/3/85, p. A20.

34. "Slapping Down the Mosquito," *Time,* 7/13/87, p. 56. See Mark Whiteside to Kenneth Robin, 8/4/86, JW papers, OA 18329/AIDS: Dr. Mark Whiteside.

35. Aaron Fink, "A Possible Explanation for Heterosexual Male Infection with AIDS," *NEJM,* 315:18, 10/30/86, p. 1167.

36. Harold Ginzburg, "Intravenous Drug Users and the Acquired Immune Deficiency Syndrome," *PHR,* 3–4/84, v. 99, pp. 206–12.

37. Matt Clark, Mariana Gosnell, and Mary Hager, "Women and AIDS," *Newsweek,* 7/14/86, p. 60.

38. Ibid., p. 62.

39. Crystal Nix, "More and More AIDS Cases Found Among Drug Abusers," *NYT,* 10/20/85, p. 51.

40. B. F. Polk, "Female-to-Male Transmission of AIDS," *JAMA,* v. 245, 1985, pp. 3177–78; and "Heterosexual Transmission of Human T-Lymphotropic Virus Type III/Lymphadenopathy-Associated Virus," *Morbidity and Mortality Weekly Report,* v. 34, 1985, pp. 561–63.

41. Joseph Bove, "Transfusion-Associated Hepatitis and AIDS," *NEJM,* 317:4, 7/23/87, pp. 242–44.

42. James Mason, "Statement Before the Committee on Foreign Relations, United States Senate," 12/9/87, RS papers, OA 16784: AIDS/Testimony, folder 1/4.

43. See Charles Rosenberg, *The Cholera Years* (Chicago: University of Chicago Press, 1962).

44. See William Coleman, *Death Is a Social Disease* (Madison: University of Wisconsin Press, 1982).

45. "The Backlash Builds Against AIDS," *U.S. News and World Report,* 11/4/85, p. 9.

46. Stephen Joseph, *Dragon Within the Gates* (New York: Carroll and Graf, 1992), p. 105.

47. Ibid., p. 106.

48. Ibid., p. 102.

49. Katie Leishman, "Heterosexuals and AIDS," *The Atlantic Monthly,* 2/87, p. 58.

50. "How-To Pamphlet on Drug Use Attacked by Hahn, Antonovich," *Los Angeles Times,* 8/22/85, p. B1.

51. See Brandt, *No Magic Bullet* (New York: Oxford University Press, 1985).

52. "Pentagon AIDS Test That Sparked Furor," *U.S. News and World Report,* 9/9/85, p. 12.

53. Philip Hilts, "The Advocate for AIDS Testing: Major Robert Redfield Battling the Disease in the Army's Ranks," *WP,* 12/27/86, p. C1. See also Donald Burke, John Brundage, et al., "Human Immunodeficiency Virus Infections Among Civilian Applicants for United States Military Service, October 1985 to March 1986," *NEJM,* 317:3, 7/16/87, pp. 131–36.

54. Jerry Adler and Nikki Finke Greenberg, "Trying to Lock Out AIDS," *Newsweek,* 9/16/85, p. 65.

55. James Oleske, Anthony Minnefor, et al., "Immune Deficiency Syndrome in Children," *JAMA,* 249:17, 5/6/83, p. 2345. See in the same issue Arye Rubenstein, Marc Sicklick, et al., "Acquired Immunodeficiency with Reversed T4/T8 Ratios in Infants Born to Promiscuous and Drug-Addicted Mothers," pp. 2350–56.

56. See Jean Seligman, Susan Katz, et al., "Babies Born with AIDS," *Newsweek,* 9/22/86, p. 70.

57. Quoted in Walter Isaacson, "Hunting for the Hidden Killers, *Time,* 7/4/83, p. 55.

58. K. Leishman, "A Crisis in Public Health," *Atlantic Monthly,* v. 256, 10/85, p. 19.

59. Carol Levine, "In and Out of the Hospital," Lawrence O. Gostin, ed., *AIDS and the Health Care System* (New Haven: Yale University Press, 1990), pp. 51–53.

60. David Weinberg and Henry Murray, "Coping with AIDS: The Special Problems of New York City," *NEJM*, 317:23, 12/3/87, pp. 1469–72.

61. Statement by Daniel Leicht before the Labor and Health and Human Services Subcommittee of the Senate Appropriations Committee, 9/26/85, RS papers, OA 16630/WGHPA 10/13, pp. 5–9.

62. K. Leishman, "A Crisis in Public Health," p. 19.

63. Matt Clark, Fred Coleman, et al., "AIDS Exiles in Paris," *Newsweek*, 8/5/85, p. 71.

64. Ibid.

65. Laurence Zuckerman, "Open Season on Gays," *Time*, 131:10, 3/7/88, pp. 24–26; John Balzar, "The Times Poll: American Views of Gays: Disapproval, Sympathy," *LAT*, 12/20/85, p. A1.

66. Zuckerman, "Open Season on Gays."

67. John Balzar, "The Times Poll: Tough New Government Action on AIDS Backed," *LAT*, 12/19/85, p. 1.

68. Barbara Amiel, "AIDS and the Rights of the Well," *MacLean's*, 9/30/85, p. 11.

69. Patrick Fagan, "Report on AIDS," RS papers, OA 16784/Sex/Education 2/5.

70. Roy McCloughry and Carol Bebawi, Grove Ethical Studies No. 64, *AIDS: A Christian Response* (Bramcote, U.K.: Grove Books, 1987), pp. 4, 5, and 16.

71. David Kirp, "AIDS and Ostracism," *Christian Science Monitor*, 9/9/85, p. 20.

72. Ibid.

73. Randy Frame, "The Church's Response to AIDS," *Christianity Today*, 11/22/85.

74. David Gelman, Pamela Abramson, et al., "The Social Fallout from an Epidemic," *Newsweek*, 8/12/85, p. 29.

75. William Haseltine, "To Seek Origins of AIDS in Africa Is Not to Cast Blame for It," *NYT*, 11/26/85, p. A26.

76. Editorial, "A Social Disease," *The Nation*, 9/14/85, p. 195.

77. Robert Bazell, "We're All Haitians Now: Waking Up to AIDS," *TNR*, 1985, 3rd page.

78. Gina Kolata, "Mathematical Model Predicts AIDS Spread: The AIDS Epidemic Among Heterosexuals May Die Out of Its Own Accord," *Science*, v. 235, 3/20/87, pp. 1464–65.

79. Ibid., p. 1464.

80. Tom Morgenthau, Mary Hager, et al., "Future Shock," *Newsweek*, 11/24/86, p. 32.

81. J. W. Pape, B. Liautaud, et al., "Characteristics of the Acquired Immunodeficiency Syndrome in Haiti," *NEJM*, v. 309, 10/20/83, pp. 945–50.

82. C. Wallis, "AIDS: A Growing Threat," *Time*, 8/12/85, p. 45.

83. P. Nicholas, J. Masci, et al., "Immune Competence in Haitians Living in New York," *NEJM*, 309:19, 11/10/83, p. 1187; Jeffrey Vieira, Elliot Frank, et al., "Acquired Immune Deficiency in Haitians," *NEJM*, 308:3, 1/20/83, p. 125.

84. Lawrence Altman, "The Confusing Haitian Connection to AIDS," *NYT*, 8/16/83, p. C2.

85. See Edward Hooper, *The River* (Boston: Little, Brown, and Company, 1999), pp. 80–82. Antwerp researcher Peter Piot agreed with this hypothesis. See Wallis, "AIDS: A Growing Threat," 5th page, p. 45.

86. As quoted in Hooper, *The River*, p. 74.

87. Ibid., p. 75.

88. Jaime Olle-Goig, "Groups at High Risk for AIDS," *NEJM*, 311:2, 7/12/84.

89. Hooper, *The River*, p. 80.

90. "The African Connection," *The Economist*, 2/1/86, p. 80.

91. Hooper, *The River*, p. 91.

92. Ibid., p. 97.

93. "Africa's Latest Torment: AIDS," *U.S. News and World Report,* 12/23/85, p. 8.

94. Rod Nordland, Ray Wilkinson, and Ruth Marshall, "Africa in the Plague Years," *Newsweek,* 11/24/86, p. 44.

95. Ibid., p. 47.

96. Ibid.

Chapter 3

1. See "Scientist Says Interferon May Be Linked to AIDS," *NYT,* 5/22/83, p. C4

2. Joseph Sonnabend, Steven Witkin, and David Purtilo, "Acquired Immunodeficiency Syndrome, Opportunistic Infections, and Malignancies in Male Homosexuals," *JAMA,* 249:17, 5/6/83, pp. 2370–74. See also "Herpes Virus May Have Role in AIDS," *American Family Physician,* 27:4, 4/83, pp. 268–69; and Donald Francis, James Curran, and Myron Essex, "Epidemic Acquired Immune Deficiency Syndrome: Epidemiologic Evidence for a Transmissible Agent," *Journal of the National Cancer Institute,* v. 71, 7/83, pp. 1–4.

3. A helpful discussion of the early pathogenic theories of AIDS can be found in Barry Schoub, *AIDS and HIV in Perspective,* 2nd ed. (New York: Cambridge University Press, 1994), particularly pp. 1–9.

4. Seth Roberts, "Lab Rat," *Spy,* 7/90.

5. Ibid., 2nd page.

6. Philip Hilts, "Cancer Virus Increasingly Seen as Most Likely Cause of AIDS," *WP,* 9/2/83, p. A2.

7. Luc Montagnier, *Virus* (New York: Norton, 2000), pp. 55–56. The reader should note that much significance was attached to Gallo's efforts to incorporate the Montagnier virus into his general HTLV model. Gallo claimed that he read the abstract to Montagnier over the phone, who approved its wording. See Robert Gallo, *Virus Hunting* (New York: Basic Books, 1991), p. 151.

8. Jean Marx, "Strong New Candidate for AIDS Agent," *Science,* v. 224, 5/4/84, p. 475.

9. Steve Connor and Sharon Kingman, *The Search for the Virus,* 2nd ed. (New York: Viking, 1989), p. 41.

10. Ibid., p. 51.

11. Montagnier and Gallo published a whitewashed chronology of HIV's discovery in "AIDS in 1988," *Scientific American,* 259:4, 10/88, pp. 41–48.

12. Montagnier, *Virus,* p. 82.

13. For more on the SIV to HIV jump, see Max Essex and Phyllis Kanki, "The Origins of the AIDS Virus," *Scientific American,* 10/88, pp. 64–71.

14. For a helpful description of the viral replication mechanism, see ibid., pp. 88–95.

15. Thomas Merigan, "What Are We Going to Do About AIDS and HTLV-III/LAV Infection?" *NEJM,* 311:20, 11/15/84, p. 1312.

16. Lewis Thomas, "AIDS: An Unknown Distance Still to Go," *Scientific American,* 10/88, p. 152.

17. Thomas Matthews and Dani Bolognesi, "AIDS Vaccines," *Scientific American,* 10/88, pp. 122–24.

18. See S. Broder and Robert Gallo, "A Pathogenic Retrovirus Linked to AIDS," *NEJM,* 1984, pp. 1292–97.

19. Matt Clark, David Gonzales, and Mary Hager, "The Mosquito AIDS Scare," *Newsweek,* 7/14/87, p. 47.

20. Robert Sassone to Gary Bauer, 10/5/87, GB papers, OA 19222/AIDS 3/3.

21. Katie Leishman, "AIDS and Insects," *The Atlantic,* 9/87, p. 72.

Chapter 4

1. See Lindsy Van Gelder and Pam Bandt, "AIDS on Campus," *Rolling Stone,* v. 483, p. 89.
2. "AIDS and Public Policy," *National Review,* 7/8/83, p. 796.
3. Eugene Clark, "The Deadly Silence: AIDS and Social Censorship," *Crisis,* 5/87, pp. 35, 37.
4. Ibid., p. 38.
5. Quoted in Michael Doan, "Charges of Media 'Cover-Up': Jerry Falwell's anti-AIDS Drive," *U.S. News and World Report,* 5/4/87, p. 12.
6. Quoted in Matt Clark, Mariana Gosness, et al., "AIDS," *Newsweek,* 8/12/85, p. 20. Buchanan had harbored antigay sentiment for some time. As early as 1977, he had written: "Homosexuality is not a civil right. Its rise almost always is accompanied, as in the Weimar Republic, with a decay of society and a collapse of its basic cinder block, the family." Quoted in "The Other Minority," *TNR,* 206:13, 3/30/92, p. 7.
7. Quoted in Robert Scheer, " 'We are Not Lepers:' AIDS Stigma Hampering a Solution," *LAT,* 11/28/86, p. A1.
8. Tom Sharratt, "Preacher Anderton Thunders Against the Gays," *The Guardian,* 12/12/86.
9. Quoted in "Stigmatizing the Victim," *The Nation,* 242:14, 4/12/86, p. 505.
10. Phyllis Schlafly, "The 'Why' Book That Stopped Chicago's Gay Rights Bill," *New York City Tribune,* 9/10/86.
11. Quoted in " 'The Mob' Fights Back," in Arthur Kahn, *AIDS: The Winter War* (Philadelphia: Temple University Press, 1993), chapter 1.
12. Jane Gross, "Homosexuals Stepping Up AIDS Education," *NYT,* 9/22/85, p. A1.
13. As quoted in Mickey Kaus, Mary Hager, et al., "The 'Small Health Problem' of AIDS," *Newsweek,* 7/13/87, p. 46.
14. See Aric Press and Ann McDaniel, "A Victory for AIDS Victims," *Newsweek,* 3/16/87, p. 33.
15. Ted Vollmer, "Anti-AIDS Brochure on 'Safe' Sex Draws Fire," *LAT,* 8/28/85, p. B1.
16. "AIDS, Nature, and the Nature of AIDS," *National Review,* 11/1/85, p. 18.
17. Marvin Vaughan and James Li, "Prevention of AIDS: Lessons from Osler," *NEJM,* 6/12/86, as reprinted in Loren Clarke and Malcolm Potts, *The AIDS Reader* (Brookline Village, Md.: Branden Publishers, 1988), p. 267.
18. Stephen Doig, *Miami Herald,* 1/31/84, p. A4.
19. William Dannemeyer, "Dannemeyer Outlines His Views," *LAT,* 2/8/86, p. B2.
20. Quoted in Fred Barnes, "The Politics of AIDS," *TNR,* 11/4/85, p. 12.
21. David Reyes and Marlene Cimons, "Gays Assail Dannemeyer for Hiring Researcher," *LAT,* 8/20/85, p. B1.
22. As quoted in Barnes, "The Politics of AIDS," p. 13.
23. Alessandra Stanley, "AIDS Becomes a Political Issue," *Time,* 3/23/87, p. 24.
24. Kerby Anderson, "Quarantine for AIDS," *Lampasas Dispatch Record,* 11/11/85.
25. Quoted in "How Republicans 'Spread' AIDS," *Harpers,* v. 276, 2/88, p. 26.
26. "Scourge of a New Disease," *NYT,* 5/15/83, p. D20; "The Fear of AIDS," *NYT,* 6/25/83, p. A22.
27. David Talbot and Larry Bush, "At Risk," *Mother Jones,* 4/85, p. 30.
28. Ibid., p. 31.
29. Robert Pear, "Health Chief Calls AIDS Battle 'No. 1 Priority,' " *NYT,* 5/25/83, p. A1.
30. "Mrs. Heckler Asks More AIDS Funds," *NYT,* 8/18/83, p. A19.
31. Ibid.
32. William Roper, "What Should the Federal Government Do to Deal with the Problem of AIDS?" RS papers, OA 16630: WGHPA 5/13, p. 5.

33. "Briefing Material for Domestic Policy Council Working Group on Health Policy: Past Present and Future Cost of AIDS," 10/17/85, RS Papers, OA 16630:WGHPA 10/13, p. 1. Also, GAO, *AIDS: Views on the Administration's Fiscal Year 1989 Public Health Service Budget,* GAO/HRD-88-104BR, 6/88, p. 16.

34. Pear, "Health Chief Calls AIDS Battle 'No. 1 Priority,' " p. A1.

35. Gina Kolata, "Congress: NIH Opens Coffers for AIDS," *Science,* v. 221, 7/19/83, p. 436.

36. Barbara Culliton, "AIDS Amendment Angers Cancer Institute," *Science,* v. 226, 11/30/84, p. 1056.

37. Talbot and Bush, "At Risk," p. 32.

38. See, for example, "Minutes of the Domestic Policy Council," 9/11/85, RS papers, OA 16630:WGHPA 6/13.

39. See "Coolfont Report: A PHS Plan for Prevention and Control of AIDS and the AIDS Virus," *PHR,* v. 101, 7–8/86, pp. 341–48.

40. "Minutes of the Domestic Policy Council," 1/13/87, RS papers, OA16785: AIDS 3 5/5.

41. Edwin Meese III, "AIDS Education," 2/11/87, GB papers, OA19363: AIDS Material/ Family Material 2/2.

42. "Minutes of the Domestic Policy Council," 12/19/85, RS papers, OA 16630:WGHPA 5/13.

43. "Remarks by the President to the American Foundation for AIDS Research Awards Dinner," 5/31/87, RS papers, OA 16629: HPWG: AIDS #2 2/6.

44. The DPC expressed concern over the commission overstepping its bounds when it voted to recommend its establishment. See Ralph Bledsoe, "AIDS in America," 4/29/87, KC papers, Box 8: AIDS: Presidential Decision Memo, p. 5.

45. "Reagan's AIDS Panel: Who the Members Are," *NYT,* 7/24/87, p. A12.

46. "The Reagan AIDS Strategy in Ruins," *NYT,* 10/11/87, p. D26.

47. Quoted in Colleen O'Connor and Mary Hager, "Koop Makes Waves in His War on AIDS," *Newsweek,* 3/2/87, p. 31.

48. C. Everett Koop, "Surgeon General's Report on Acquired Immune Deficiency Syndrome," *PHR,* v. 102, 1–2/87, pp. 1–3.

49. William Dannemeyer, "Summary of Recommendations," RS papers, OA 16785: AIDS 3 1/5.

50. Ibid.

51. "Minutes of the Domestic Policy Council," 1/21/87, RS papers, OA 16785: AIDS 3 5/5, p. 2.

52. Sweet to Koop, 1/14/86, RS papers, OA 16630: WGHPA 10/13.

53. David Whitman, "C. Everett Koop Takes on Intractable Issues as Surgeon General— But He's Also Made Enemies," *U.S. News and World Report,* 5/25/87, p. 27.

54. "What's Wrong with Sex Education," *The Phyllis Schlafly Report,* 14:7, 2/81. p. 1.

55. "School-Based Sex Clinics vs. Sex Respect," *The Phyllis Schlafly Report,* 19:11, 6/86, p. 1.

56. Schlafly to Mart T., White House Memo, 12/19/86, RS papers, OA 16784: AIDS Testing 1/4.

57. See, for example, William Bennett, *AIDS and the Education of Our Children: A Guide for Parents and Teachers* (Washington, D.C.: GPO, 1987), pp. 9–11.

58. Robert Redfield and Wanda Kay Franz, *AIDS and Young People* (Washington, D.C.: Regnery-Gateway, 1987), 2nd printing, p. 32.

59. Ibid., p. 35.

60. Julia Reed, James Hildreth, and Kathleen McAuliffe, "The Hot New Politics of AIDS," *U.S. News and World Report,* 3/30/87, p. 30.

61. John Leo, "Sex and Schools," *Time,* 11/24/86, p. 56.

62. R. Valdiserri, L. C. Leviton, et al., "Variables Influencing Condom Use in a Cohort of Gay and Bisexual Men," *AJPH,* v. 78, 1988, pp. 801–5.

63. See R. Valdiserri, L. C. Leviton, et al., "AIDS Prevention in Homosexual and Bisexual Men," *AIDS,* v. 3, 1989, pp. 21–26.

64. See Allan Brandt, *No Magic Bullet* (New York: Oxford University Press, 1985).

65. Vernon Mark, "On Condoms and AIDS," RS papers, OA 16784: Sex/Education 2/5.

66. Kaye Wellings, "AIDS and the Condom," *British Medical Journal,* v. 293, 11/15/86, p. 1259. See also M. Conant, D. Hardy, et al., "Condoms Prevent Transmission of AIDS Associated Retrovirus," *JAMA,* 1986, v. 255, p. 1706.

67. Ibid.

68. United States Centers for Disease Control, *What You Should Know About AIDS* (Washington, D.C.: GPO, 1987).

69. Theresa Crenshaw, "America Responds to AIDS," RS papers, OA 16784: AIDS/Publications 1/2.

70. Bauer to Koop, date unknown, RS papers, OA 16784: AIDS/Klenk 1/2.

71. Memo beginning "The brochure *What You Should Know About AIDS,*" RS papers, OA 16784: AIDS/Publications 1/2.

72. For helpful details on the administration's complete education efforts, particularly through the PHS and the CDC, see U.S. GAO, *AIDS Education: Activities Aimed at the General Public Implemented Slowly,* GAO/HRD-89-21, pp. 1–5.

73. U.S. Surgeon General's Office, *Understanding AIDS,* 1988, HHS publication (CDC) HHS-88-8404.

74. Chris Mondics, "N.J. Panel Makes AIDS Transmittal a Felony," *Bergen Record,* 3/29/88, p. A1.

75. Ann Gregor, "Harsh Measures: The Dispute over Tighter AIDS Regulations," *MacLean's,* 10/31/88, p. 55.

76. Lee Harris, "Official in Lynwood Calls for Enactment of AIDS Quarantine," *LAT,* 8/22/85, p. I1.

77. Ibid.

78. Ehrlich, p. 92.

79. Knudson, p. A13.

80. Philip Boffey, "Pentagon: Of AIDS and the Lack of Confidentiality," *NYT,* 8/10/85, p. A7.

81. For a detailed description of the tests, see AMA Council on Scientific Affairs, "Status Report on the Acquired Immunodeficiency Syndrome: Human T cell Lymphotropic Virus Type III Testing," *JAMA,* 254:10, 9/13/85, pp. 1342–45.

82. See J. Silberner, "AIDS Blood Test: Qualified Test," *Science News,* v. 128, 8/10/85, p. 84.

83. See J. Silberner, "AIDS Blood Screen Approved," *Science News,* v. 127, 3/9/85, p. 148.

84. Ronald Sullivan, "Blood Center Fears Impact of AIDS Test," *NYT,* 2/14/85, p. B1.

85. See Report, "Conference on the Role of AIDS Virus Antibody Testing in the Prevention and Control of AIDS, 2/24–25/87, Appendix I," RS papers, OS 16784: AIDS Testing 4/4. Also, Michael Marmor, "Second AIDS Tests Increase Accuracy Dramatically," *NYT,* 5/23/87, p. A26. Marmor was an AIDS researcher at NYU Hospital.

86. Burton Lee to George Bush, 6/2/87, VP Records, Chief of Staff Papers, Craig Fuller: OA/ID 14278.

87. Isabel Wilkerson, "AMA Urges Breach to Privacy to Warn Potential AIDS Victims," *NYT,* 7/1/88, p. A1.

88. James Goedert, "What Is Safe Sex? Suggested Standards Linked to Testing for Human Immunodeficiency Virus," *NEJM,* 316:21, 5/21/87, pp. 1339–41.

89. See Frank Rhame and Dennis Maki, "The Case for Wider Use of Testing for HIV Infection," *NEJM,* 320:16, 5/11/89, pp. 1248–54.

90. See Tim Beardsley, "AIDS and the Election," *Scientific American,* 10/88, p. 14.

91. Denise Hughes to George Bush, 6/6/87, VP Records, Correspondence Office, AIDS: OA/ID 15310 1/2.

92. Lee to Bush, 6/2/87, VP Records, Chief of Staff Papers, Craig Fuller: OA/ID 14278.

93. Gary Bauer, "The Case for Routine Testing," JW papers, OA 18329: AIDS: Testing; Gary. Also Bauer to Editor of the *New York Times,* 5/21/87, GB Papers, OA 19222: AIDS 3/3.

94. James Warner to Domestic Policy Counsel, "On the Issue of Testing for AIDS," 4/8/87, JW papers, OA 18329: AIDS: Memo Re: Accuracy of Testing.

95. The president outlined his testing policy in a speech before AmFAR on 5/31/87. See Beryl Sprinkel to Otis Bowen, 7/20/87, GB Papers, OA 19222: AIDS 3/3.

96. Officially, the nation reported only 102 cases of AIDS by 1987, but this claim almost certainly was too low. See "Those Who Endanger the People," *Newsweek,* 9/7/87, p. 41.

97. Chandler Burr, "Cuba and AIDS: Traditional Epidemiology Solved the AIDS Crisis in Cuba Before It Began," *National Review,* 49:18, 9/29/97, pp. 42–46.

98. Ibid.

99. Koop to Robert Wilson, 4/13/87, GB papers, OA 19222: AIDS 3/3.

100. AP, "Pre-Pregnancy Test Urged," 3/25/87, 9:12 EST.

101. "Quarantining Will Help No One: Interview with AIDS Expert and Nobel Laureate David Baltimore," *U.S. News and World Report,* 1/12/87, p. 70.

102. Even reputable medical journals succumbed to the bombast, with the illustrious *New England Journal of Medicine* reporting in 1988 that the cost of universal screening would approach $40,000 per detected AIDS case, while most previous estimates had put the cost at less than half that. Robin Weiss and Samuel Thierr, "HIV Testing Is the Answer—What's the Question?" *NEJM,* 319:15, 10/13/88, pp. 1010–13.

103. "AIDS: Politics and Science," *NEJM,* 318:7, 2/18/88, p. 445.

104. Tamar Jacoby, "Who Will Pay the AIDS Bill?" *Newsweek,* 4/11/88, p. 71.

105. For details on the development of Blue Cross plans, see Robert Cunningham, *The Blues: A History of the Blue Cross and Blue Shield System* (DeKalb: Northern Illinois University Press, 1997).

106. Joan Hamilton and Susan Garland, "Insurers Pass the Buck on AIDS Patients," *Business Week,* 3/28/88, p. 27.

107. Robert Pear, "Pro and Con: The Costs of an Epidemic; AIDS: Should Insurers Be Able to Test?" *NYT,* 5/17/87, p. D7.

108. Ted Gest, "AIDS Triggers Painful Legal Battles," *U.S. News and World Report,* 3/24/86, p. 73.

109. See Joan Hamilton, Julie Flynn, et al., "The AIDS Epidemic and Business," *Business Week,* 3/23/87, p. 122.

110. AP, "Senate Votes to Let Insurers in Capital Reject AIDS Clients," 10/2/87.

111. "Dukakis Ends AIDS Test Ban As State Insurance Aide Quits," *NYT,* 7/11/87, p. A12.

112. "Talking Points for Dr. MacDonald, Report of the Presidential Commissions on Human Immunodeficiency Virus Epidemic," 6/26/88, DM papers, OH 16757: "Misc. Notes—Grossman."

113. "No Comforts," *The Economist,* 6/11/88, p. 26.

114. National AIDS Network, "Will Reports Lead to National Policy?" *Network News,* 2:11, 6/15/88, p. 1.

115. "The President's Ten Point Action Plan Against HIV Infection," 12/31/88, DM papers, OA 16758: "Williams Correspondence."

116. Institute of Medicine, *Confronting AIDS: Directions for Public Health, Health Care, and Research* (Washington, D.C.: 1986).

117. "Remarks by the President to the College of Physicians of Philadelphia," 4/1/87, DM papers, OA 16756: HIV (1).

118. Kathy Facklemann, ed., "An AIDS Battle Plan," *Perspectives on Medicine and Health*, 6/13/88, p. 2.

119. Herbits to MacDonald, 7/18/88, DM papers, OH 16757: "Response to Recommendations 14 July 1988."

120. "Facing the AIDS Onslaught," *BG*, 12/7/88, p. A14.

Chapter 5

1. Michael Callen and Daniel Turner, "A History of the PWA Self-Empowerment Movement," in *Surviving and Thriving with AIDS: Collected Wisdom*, vol. II, ed. Michael Callen (New York: People With AIDS Coalition, 1988), pp. 288–93.

2. See Martha Engel, "Private NW Clinic Has Support Plan for Victims of AIDS," *WP*, 9/22/83, p. DC4. For biographical details on Graham, see also Madeleine Blais, "I Never Knew Whether I Could Let Go," *WP Magazine*, 1/26/92, pp. 8–25.

3. See Stephen Morin and Walter Batchelor, "Responding to the Psychological Crisis of AIDS," *PHR*, v. 99, 1–2/84, pp. 4–9.

4. Nancy Stoller, *Lessons from the Damned* (New York: Routledge, 1998), pp. 33–38.

5. Maureen Dowd, "For Victims of AIDS, Support in a Lonely Siege," *NYT*, 12/5/83, p. B1.

6. Quoted in Dennis Altman, *AIDS in the Mind of America* (New York: Anchor Books, 1987), p. 85.

7. See Peter Arno, "The Nonprofit Sector's Response to the AIDS Epidemic: Community-Based Services in San Francisco," *AJPH*, 76:11, 11/86, pp. 1325–30.

8. "Some Encouraging News About AIDS," *Newsweek*, 11/30/87, p. 62.

9. On dementia, see Erica Goode and Joanne Silberner, "AIDS Attacking the Brain," *U.S. News and World Report*, 9/7/87, p. 48.

10. Jean Seligman, Peter McKillop, et al., "A Very Risky Business," *Newsweek*, 11/20/89, p. 82.

11. Philip Boffey, "Doctors Who Shun AIDS Patients Are Assailed by Surgeon General," *NYT*, 9/10/87, p. A1.

12. Deborah Ibert, "A Dump for AIDS Patients: Hospital in Newark Says It's Swamped," *Bergen Record*, 10/30/87, p. A1.

13. See "Private Hospital to Treat AIDS Closes After Loss of $8 Million," *NYT*, 12/13/87, p. A58.

14. Alfonso Narvaez, "Newark Hospitals Seek Unit for AIDS Treatment," *NYT*, 7/21/87, p. B1.

15. Ibert, "A Dump for AIDS Patients," p. A1.

16. Statistics are from an internally published fact sheet, OPL JC papers, AIDS: Whitman-Walker: OA/ID 08403.

17. See Phil Kayal, *Bearing Witness: Gay Men's Health Crisis and the Politics of AIDS* (Boulder: Westview Press, 1992), pp. 192–95.

18. Armistead Maupin, "Putting Sex in Its Place," in Leon Nungesser, ed., *Epidemic of Courage: Facing AIDS in America* (New York: St. Martin's Press), p. 207.

19. Larry Kramer, "Equal to Murderers," *New York Native*, v. 95, 8/12/84.

20. Larry Kramer, "An Open Letter to Richard Dunne," *New York Native*, v. 197, 1/26/87.

21. Stephen Smith, "Devastating Moment for PWA's," *The Washington Blade*, 1/10/92, p. 32.

22. Eloise Salholz, Tony Clifton, et al., "The Future of Gay America," *Newsweek*, 115:11, 3/12/90, pp. 20–26.

23. Arthur David Kahn, *AIDS: The Winter War,* (Philadelphia: Temple University Press, 1993), pp. 4–7.

24. David Friedman, "Larry Kramer's Cool," *Newsday*, 10/20/92, p. 60.

25. Salholz, Clifton, et al., "The Future of Gay America," p. 23.

26. Kramer, *Reports from the Holocaust,* p. 31.

27. Ibid.

28. Larry Kramer, "GMHC Newsletter," no. 2, 2/83.

29. See Marvin Bailey, "Community-Based Organizations and CDC as Partners in HIV Education and Prevention," *PHR,* v. 106, 11–12/91, pp. 702–8.

30. William Deresiewicz, "Against All Odds: Grassroots Minority Groups Fight AIDS," *Health/PAC Bulletin,* Spring 1988, p. 5.

31. Ibid., p. 8.

32. Andrew Sullivan, "Gay Life, Gay Death," *TNR,* 203:24, 12/17/90, p. 21.

33. Margaret Nichols, "Bringing the Terror of AIDS Down to a Human Level," *NYT,* 1/26/86, p. NJ22.

34. Stoller, *Lessons from the Damned,* p. 11.

35. Eloise Salholz, Lucille Beachy, et al., "The Power and the Pride," *Newsweek,* 121:25, 6/21/93, p. 55.

36. Stoller, *Lessons from the Damned,* p. 20.

37. Benjamin Heim Shepard, *White Nights and Ascending Shadows: An Oral History of the San Francisco AIDS Epidemic* (Washington, D.C.: Cassell, 1997), p. 168.

38. For an alternative discussion of the participation of lesbians in the AIDS self-help movement, see Dennis Altman, *AIDS in the Mind of America* (New York: Anchor Books/ Doubleday, 1986), pp. 93–95.

39. Susan Vaughn, "Search for Cure Fuels Scientist's Drive," *LAT,* 12/31/2000, p. W1.

40. Geraldine Baum, "A Star in the AIDS War," *LAT,* 3/21/90, p. E1.

41. Jennet Conant, "The Fashionable Charity," *Newsweek,* 12/28/87, p. 54.

42. Paul Rudnick, "Now It's AIDS Inc.," *Time,* 148:29, 12/30/96, p. 86.

43. David Seidner, "The Red Ribbon," *New Yorker,* 68:52, 2/15/93, p. 31.

44. Conant, 12/28/87, p. 54.

45. Cleve Jones, *Stitching a Revolution* (San Francisco: HarperSanFrancisco, 2000), pp. 122–23.

46. "Memorial Quilt Rolls Out," *NYT,* 10/12/87, p. D11.

47. Andrew Sullivan, "Quilt," *TNR,* 207:6, 11/2/92, reprinted in Douglas Feldman and Julia Wang Miller, *The AIDS Crisis: A Documentary History* (Westport, Conn.: Greenwood, 1998), p. 152.

48. *The Normal Heart* was as much a work of politics as it was a work of art. Frank Rich, the *New York Times*'s theater critic, observed, "The playwright starts off angry, soon gets furious and skyrockets into sheer rage." From "Theater: 'The Normal Heart,' " *NYT,* 4/22/85, p. C17.

49. See Mark Miller, "The Selling of Philadelphia," *Newsweek,* 122:25, 12/20/93, p. 99.

50. Robert Koehler, "Normal Heart Stirs Up the Heartland," *LAT,* 12/3/89, p. 41 (Calendar section).

51. Catherine Woodard, "Cuomo Defends Archdiocese on AIDS Care," *Newsday,* 1/10/90, p. 6.

52. Peter Dworkin and Scott Minerbrook, "The AIDS Threat to Teenagers," *U.S. News and World Report,* 107:16, 10/23/89, p. 29.

53. AP, "Vatican Firms Its Stand on Homosexuals: Orders Bishops to Attack 'Sinful' Acts, Oppose Acceptance," *LAT,* 10/30/86, p. A2.

54. "Excerpts from Statement on AIDS and Condoms by Catholic Conference," *NYT,* 12/11/87, p. D17.

55. William Montalbano, "AIDS Conference Hears Papal Appeal for Unity," *LAT,* 11/16/89, p. A7.

56. Malcolm Gray, Anne Steacy, and Larry Black, "AIDS and the Priesthood," *MacLean's*, 2/23/87, p. 43.

57. Kenneth Woodward, Jane Whitmore, et al., "Gays in the Clergy," *Newsweek*, 2/23/87, p. 58.

58. Gray, Steacy, and Black, p. 43.

59. Andrew Sullivan, *Love Undetectable* (London: Chatto and Windus), p. 44.

60. Peter Steinfels, "Southern Baptists Condemn Homosexuality as 'Depraved,' " *NYT*, 6/17/88, p. B6.

61. Ibid.

62. Randy Shilts, "Gay Nuptials and Public Health," *San Francisco Chronicle*, 10/30/89, p. A4.

63. Americans for a Sound AIDS/HIV Policy, *To the Challenge of AIDS/HIV* (MAP International), p. 12.

64. Bishop Swing to George Bush, "Personal Comments," VP Records, Domestic Policy Office 87–88: AIDS Domestic Policy Council, OA/ID 15224.

65. Marjorie Hyer, "Bishop Urges Church Action on AIDS Care," *WP*, 10/31/86, p. A16.

66. Among AmFAR grants recipients in a typical month were an AZT trial study, a pilot study of aerosolized pentamidine, a study of acupuncture, a clinical trial of newly developed antibiotics useful in treatment of opportunistic infections. See "AmFAR Awards Nearly $1 Million to Community-Based Clinical Trial Centers Testing Promising AIDS/HIV Treatments," *AmFAR News Release*, 8/14/90, OFL JC Papers, AIDS-AmFAR: OA/ID 08403. See also David Firestone, "GMHC's New Six-Story Home Is a Symbol of 'Success' for Service Organizations That Would Rather Go Out of Business," *Newsday*, 12/29/88, part II, p. 4.

67. See Jeanne Braham and Pamela Paterson, *Starry, Starry Night: Provincetown's Response to the AIDS Epidemic* (Cambridge, Mass.: Lumen Editions, 1998), pp. 1–5.

68. Rifka Rosenwein, "Associates Raising Money to Fund Suits over AIDS," *Manhattan Lawyer*, 5/31/88, p. 4.

69. As quoted in Arthur Kahn, *AIDS: The Winter War* (Philadelphia: Temple University Press, 1993), p. 4.

70. Victor Zonana, "AIDS Overwhelming San Francisco System," *LAT*, 5/12/89, p. A3.

71. Quoted in Robert Scheer, " 'We Are Not Lepers': AIDS Stigma Hampering a Solution," *LAT*, 11/28/86, p. A1.

72. Christopher Sherman, "My Suggestions for Those Diagnosed with AIDS," in Michael Callen, Jane Rosett, and Richard Dworkin, eds., *Surviving and Thriving with AIDS*, vol. 2, (New York: People with AIDS Coalition, 1988) p. 17.

73. Larry Kramer, *Reports from the Holocaust*, p. 23.

Chapter 6

1. "Ozone Tops AIDS: Ozone Blood Treatment Cures AIDS Victims in Germany, No Mention in U.S. Media," *Now What*, no. 1, 3/87.

2. Deborah Ibert, "Bogus Cures for AIDS Abound," *Bergen Record*, 10/11/87, p. A1.

3. Cory SerVaas, "Did This Doctor Cure His AIDS?" *Saturday Evening Post*, 10/86, p. 60.

4. "Inside the Illegal AIDS Drug Trade," *Newsweek*, 8/15/88, p. 41.

5. See Kent Sepkowitz, "AIDS—The First Twenty Years," *NEJM*, 344:23, 6/7/01, p. 1766.

6. See Terence Monmaney, "Kids with AIDS," *Newsweek*, 9/7/87, p. 56.

7. Andrew Veitch, "New Hope of Cure of AIDS," *The Guardian*, 9/26/84.

8. The 721 in the substance's name came from a semimythologized optimal ratio of 7 parts neutralipids, 2 parts phosphatidylcholine, and 1 part phosphitydaletheanolamine. See Mi-

chael Callen and Joseph Sonnabend, "A Word of Caution to Egg Lipid Purchasers," in Michael Callen, Jane Rosett, and Richard Dworkin, eds., *Surviving and Thriving with AIDS: Collected Wisdom,* vol. 2, (New York City: People with AIDS Coalition, 1988), p. 99.

9. It was HPA-23 for which Rock Hudson had traveled to France shortly before he died.

10. Laurie Rich and Reginald Rhein, "Weapons Against a Modern Scourge," *Chemical Week,* 5/6/87, pp. 48–51.

11. Robert Hanley, "Tragedy Spurs Demand for New Drugs, Products; AIDS Creates Niches for Medical Firms," *LAT,* 12/11/86, p. D1. See also Erik Calonius, "The Stock Play in AIDS Drugs," *Newsweek,* 11/3/86, pp. 48–49.

12. Ibert, "Bogus Cures for AIDS Abound," p. A1.

13. Stephen Morin and Walter Batchelor, "Responding to the Psychological Crisis of AIDS," *PHR,* v. 99, 1–2/84, pp. 4–9.

14. Donald Riesenberg and Charles Marwick, "Anti-AIDS Agents Show Varying Early Results in Vitro and in Vivo," *JAMA,* 254:18, 11/8/85, pp. 2521–29.

15. See Arthur Kahn, *AIDS: The Winter War* (Philadelphia: Temple University Press, 1993), p. 15.

16. See Riesenberg and Marwick, "Anti-AIDS Agents Show Varying Early Results," p. 2521; and Barry Schoub, *HIV and AIDS in Perspective,* 2nd ed. (New York: Cambridge University Press, 1994), especially chapter 6.

17. Sandra Boodman, "Victims Hail Distribution of AZT: Optimism Guarded About AIDS Drug's Long-Term Effectiveness," *WP,* 9/20/86, p. A7.

18. See Matt Clark and Mariana Gosnell, "Uproar over AIDS Drugs: Are Government Tests Going Too Slowly?" *Newsweek,* 4/6/87, p. 24.

19. See Peter Arno and Douglas Shenson, "Testimony Before the National Commission on AIDS," Washington, D.C., November, 1989, in AIDS Hearings, Box 1: Folder "T&S 8/30/89–1/25/90."

20. Quoted in Kahn, *AIDS: The Winter War,* p. 12.

21. See Barbara Culliton, "AZT Reverses AIDS Dementia in Children," *Science,* v. 246, 10/6/89, p. 21.

22. Larry Thompson, "Progress Against AIDS: Work Proceeds Amid Guarded Optimism," *WP,* 12/30/86, p. Z6.

23. "Excerpts of Remarks for Vice President George Bush," 7/21/87, OPD WE papers, AIDS Research:OA/ID 07496.

24. Peter Hutt, as quoted in Peter Arno and Karyn Feiden, *Against the Odds: The Story of the AIDS Drug Development, Politics and Profits* (New York: HarperCollins, 1992), p. 28.

25. For more on FDA trials, see Schoub, *HIV and AIDS in Perspective,* pp. 174–75.

26. Quoted in Arno and Feiden, *Against the Odds* p. 31.

27. See Mary Graham, "The Quiet Drug Revolution," *The Atlantic,* 1/91, pp. 34–40.

28. See Rich and Rhein, "Weapons Against a Modern Scourge," pp. 48–49.

29. As quoted in Kahn, *AIDS: The Winter War,* p. 166.

30. Michael Specter, "Public Nuisance," *New Yorker,* 5/13/02, p. 59.

31. Kramer, "An Open Letter to Dr. Anthony Fauci," *San Francisco Examiner,* 1/26/88, reprinted in *Notes from the Holocaust,* pp. 193–94.

32. Specter, "Public Nuisance," p. 58.

33. Jason DeParle, "Rude, Rash, Effective, ACT-UP Shifts AIDS Policy," *NYT,* 1/3/90, p. B1.

34. See Robert Houston, "Unfair Aspects of a Study for NCI on Alternative Cancer Therapies," *Townsend Letter for Doctors,* 1/90, pp. 66–68.

35. Lederer to Fauci, 1/31/90, NCAIDS papers, RG220, Correspondence Box 2, Folder L.

36. Jim Eigo, "Address to the AIDS Commission," AIDS Hearings papers, box 1, Testimony and Statements, 8/30/89–1/25/90.

37. See Kahn, *AIDS: The Winter War,* p. 10.

38. See Daniel Greenberg, "Putting Drugs on a Fasttrack May Hurt Research," *U.S. News and World Report,* 3/23/87, p. 76.

39. Joseph Palca, "AIDS Drug Trials Enter New Age," *Science,* v. 246, 10/6/89, p. 21.

40. See "AIDS: Out of Sight," *The Economist,* 10/8/88, p. 59.

41. Greenberg, "Putting Drugs on a Fasttrack May Hurt Research," p. 76.

42. Arno and Feiden, *Against the Odds,* p. 101.

43. Ibid., p. 102.

44. Frank Young, "Testimony Before the Committee on Labor and Human Resources, United States Senate," 7/13/88, p. 13, DM papers, OA 19046: "Dr. Mac's Book 3," 4/6.

45. Arno and Feiden, *Against the Odds,* p. 102.

46. Young, "Testimony," 7/13/88, p. 15.

47. Arno and Feiden, *Against the Odds,* p. 161.

48. Ibid., p. 107.

49. See "T cell Testing Recommendations Affect Planning Activities," *Intergovernmental AIDS Reports,* 2:2, 7–8/89, p. 1.

50. See Victor Zonana, "Network Set to Import Drugs That Are Not Approved by FDA," *LAT,* 3/7/89, p. A3.

51. Gina Kolata, "U.S. To Expand Uses of AIDS Medicines," *NYT,* 5/19/90, p. A8.

52. Quoted in Derek Link, "Fighting for Fair Access: DDI and Parallel Track Alternatives," *Gay Community News,* 17:25, 1/7–13/90.

53. Larry Kramer, "A Call to Riot," reprinted in *Notes from the Holocaust,* p. 315.

54. G. Steven Rose to National Commission on AIDS, 1/8/90, RG220, NCAIDS, Correspondence M-R, Box1: folder R.

55. National Commission on AIDS, "HIV Research and Drug Development," Draft of Report Number Three, 8/21/90, pp. 4–5, RG220, NCAIDS, Correspondence, Box 1/ Folder C.

56. See Anthony Fauci, "Background Statement for National Commission on AIDS, 5/7/90, pp. 7–8, RG220, AIDS Hearings, Box 1/ T&S, 8/30/89–1/25/90.

57. Specter, "Public Nuisance," p. 64.

58. Ibid., p. 63.

59. Ibid., p. 65.

60. T. Vollmer, "How Far with the Politics of Anger?" *San Francisco Sentinel,* 6/28/90, as quoted in Robert Wachter, "AIDS, Activism, and the Politics of Health," *NEJM,* 326:2, 1/9/92, p. 130.

61. Sullivan, "Gay Life, Gay Death," p. 21.

62. "Out and About," *The Economist,* 320:7717, 7/27/91, p. 21.

Chapter 7

1. See, Philip Elmer-Dewitt, "How Safe Is Sex?" *Time,* 138:21, 11/25/91, p. 73.

2. Ibid., p. 72.

3. Lisa Levitt Ryckman, "The 2nd Wave of the AIDS Epidemic Begins to Stalk a New Generation," *LAT,* 7/21/91, p. A27. See also James Curran, Harold Jaffe, et al., "Epidemiology of HIV Infection and AIDS in the United States," *Science,* v. 239, 2/5/88, p. 239.

4. See AIDS Program, Center for Infectious Diseases, CDC, "AIDS and Human Immunodeficiency Virus Infection in the United States: 1988 Update," Table 2, "Racial/Ethnic Distribution of the U.S. Population Compared to AIDS Cases, 1981–1988.

5. See "Report of the Second Public Health Service AIDS Prevention and Control Conference," *PHR,* v. 103, 11/88, pp. 91–94.

6. James Warner, "Estimating the Extent of HIV Infection," Memorandum for Health Policy Working Group, RS papers, 9/2/87, OA/6785: AIDS/Bauer, 1/2.

7. Stephen Joseph, *Dragon Within the Gates* (New York: Carroll and Graf, 1992), p. 121. See also early reporting on the IV epidemic in Ronald Sullivan, "In City, AIDS Affecting Drug Users More Often," *NYT*, 10/21/84, p. A42.

8. Stephen Joseph, *Dragon Within the Gates*, p. 123.

9. As quoted in Naomi Freundlich, "Now That AIDS Is Treatable, Who'll Pay the Crushing Cost?" *Business Week*, 9/11/89, p. 115.

10. Stephen Joseph, "How Great Is the TB Threat This Time?" *Newsday*, 2/15/88, p. 45.

11. James Baker, Nadine Joseph, et al., "Needing a Place to Die," *Newsweek*, 4/4/88, p. 24.

12. Ibid.

13. Francis Clines, "Via Addict Needles, AIDS Spreads in Edinburgh," *NYT*, 1/4/87, p. A8. See also Jennifer Foote, "AIDS, Ireland and the Church," *Newsweek*, 9/17/90, p. 44.

14. Don Schanche, "AIDS Increase in Caribbean Alarms Experts," *LAT*, 5/29/89, p. A1.

15. Tom Morganthau, Mark Miller, and Renee Michael, "The New Panic in Needle Park: AIDS," *Newsweek*, 4/13/88, p. 63.

16. Charles Schuster, "Intravenous Drug Use and AIDS Prevention," *PHR*, v. 103, 5–6/88, p. 26

17. Judy Foreman, "AIDS Panel Chief Paints Dire Future," *BG*, 11/19/88, p. A8.

18. Lewis Schrager, Gerald Friedland, Cheryl Feiner, and Patricia Kahl, "Demographic Characteristics, Drug Use, and Sexual Behavior of IV Drug Users with AIDS in Bronx, New York," *PHR*, v. 106, 1–2/91, pp. 78–84.

19. Stephen Joseph, *Dragon at the Gates*, pp. 114–15.

20. Ibid., p. 114.

21. Joseph's exact words describing this phenomenon are as follows: "It is likely that many cases of AIDS and AIDS deaths among drug addicts went unrecognized early in the epidemic, leaving the impression that the curve of infection among IV drug users lagged further behind that of gay men than it actually did" (p. 115).

22. See B. R. Edlin, S. Faruque, et al., "Intersecting Epidemics—Crack Cocaine Use and HIV Infection Among Inner-City Adults," *NEJM*, v. 331, 11/24/94, pp. 1422–27.

23. John Tierney, "Urban Epidemic: Addicts and AIDS," *NYT*, 12/16/90, p. A1.

24. "The AIDS Plague Spreads," *The Economist*, 7/15/89, p. 23.

25. Tierney, "Urban Epidemic."

26. Catherine Dressler, "Women Speak Out on Effects of AIDS," *LAT*, 10/29/89, p. E7.

27. Tierney, "Urban Epidemic."

28. William Schwartz, "Drug Addicts with Dirty Needles," *The Nation*, 6/20/87, p. 843.

29. Ibid.

30. See David Musto, *The American Disease: Origins of Narcotics Control* (New York: Oxford University Press, 1987).

31. Institute of Medicine, *Confronting AIDS: Directions for Public Health and Research* (Washington, D.C.: National Academy Press, 1986), p. 12.

32. "Report of the Workgroup on Intravenous Drug Abuse," from "Report of the Second Pubic Health Service AIDS Prevention and Control Conference," *PHR*, v. 103, 11/88, pp. 66–67.

33. See, for example, Robert Cohen, "Testimony Before the National Commission on AIDS," 8/17/90, New York, New York, AIDS Hearings Papers, Box 2: "Testimony and Statements, September 17–18, 1990."

34. Ibid.

35. See Musto, *The American Disease*, particularly chapter 12.

36. The study, conducted by Edward Kaplan, professor of policy modeling at Yale, was deemed conservative in its estimates—most likely the reduction rate was substantially higher. GAO, *Needle Exchange Programs: Research Suggests Promise as an AIDS Prevention Strategy*, GAO/HRD-93-60, 3/93, particularly appendix III.

37. "Assembly Minority Opposes Giving Addicts Free Needles," *NYT*, 2/18/88, p. B11.

38. Bruce Lambert, "The Free-Needle Program Is Under Way and Under Fire," *NYT*, 11/13/88, p. D6.

39. David Kirp and Ronald Bayer, "Needles and Race," *Atlantic*, 272:1, 7/93, p. 39.

40. Catherine Woodard, "AIDS Experts: Policy on Needles 'Genocide,' " *Newsday*, 6/8/90, p. 2.

41. See Thomson Prentice, "New Needle Swaps to Help Curb AIDS," *The Times of London*, 12/19/86.

42. June Osborn, "AIDS: Politics and Science," *NEJM*, 318:7, 2/18/88, p. 446.

43. Jeffrey Schmalz, "Addicts to Get Needles in Plan to Curb AIDS," *NYT*, 1/31/88, p. A1.

44. "Realism on AIDS," *The Nation*, 2/13/88, p. 1.

45. "Teens: The Rising Risk of AIDS," *Time*, 138:9, 9/2/91.

46. Allan Gold, "Bostonians Split on Mayor's Idea of Needle Swap," *BG*, 3/24/88, p. A16.

47. Paul Majendie, "As AIDS Strikes Catholic Ireland, a Dispute Erupts over Limited Sale of Condoms," *LAT*, 11/26/89, p. A11.

48. Robert Suro, "Vatican and the AIDS Fight: Amid Worry, Papal Reticence," *NYT*, 1/29/88, p. A1.

49. San Francisco AIDS Foundation, "The Adventures of Bleachman," 1988, reprinted in GAO, *AIDS Education: Reaching Populations at Higher Risk*, GAO/PEMD-88-35, 9/88, p. 51.

50. Allan Gold, "Crisis Spurs Shift in Program for Addicts," *NYT*, 4/27/88, p. A16.

51. Lewis Schrager, Gerald Friedland, Cheryl Feiner, and Patricia Kahl, "Demographic Characteristics, Drug Use, and Sexual Behavior of IV Drug Users with AIDS in Bronx, New York," *PHR*, v. 106, 1–2/91, p. 78. Also, Donald Hopkins, "AIDS in Minority Populations in the United States," *PHR*, v. 102, 11–12/97, p. 677.

52. See ibid. Also, Vickie Mays and Susan Cochran, "Acquired Immunodeficiency Syndrome and Black Americans: Special Psychosocial Issues," *PHR*, v. 102, 3–4/87, p. 224.

53. Charles Stewart, "Double Jeopardy: Black, Gay (and Invisible)," *The New Republic*, 205:23, 12/2/91, p. 14.

54. Kevin Leary, "Koop Warns Minorities Not to 'Politicize' AIDS," *San Francisco Chronicle*, 11/10/89, p. A3. See also Robert Schilling, Steven Schinke, et al., "Developing Strategies for AIDS Prevention Research with Black and Hispanic Drug Users," *PHR*, v. 104, 1–2/89, pp. 2–11.

55. Mays and Cochran, "Acquired Immunodeficiency Syndrome and Black Americans: Special Psychosocial Issues," pp. 224–31.

56. James Baker, Regina Elam, et al., "Joining the AIDS Fight," *Newsweek*, 4/17/89, p. 26.

57. Ibid.

58. Quoted in Andrew Sullivan, "Gay Life, Gay Death," *The New Republic*, 203:24, 12/17/90, p. 22.

59. Quoted in Clarence Page, "Deathly Silence," *The New Republic*, 205:23, 12/2/91, p. 15.

60. Quoted in ibid., p. 17.

61. Joseph, *Dragon Within the Gates*, p. 113.

62. For more on the Tuskegee syphilis study, see James Jones, *Bad Blood* (New York: The Free Press, 1981).

63. As quoted in David Holmberg, "Outrage over Needle Program; Black Leaders Protest Plan to Slow Spread of AIDS," *Newsday*, 10/13/88, p. 9.

64. Joseph, *Dragon Within the Gates*, p. 125.

65. See images in GAO, *AIDS Education: Reaching Populations at Higher Risk*, GAO/PEMD-88-35, 9/88, pp. 40–44.

66. Tim Padgett, "Waking Up to a Nightmare," *Newsweek*, 12/5/88, p. 24.

67. Gerardo Marin, "AIDS Prevention Among Hispanics: Needs, Risk Behaviors, and Cultural Values," *PHR,* v. 104, 9–10/89, p. 412.
68. See ibid., pp. 413–15.
69. Padgett, "Waking Up to a Nightmare," p. 24.
70. Ibid.
71. Marin, "AIDS Prevention Among Hispanics," p. 413.
72. Ibid., p. 412.
73. For statistics, see Isabel Suliveres, "Testimony Offered at the National AIDS Commission Hearing in Puerto Rico," 11/27/90, RG 220, NC AIDS papers, AIDS Hearings Box 1: "Testimony and Statements, 12/9–10/91."
74. Ron Howell, "AIDS in Puerto Rico," *Newsday,* 12/11/90, p. 55.
75. Charles Hughes to Maureen Byrnes, 11/29/90, RG 220, NC AIDS papers, AIDS Hearings Box 1: "Testimony and Statements 12/9–10/91."
76. Ibid.
77. Nancy Neveloff Dubler, "Testimony for the National Commission on Acquired Immune Deficiency Syndrome," 11/2/89, AIDS Hearings papers, Box 1: Testimony and Statements, 8/30/89–1/25/90.
78. Heather Rhoads, "The New Death Row," *The Progressive,* 9/91, p. 18.
79. Jon Nordheimer, "Medical Officials Worry About AIDS in Prisons," *NYT,* 8/11/85, p. A22.
80. Sara Polonsky, Sandra Kerr, et al., "HIV Prevention in Prisons and Jails: Obstacles and Opportunities," *PHR,* v. 109, 9–10/94, pp. 615–20.
81. Rhoads, "The New Death Row," p. 18.
82. Ibid., p. 23.
83. Larry Johnson, "Biographical Statement," 7/19/90, NC AIDS papers, RG 220, "Records Relating to Hearings on HIV and AIDS, Box 2: "Testimony and Statements, 9/17–18/90."
84. Alexa Freeman, "Alabama Prison Policies and Practices on AIDS," Testimony before the National Commission on AIDS, 8/17/90, NC AIDS papers, RG 220, "Records Relating to Hearings on HIV and AIDS, Box 2: "Testimony and Statements, 9/17–18/90."
85. Mike Arrington, "On Being HIV Positive in Alabama's Doc," NC AIDS papers, RG 220, "Records Relating to Hearings on HIV and AIDS, Box 2: "Testimony and Statements, 9/17–18/90."
86. Rhoads, p. 20.
87. M. E. Malone and Elizabeth Neuffer, "AIDS on Rise in Prisons," *BG,* 3/29/92, p. A1.
88. J. Michael Quinlan, "Mandatory Testing for HIV in Federal Prisons," *NEJM,* 320:5, 2/2/89, p. 316.
89. See, for example, Adam Starchild, "How Prisons Punish AIDS Victims," *NYT,* 6/7/88, op-ed page.
90. From an anonymous letter to Judy Greenspan, found in NC AIDS papers, AIDS Hearings, Box 2: "Testimony and Statements, 9/17–18/90."
91. Ibid.
92. As described in Nancy Neveloff Dubler, "Testimony to the National Commission on Acquired Immune Deficiency Syndrome," 11/2/89, from NC AIDS papers, AIDS Hearings, Box 1: "Testimony and Statements, 8/30/89–1/25/90."
93. Quoted in Judy Greenspan, "Testimony Before the National Commission on AIDS on Behalf of Prisoners with HIV Disease/AIDS," NC AIDS papers, AIDS Hearings, Box 2: "Testimony and Statements, 9/17–18/90."
94. Juan Rivera, "The Haven II," NC AIDS papers, Aids Hearings, Box 2: "Testimony and Statements, 9/17–18/90."
95. Alexa Freeman, "Alabama Prison Policies and Practices on AIDS," NC AIDS papers, Box 2: "Testimony and Statements, 9/17–18/90."

96. All statistics on sexual and drug-related activity are from Sara Polonsky, Sandra Kerr, et al., "HIV Prevention in Prisons and Jails: Obstacles and Opportunities," *PHR*, v. 109, pp. 615–20.

97. Juan Rivera, "The Haven II," NC AIDS papers, Aids Hearings, Box 2: "Testimony and Statements, 9/17–18/90."

98. Polonsky, Kerr, et al., "HIV Prevention in Prisons and Jails: Obstacles and Opportunities," pp. 620–22.

99. GAO, *Pediatric AIDS: Health and Social Service Needs of Infants and Children,* GAO/HRD-89-96, p. 1.

100. "Report of the Second Public Health Service AIDS Prevention and Control Conference," *PHR*, v. 103, 11/88, pp. 94–96.

101. See L. Thiry, S. Sprecher-Goldberger, et al., "Isolation of AIDS Virus from Cell-Free Breast Milk of Three Healthy Virus Carriers," *The Lancet*, 10/19/85, as reprinted in *The AIDS Reader*, 2nd ed., pp. 252–53.

102. Art Levine and Scott Minerbrook, "AIDS and the Innocents," *U.S. News and World Report*, 2/1/88, p. 49.

103. Ibid.

104. Ibid.

Chapter 8

1. Estimates varied, although many AIDS watchers had the greatest confidence in those generated by Scitovsky and Rice. See Anne Scitovsky and Dorothy Rice, "Estimates of the Direct and Indirect Costs of Acquired Immunodeficiency Syndrome in the United States," *PHR*, v. 102, 1–2/87, pp. 5–16. For per capita spending, see Fred Hollinger, "Updated Forecasts of the Costs of Medical Care for Persons with AIDS, 1989–93," *PHR*, v. 105, 1–2/90, pp. 1–12. Also Harris Collingwood, "What AIDS Will Cost Insurers," *Business Week,* 1/11/88, p. 49; and David Bloom and Geoffrey Carliner, "The Economic Impact of AIDS in the United States," *Science,* v. 239, 2/5/88, pp. 604–9.

2. Bloom and Carliner, "The Economic Impact of AIDS," p. 606.

3. David Rogers, "Federal Spending on AIDS: How Much Is Enough?" *NEJM,* 320:24, 6/15/89, pp. 1623–24.

4. Statistics from "Cost of Financing of HIV Infection," 4/28/89, CEA RS papers, Working Group on Health Policy/AIDS: OA/ID 03686. See also Philip Lee, "Statement Before the National Commission on AIDS," 11/3/89, NC AIDS papers, AIDS Hearings, Box 1: "Testimony and Statements 8/30/89–1/25/90."

5. Jesse Green and Peter Arno, "The Medicaidization of AIDS: Implications of the AIDS Payor Mix for Access and Quality," NC AIDS papers, Box 1: "Testimony and Statements 8/30/89–1/25/90," p. 2.

6. Tamar Jacoby, "Who Will Pay the AIDS Bill?" *Newsweek,* 4/11/88, p. 71.

7. Joan Hamilton, "Where Insurers Are Showing Little Mercy," *Business Week,* 11/21/88, p. 86.

8. Michael Winerip, "The Cost Crisis in Health Care Strikes Home," *NYT,* 6/20/93, p. A29.

9. Robert Pear, "Study Finds Most Health Insurers Screen Applicants for AIDS Virus," *NYT,* 2/18/88, p. A1.

10. Jacoby, "Who Will Pay the AIDS Bill?" p. 71.

11. All statistics from Green and Arno, "The Medicaidization of AIDS." See also Richard Conviser, "Testimony on Medicaid and the HIV Epidemic," Testimony before the Subcommittee on Health and Environment, Committee on Energy and Commerce, U.S. House of Representatives, 2/27/90.

12. NC AIDS, "Report Number One" (draft), 12/5/89, p. 4. OLA CA papers, AIDS Committee: OA/ID 05945.

13. Conviser, "Testimony," p. 5.

14. Ibid., p. 4. See also Martha McKinney, Melanie Wieland, et al., "States' Responses to Title II of the Ryan White CARE Act," *PHR*, v. 108, 1–2/93, pp. 4–11.

15. Catherine Woodard, "Bill on Private Insurance for AIDS," *Newsday*, 3/13/90, p. 17.

16. "Interview between 'Marc' and Michael Callen," Halloween, 1987, in Michael Callen, ed., *Surviving and Thriving with AIDS: Collected Wisdom*, vol. 2 (New York: People With AIDS Coalition, 1988), pp. 145–46.

17. See Robert Parrish, "Statement Before the House Energy and Commerce Committee, Subcommittee on Health and the Environment," 2/27/90, PPI papers, Box 22: "Medicaid and HIV Hearings."

18. "Statement of Philip Fornaci Before the National AIDS Commission," 12/9/91, NC AIDS papers, Box 3: "Testimony and Statements," 12/9–10/91, 3/3.

19. Irvin Molotsky, "Congress Passes Compromise AIDS Bill," *NYT*, 10/14/88.

20. Kennedy to Osborn, 2/5/90, NC AIDS papers, Correspondence 1989–93, A-F, Box 1: Folder C.

21. "Opening Statement of Congressman Henry Waxman at Hearings on AIDS and Medicaid," 2/27/90, PPI papers, Box 22: "Medicaid and HIV Hearings."

22. "Statement of Administration Policy" (HR 4785), 6/12/90, DPC papers, AIDS: OA/ID 04807 1/3. Also "Fact Sheet HIV/AIDS: Ryan White Comprehensive AIDS Services," OPD JK papers, AIDS Federal Efforts and Legislation: OA/ID 06961.

23. Philip Hilts, "$2.9 Billion Bill for AIDS Relief Gains in Senate," *NYT*, 5/16/90, p. A1.

24. Philip Hilts, "Senate Panel Approves a Major Cut in AIDS Relief for Cities," *NYT*, 10/11/90, p. D23.

25. Jack Sirica, "Senate Unit Cuts AIDS Funding: Reduces $882 Million in Bill to $110 Million," *Newsday*, 9/13/90, p. 6.

26. See Stephen Brown, Katherine Marconi, et al., "First Year of AIDS Services Delivery Under Title I of Ryan White CARE Act," *PHR*, v. 107, 9–10/92, pp. 491–99.

27. Martha McKinney, Melanie Wieland, et al., "States' Responses to Title II of the Ryan White CARE Act," *PHR*, v. 108, 1–2/93, pp. 4–11.

28. "Remarks for Vice President George Bush, Third International Conference on AIDS," 6/1/87, VP Records, Press Office: AIDS, OA/ID 14922.

29. Marcia Angell, "A Dual Approach to the AIDS Epidemic," *NEJM*, 324:21, 5/23/91, p. 1500.

30. Stephen Joseph, "Quarantine: Sometimes a Duty," *NYT*, 2/10/90, p. A25. Joseph had been appalled at a recently exposed case of a California man, knowing that he was infected with HIV, repeatedly selling his blood for transfusion.

31. David Rogers and June Osborn, "Another Approach to the AIDS Epidemic," *NEJM*, 325:11, 9/12/91, p. 806. Also, GAO, *AIDS-Prevention Programs: High-Risk Groups Still Prove Hard to Reach*, GAO/HRD-91-52.

32. "Remarks for Vice President George Bush," 6/1/87, p. 4.

33. Mike Clary, "Florida's Dilemma with AIDS-Infected Health Workers Stirs National Attention," *LAT*, 6/9/91, p. A21.

34. Mike Clary, "AIDS Victim Infected by Dentist Dies," *LAT*, 12/9/91, p. A4.

35. Quoted in Intergovernmental Health Policy Project, "Testing Health Care Workers: The Debate Continues; Everett Koop 'Sets the Record Straight,' " *Intergovernmental AIDS Reports*, 10/91, p. 4.

36. Gerry Studds, "Revealing Health Workers' HIV Status Costs," *Boston Sunday Herald*, 10/27/91.

37. See Michael Paulson, "Rep. Studds Resists AIDS Test Plea by Bergalis," *The South Boston Patriot Ledger,* 9/27/91.

38. "Comments of David Barr, Assistant Director of Policy of the Gay Men's Health Crisis to the National Commission on AIDS," 11/5/91, NC AIDS papers, AIDS Hearings, Box 3: "Testimony and Statements," 12/9–10/91, 3/3.

39. See Intergovernmental Health Policy Project, "1989 Legislative Overview," *Intergovernmental AIDS Reports,* 1/90.

40. See, for example, "Immigrants with AIDS Would Only Burden U.S.," *Macon (Ga.) Telegraph,* 2/24/91, p. 48.

41. The Nevada program was passed after the Chicken Ranch brothel voluntarily began requiring all patrons to wear condoms, resulting in a zero AIDS transmission rate as well as a 95 percent drop-off in cases of gonorrhea among the prostitutes. See Bob Baker, "Study of Brothel Prostitutes Finds Little Venereal Disease," *LAT,* 8/26/91, p. A3.

42. Ruth Faden and Nancy Kass, "Health Insurance and AIDS: The Status of State Regulatory Activity," *AJPH,* 78:4, 4/88, pp. 437–39.

43. "Comments of David Barr," 11/5/91, p. 1.

44. Gary Noble, William Parra, and Priscilla Holman, "Organizational Structure and Resources of CDC's HIV-AIDS Prevention Program," *PHR,* v. 106, 11–12/91, pp. 604–7. Also, CDC, "Information/Education Plan to Prevent and Control AIDS in the United States," 2/18/87, RS papers, OA 16784: "AIDS General," 1/2.

45. George Bush, "AIDS-Education," 6/13/88, VP Records Press Office: "Kristen Clark Taylor, AIDS," OA/ID 14958.

46. Peter Smith, "Homeless with AIDS Desperately Need Supportive Housing," *NYT,* 4/30/90, p. A16.

47. "Statement of the American Hospital Association on the AIDS Housing Opportunity ACT, H.R. 3423," Testimony before the Subcommittee on Housing and Community Development, House Committee on Banking, Finance, and Urban Affairs, 3/21/90, NC AIDS papers, AIDS Hearings, Box 1: "Testimony and Statements," 8/30/89–1/25/90.

48. Ervin Marrero, Untitled letter, NC AIDS papers, Correspondence, Box 3: folder N.

49. Ibid.

50. Barry Bianchi, "Testimony to the Housing Subcommittee on Banking, Finance, and Urban Affairs," 3/21/90, p. 4, NC AIDS papers, AIDS Hearings, Box 1: "Testimony and Statements," 8/30/89–1/25/91.

51. Robert Greenwald, "Statement on AIDS Housing Opportunities for the National Commission on AIDS," 3/2/92 NC AIDS papers, AIDS Hearings, Box 3: "Testimony and Statements," 1/14/92.

52. Jim Graham, "Testimony to the Housing Subcommittee on Banking, Finance, and Urban Affairs," 3/21/90, NC AIDS papers, AIDS Hearings, Box 1: "Testimony and Statements," 8/30/89–1/25/91.

53. Bianchi, 3/21/90, p. 6.

54. Greenwald, 3/2/92, p. 5.

55. See Testimony of Anna Kondrates, "Hearing of the National Commission on AIDS," 3/3/92, NC AIDS papers, AIDS Hearings, Box 3: "Testimony and Statements," 1/14/92.

56. Greenwald, 3/2/92, p. 6.

57. "Remarks by the President in Address to National Leadership Coalition on AIDS," 3/29/90, Office of the First Lady, Jean Becker papers, AIDS: OA/ID 07494.

58. See Johnson to Bush, 1/14/92, Office of Cabinet Affairs, Daniel Casse papers, AIDS Commission: OA/ID 07133. Johnson's letter reads with some drama: "In the last two months I have switched games, from basketball to, I guess, the biggest game of all—life and death."

59. Scott Harris and Stephanie Chavez, "Calls Flood AIDS Hot Lines, Clinics After Announcement," *LAT,* 11/9/91, p. A1. Many people were initially skeptical of Johnson's claims to have contracted the disease through heterosexual intercourse. Johnson's response was to emphasize his own promiscuity, or possibly virility: "I confess that after I arrived in L.A. in 1979, I did my best to accommodate as many women as I could—most of them through unprotected sex." Associated Press, "Magic Blames Weakness in Numbers," *LAT,* 11/13/91, p. C1.

60. Henry Waxman, "Perspective on AIDS: Can Magic Lead Where Two Presidents Wouldn't?" *LAT,* 11/10/91, p. M5.

61. "News from the Office of Congressman Gerry E. Studds," 5/7/92, NC AIDS papers, Correspondence, Box 4: Folder S.

62. Marlene Cimons, "Boost in AIDS Research Funding Urged: Health Panel Asks Government to Raise Federal Agency's $804 Million Budget by 25%," *LAT,* 3/8/91, p. A25.

63. "Statement on the Meeting Between the National Commission on AIDS and the Secretary of Health and Human Services," 6/25/92, OCA JL papers, AIDS: OA/ID 07867.

64. Philip Hilts, "National AIDS Panel Says Administration Has Not Done Enough," *NYT,* 6/26/92, p. A18.

65. Waxman, "Perspective," 11/10/91.

66. Johnson to Bush, 1/14/92.

67. "HIV/AIDS Versus Cancer Spending," 2/7/92. OLA JK papers, AIDS: OA/ID 07244.

68. From PHS staff estimates. See Jeff Blend and Peter Nakahata, "Memorandum for the Director," 8/4/92, OPD JK papers, AIDS Federal Effort-Legislation: OA/ID 00961.

69. "Investment in AIDS Research by the Administration," 9/12/91, CS JS papers, AIDS: CF/OA 00470.

70. Michael Fumento, "The Magic's Gone," *National Review,* 44:20, 10/19/92, p. 49.

71. See National Commission on AIDS, *Mobilizing America's Response to AIDS: Recommendations to President Clinton,* 1/22/93, NC AIDS papers, Box 1: folder C.

Chapter 9

1. Mortimer Zuckerman, "Epidemics and Delusions," *U.S. News and World Report,* 107:19, 11/13/89, p. 92; Geoffrey Cowley, Mary Hager, and Ruth Marshall, "AIDS: The Next Ten Years," *Newsweek,* 115:26, 6/25/90, p. 20.

2. Sandy Rovner, "Can AIDS Travel from Women to Men?" *WP,* 1/8/86, p. 11 ("Health" Section). The Oprah Winfrey incident is recounted in an untitled article dated 11/2/98 on Michael Fumento's Web site, www.mfumento.com.

3. "Modeling Calamity," *Science News,* 1988, p. 26.

4. Geoffrey Cowley, Mary Hager, and Ruth Marshall, "AIDS: The Next Ten Years," *Newsweek,* 115:26, 6/25/90, p. 20.

5. Connie Leslie, Tim Padgett, Pat Wingert, and Mary Hager, "Amid the Ivy, Cases of AIDS," *Newsweek,* 11/14/88, p. 65.

6. Described in Michael Fumento, *The Myth of Heterosexual AIDS* (New York: Basic Books, 1991), pp. 7–8.

7. William Masters, Virginia Johnson, and Robert Kolodny, *Crisis: Heterosexual Behavior in the Age of AIDS* (New York: Grove Press, 1988), p. 3.

8. Ibid., p. 7.

9. Ibid., p. 22.

10. See excerpted sections and comments "Sex in the Age of AIDS," *Newsweek,* 3/14/88, pp. 45–50.

11. "Cold Comfort on AIDS," *The Economist,* 3/12/88, p. 14.

12. Quoted in Philip Boffey, "Therapists Say Heterosexual AIDS Is 'Rampant,' " *NYT,* 3/6/88, p. A38; and "Masters and Johnson AIDS Controversy Grows; Researchers Dismiss Findings as Unfounded," *Bergen Record,* 3/8/88, p. A3.

13. See Lawrence Altman, "Expert Sees No Sign of Heterosexual Outbreak," *NYT,* 6/5/87, p. A17.

14. As quoted in Mickey Kaus, Mary Hager, et al., "The 'Small Health Problem' of AIDS," *Newsweek,* 6/13/87, p. 46.

15. As quoted in Steven Findlay, "AIDS Is Not Exploding in the General Population," *U.S. News and World Report,* 2/29/88, p. 58.

16. Mary Cronin, "How to Block a Killer's Path," *Time,* 1/30/89, p. 60.

17. "Excerpts from Report of Commission on AIDS," *NYT,* 2/25/88, p. B7.

18. Ibid.

19. From the Web site of Michael Fumento, 2/2/98, www.mfumento.com.

20. See Stephen Joseph, *Dragon Within the Gates* (New York: Carroll and Graf, 1992) pp. 136–38.

21. See Joe Queenan, "Straight Talk About AIDS," *Forbes,* 6/26/89, p. 41.

22. Fumento, *The Myth of Heterosexual AIDS,* p. 16.

23. Ibid., pp. 16–17.

24. As quoted in ibid., p. 18.

25. Ibid., p. 21.

26. Ibid., p. 30.

27. Ibid., p. 32.

28. Alfred Kinsey, *Sexual Behavior in the Human Male* (Philadelphia: W. B. Saunders, 1948). See also Michael Fumento, "How Many Gays?" *National Review,* 45:8, 4/26/93, pp. 28–29. The National Opinion Research Center at the University of Chicago estimated that 2.8 percent of men were exclusively homosexual, and 2.5 percent of women. See Patrick Rogers, "How Many Gays Are There?" *Newsweek,* 121:7, 2/15/93, p. 46.

29. Ibid., p. 29.

30. Michael Fumento, "Good Cause," *National* Review, 44:14, 7/20/92, p. 15.

31. See Mona Charen, "The Curious Ways of AIDS Activists," *Newsday,* 1/22/92.

32. Select Committee on Children, Youth, and Families, 102nd Congress, *A Decade of Denial: Teens and AIDS in America: Minority Report,* pp. 1–3, OPP JK papers, AIDS Government Background, OA/ID 06961, 3/3.

33. Andrew Sullivan, *Love Undetectable: Notes on Friendship, Sex, and Survival* (New York: Knopf, 1998).

34. Ibid., p. 61.

35. See Michael Fumento, "Media, AIDS, and Truth," *National Review,* 6/21/93, pp. 45–47.

36. Michael Fumento, "Exploding Myths," *National Review,* 45:24, 12/13/93, pp. 42–43.

37. Reprinted in "I Agree," *Forbes,* 7/10/89, pp. 20–21.

38. "Medical Correctness," *National Review,* 45:5, 3/15/93, p. 19.

39. GAO, *Defense Health Care: Effects of AIDS in the Military,* GAO/HRD-90-39, 2/90, pp. 2–4.

40. Quoted in Earl Lane, "Invisible Epidemic" AIDS Seen as a Clout Issue," *Newsday,* 2/5/93, p. 26.

41. "Medical Correctness," p. 19.

42. Robert Jeffery, Gregory Burke, Thomas Schmid, and Jing Ma, "Pilot Study of AIDS Risk in the General Population," *PHR,* v. 107, 1–2/92, pp. 105–9.

43. Nancy Padian, Stephen Shiboski, and Nicholas Jewell, "Female-to-Male Transmission of Human Immunodeficiency Virus," *JAMA,* 266:12, 9/25/91, pp. 1664–67.

44. See Nancy Padian, Stephen Shiboski, and Nicholas Jewell, "The Effect of Number of Exposures on the Risk of Heterosexual HIV Transmission," *Journal of Infectious Diseases*, v. 161, 5/90, pp. 883–87.

45. Padian, Shiboski, and Jewell, "Female-to-Male Transmission," p. 1666.

46. See, for example, J. Neil Simonsen, D. William Cameron, et al., "Human Immunodeficiency Virus Infection Among Men with Sexually Transmitted Diseases," *NEJM*, 319:5, 8/4/88, pp. 274–77.

47. Quoted in Laurie Garrett, "Clue to AIDS Transmission in Africa," *Newsday*, 9/18/88, p. 13.

48. Described in Philip Hilts, "Spread of AIDS by Heterosexuals Remains Slow," *NYT*, 5/1/90, p. C1.

49. Described in Malcolm Gladwell, "Only Select," *TNR*, 208:25, 6/21/93, pp. 21–26.

50. Ibid., p. 22.

51. Peter Duesberg, "HIV Is Not the Cause of AIDS," *Science*, v. 241, 7/29/88, pp. 514–17.

52. Peter Duesberg, *Inventing the AIDS Virus* (Washington, D.C.: Regnery Publishing, 1996), p. 217.

53. Quoted in Virginia Berridge, *AIDS in the UK: The Making of Policy, 1981–1994* (Oxford, U.K.: Oxford University Press, 1996), p. 241.

54. See Tom Bethell, "Could Duesberg Be Right?" *National Review*, 44:16, 8/17/92, p. 22.

55. Quoted in Stephen Joseph, "In Search of AIDS," *National Review*, 45:12, 6/21/93, p. 71.

56. See Jerome Groopman, "The End of Etiologogy," *TNR*, 221:26, 12/27/99, pp. 28–34.

57. Joan Shenton, *Positively False: Exposing the Myths Around HIV and AIDS* (New York: St. Martin's Press, 1998), p. 157.

58. See William Schmidt, "British Paper and Science Journal Clash on AIDS," *NYT*, 12/10/93, p. A9.

59. See V. K. Agadzi, *AIDS: The African Perspective of the Killer Disease* (Accra: Ghana Universities Press, 1989), pp. 17–20. Also, "Sense and Nonsense on AIDS," *West Africa*, 2/9/87, reprinted in Loren Clarke and Malcolm Potts, eds., *The AIDS Reader* (Brookline Village, Md.: Branden Publishing, 1988), pp. 305–7.

60. Richard and Rosalind Chirimuuta, *AIDS, Africa, and Racism* (London: Free Association Books, 1989), p. 7.

61. Robert Strecker, "AIDS: Who Invented It and Why," PPI papers, Box 6: "Communities of Color/Racial Issues."

62. Ibid, p. 3.

63. Alan Cantwell Jr., *AIDS and the Doctors of Death: An Inquiry into the Origin of the AIDS Epidemic* (Los Angeles: Aries Rising Press, 1988), p. 7.

64. Ibid., p. 30.

65. Tony Brown, *Black Lies, White Lies: The Truth According to Tony Brown,* (New York: Harper, 1997), pp. 142, 146.

66. Ibid., p. 143.

Chapter 10

1. Andrew Veitch, "Society Tomorrow: The Aids That Africa Could Do Without: Immune Deficiency Disease Among African Heterosexuals," *The Guardian*, 10/31/84.

2. Colin Norman, "Politics and Science Clash on African AIDS," *Science*, v. 230, 12/6/85, pp. 1140–41.

3. Marlene Cimons, "1 Million Africans to Die of AIDS, Report Predicts," *LAT*, 12/5/86, p. A5.

4. Quoted in Lawrence Altman, "AIDS in Africa: A Pattern of Mystery," *NYT,* 11/8/85, p. A1.

5. As quoted in Laurie Garrett, "A Continent at Risk: Heterosexual Epidemic Ravaging World of Poor Resources, Education," *Newsday,* 12/26/88, p. 5.

6. Jonathan Mann, "Statement of the U.S. National AIDS Commission," 11/2/89, NC AIDS papers, AIDS Hearings, Box 1: "Testimony and Statements," 8/30/89–1/25/90.

7. GAO, *AIDS: Information on Global Dimensions and Possible Impacts,* GAO/NSIAD-88-51FS, p. 8.

8. Cited in James Brooke, "Nigeria Insists It'll Keep AIDS the Rare Exception," *NYT,* 8/9/88, p. A6.

9. See Daniel Hrdy, "Cultural Practices Contributing to the Transmission of Human Immunodeficiency Virus in Africa," in Dieter Koch-Weser and Hannelore Vanderschmidt, eds., *The Heterosexual Transmission of AIDS in Africa* (Cambridge, Mass.: Abt Books, 1988), pp. 256–57; also Albert Gunn, Nancy Hansel, et al., *AIDS in Africa* (Washington, D.C.: Foundation for Africa's Future, 1988), pp. 24–27.

10. As quoted in Kurt Shillinger, "Churches' Aid Sought for Gay Rights in Zimbabwe," *BG,* 12/8/98, p. A16.

11. Lynn James, "African Practices May Offer Insights on AIDS," *NYT,* 11/22/85, p. A34.

12. See also Hrdy, "Cultural Practices Contributing to the Transmission of Human Immunodeficiency Virus in Africa," pp. 259–60.

13. See Larry Olmstead, "AIDS a Political Issue in S. Africa; Blacks Wary of Any Contraceptive Methods," Knight-Ridder News Service, 10/9/88.

14. Quoted in Tom Masland, "Breaking the Silence," *Newsweek,* 136:3, 7/17/00, p. 30.

15. Ibid., p. 32.

16. Christopher Wren, "A Continent's Agony: A Periodic Report," *NYT,* 9/27/90, p. A12.

17. Jonathan Mann, Thomas Quinn, and Peter Piot, "Condom Use and HIV Infection Among Prostitutes in Zaire," *NEJM,* 316:6, 2/5/87, p. 345. Also, Laurie Garrett, "A Continent at Risk: Heterosexual Epidemic Ravages World of Poor Resources, Education," *Newsday,* 12/26/88, p. 5.

18. Johanna McGeary, "Death Stalks a Continent," *Time Atlantic,* 157:6, 2/12/01, pp. 44–48.

19. For more on the demography of gender roles across sub-Saharan Africa, see Panos Institute, *The Hidden Cost of AIDS: The Challenge of HIV to Development* (Washington, D.C.: The Panos Institute, 1992), particularly chapter 1.

20. Recounted in "Elizabeth," in *Positive Women: Voices of Women Living with AIDS,* ed. Andrea Rudd and Darien Taylor (Toronto: Second Story Press, 1992), pp. 64–66.

21. H. Jack Geiger, "Letter from South Africa," *PHR,* v. 110, 3–4/95, pp. 114–16.

22. "In the Heart of the Plague," *The Economist,* 3/21/87, p. 59.

23. Ibid.

24. Denise Gilgen, Catherine Campbell, Brian Williams, et al., *The Natural History of HIV/AIDS in South Africa: A Biomedical and Social Survey in Carletonville* (Braamfontein: Council for Scientific and Industrial Research), pp. 13–16.

25. McGeary, "Death Stalks a Continent," pp. 44–48.

26. Ibid.

27. Ann Giudici Fettner, "We Can't Ask Africa to See Sex As We Do," *NYT,* 11/5/90, p. A20.

28. John Tierney, "AIDS in Africa: Experts Study Role of Promiscuous Sex in the Epidemic," *NYT,* 10/19/90, p. A10.

29. Alex Shoumatoff, "In Search of the Source of AIDS," from Shoumatoff, *African Madness* (New York: Knopf, 1988), p. 171.

30. N. Clumeck, P. Van de Perre, M. Carael, et al., "Heterosexual Promiscuity Among African Patients with AIDS," *NEJM,* 313:3, 6/18/85, p. 182.

31. Blaine Harden, "Uganda Battles AIDS Epidemic: Disease Reported Rampant Among Promiscuous Heterosexuals," *WP*, 6/2/86, p. A1.

32. Sanford Ungar, "AIDS Cases in Africa: An Everyone Epidemic," *LAT*, 1/15/89.

33. Joan Kreiss, Davy Koech, et al., "AIDS Virus Infection in Nairobi Prostitutes," *NEJM*, 314:7, 2/13/86, pp. 414–18.

34. Jonathan Mann, "Sexual Practices Associated with LAV/HTLV-III Seropositivity Among Female Prostitutes in Kinshasa, Zaire," presented at the 2nd International Conference on AIDS, Paris (6/23–25/86), as cited in Brooke Grundfest Schoepf, Rukarangira wa Nkera, et al., "AIDS and Society in Central Africa: A View from Zaire," in *The Heterosexual Transmission of AIDS in Africa*, ed. Koch-Weser and Vanderschmidt. See also Jonathan Mann, James Chin, Peter Piot, and Thomas Quinn, "The International Epidemiology of AIDS," *Scientific American*, 10/88, pp. 81–90.

35. Francis Plummer, Mark Tyndall, et al., "Sexual Transmission of HIV and the Role of Sexually Transmitted Disease," in *AIDS in Africa*, ed. Max Essex, Souleymane Mboup, Phyllis Kanki, and Mbowa Kalengayi (New York: Raven Press, 1994), pp. 195–202.

36. Bea Vuylsteke, Rose Sunkutu, and Marie Laga, "Epidemiology of HIV and Sexually Transmitted Infections in Women," in *AIDS in the World*, ed. Jonathan Mann and David Tarantola (New York: Oxford University Press, 1996), pp. 101–14.

37. Gilgen, Campbell, Williams, et al., *The Natural History of HIV/AIDS*, pp. 124–25.

38. As quoted in Laurie Garrett, "Discovery: Sex and AIDS," *Newsday*, 12/27/88, p. 1.

39. Gilgen, Campbell, Williams, et al., *The Natural History of HIV/AIDS*, pp. 126–28.

40. Quoted in "Tuberculosis, HIV Co-Epidemic to Multiply Sevenfold in Asia," *PHR*, v. 110, 1–2/95, pp. 108–9.

41. Peter Piot, Johan Goeman, and Marie Laga, "The Epidemiology of HIV and AIDS in Africa," in *AIDS in Africa*, ed. Max Essex, Souleymane Mboup, Phyllis Kanki, and Mbowa Kalengayi (New York: Raven Press, 1994), p. 164.

42. "Tuberculosis Epidemic Worldwide Emergency," *PHR*, v. 111, 1–2/96, pp. 8–9.

43. See, for example, Donatella Lorch, "After Years of Ignoring AIDS Epidemic, Kenya Has Begun Facing Up to It," *NYT*, 12/18/93, p. A5.

44. Gunn, Hansel, et al., *AIDS in Africa*, pp. 33–39.

45. Quoted in Norman, "Politics and Science Clash on African AIDS," p. 1140.

46. Sheryl Ramsey, "The Tragedy of AIDS in Africa," *Newsweek*, 135:6, 2/7/00, p. 16.

47. Ibid. p. 17.

48. Johanna McGeary, "Death Stalks a Continent," *Time Atlantic*, 157:6, 2/12/01, pp. 44–53.

49. Bill Keller, "As Isolation of Racism Eases, South Africa Confronts AIDS," *NYT*, p. A1.

50. Ibid.

51. Quoted in Norman, "Politics and Science Clash on African AIDS," p. 1140.

52. As quoted in Gunn, Hansel, et al., *AIDS in Africa*, p. 31.

53. Ibid., pp. 42–45.

54. Panos Institute, *The Hidden Cost of AIDS*, pp. 30–32.

55. Quoted in McGeary, "Death Stalks a Continent," p. 45.

56. Laurie Garrett, "A Continent at Risk: Heterosexual Epidemic Ravaging World of Poor Resources, Education," *Newsday*, 12/26/88, p. 5.

57. Panos Institute, *The Hidden Cost of AIDS*, p. 43.

58. Ibid., p. 42.

59. See Robert Colebunders and Bila Kapita, "Treatments for HIV Infection," in *AIDS in Africa*, ed. Max Essex, Souleymane Mboup, Phyllis Kanki, and Mbowa Kalengayi (New York: Raven Press, 1994), pp. 423–34.

60. THETA, "Innovation or Re-Awakening? Roles of Traditional Healers in the Management and Prevention of HIV/AIDS in Uganda" (THETA, 1998), p. 29.

61. "An African Example," *The Economist*, 320:7725, 9/21/91, p. 22.

62. Gunn, Hansel, et al., *AIDS in Africa*, p. 23.

63. See H. Jack Geiger, "Letter from South Africa," *PHR*, v. 110, 3–4/95, pp. 114–16.

64. Jane Perlez, "Briton Sees AIDS Cutting Population in Parts of Africa," *NYT*, 6/22/92, p. A8.

65. Michael Specter, "Doctors Powerless as AIDS Rakes Africa," *NYT*, 8/6/98, p. A1.

66. See Rozlyn Coleman Engel, *An Analysis of the Effects of HIV/AIDS on Worker Training in Africa*, Ph.D. dissertation, Department of Economics, Columbia University, 2003.

67. Alan Whiteside, "Economic Impact in Selected Countries and the Sectoral Impact," in *AIDS in the World*, ed. Jonathan Mann and David Tarantola (New York: Oxford University Press, 1996), pp. 112–13.

68. See Tony Barnett and Piers Blaikie, "The Reality of HIV/AIDS: Three Households," in Panos Institute, *The Hidden Cost of AIDS*, pp. 96–97.

69. John Barnes and Steven Findlay, "AIDS in Africa: Ravager of Nation Builders," *U.S. News*, 6/27/88, p. 32.

70. M. Ndilu, D. Sequeira, S. Hassig, et al., "Medical, Social, and Economic Impact of HIV Infection in a Large African Factory," *IV International Conference on AIDS*, Stockholm, Sweden, 6/88, as cited in Martha Ainsworth and A. Mead Over, "The Economic Impact of AIDS on Africa," in *AIDS in Africa*, ed. Max Essex, Souleymane Mboup, Phyllis Kanki, and Mbowa Kalengayi (New York: Raven Press, 1994), pp. 561–62.

71. Kathleen Hunt, "Scenes from a Nightmare," *NYT*, 8/12/90, p. F25.

72. Data from the *Demographic Projection Model* using data from Population Division of the United Nations Department of International and Economic and Social Affairs. Cited in Carol Levine, David Michaels, and Sara Back, "Orphans of the HIV/AIDS Pandemic," in *AIDS in the World*, ed. Jonathan Mann and David Tarantola (New York: Oxford University Press, 1996), pp. 279–81.

73. GAO, *Foreign Assistance: Combating HIV/AIDS in Developing Countries*, GAO/NSI-AD-92-244, p. 9.

74. Lois McHugh, *AIDS: International Problems and Issues*, CRS Issue Brief IB87214, 10/16/89, p. 10.

75. Jonathan Mann, "Global AIDS: Epidemic at a Crossroads," 11/1/89, NC AIDS papers, AIDS Hearings, Box 1: "Testimony and Statements," 8/30/89–1/25/90.

76. GAO, *Foreign Assistance: Combating HIV/AIDS in Developing Countries*, GAO/NSI-AD-92-244, p. 31.

77. Uganda, for example, found that its greatest challenge in AIDS education was overcoming an adult illiteracy rate of 50 percent. See Gunn, Hansel, et al., *AIDS in Africa*, pp. 31–32.

Chapter 11

1. See Sabin Russell, "AIDS Cases Decline in S.F., Experts Say: Peak in 1992 Proves Prevention Programs Work," *San Francisco Chronicle*, 2/16/94, p. A1; also Lisa Krieger, "S.F. AIDS Epidemic Waning," *San Francisco Chronicle*, 2/16/94, p., A1.

2. Laurie Garrett, "Decline Seen in New HIV Cases/Evidence Epidemic May Be Peaking," *Newsday*, 11/13/95, p. A6.

3. David Kirp, "After the Band Stopped Playing," *The Nation*, 259:1, 7/4/94, p. 15.

4. See Wendy Koch, "White House Apologizes for Gay Inspection Gaffe," *Albany Times Union*, 6/15/95, p. A5.

5. Stephanie Salter, "Dr. Elders Just Wasn't Nice Enough," *San Francisco Examiner*, 12/15/94, p. A21.

6. See Michael Putzel, "Sex Talk Doomed Surgeon General: Masturbation Remark Spurs Clinton to End Elders' Stormy Career," *San Francisco Examiner,* 12/11/94, p. A1. Putzel quotes Christian Action Network president Martin Mawyer describing Elders as "a proponent of the most anti-Christian policies in the history of this nation."

7. Katherine Seelye, "Helms Puts the Brakes to a Bill Financing AIDS Treatment," *NYT,* 7/5/95, p. A12.

8. Sarah Schulman, "We Can Get There from Here," *The Nation,* 257:1, 7/5/93, p. 30.

9. See AP, "New HIV Strains Resist AIDS Drug," *NYT,* 1/1/93, p. A18.

10. Quoted in Lawrence Altman, "Deadly Strain of Tuberculosis is Spreading Fast, U.S. Finds," *NYT,* 1/24/92, p. A1.

11. Quoted in Jeff Barge, "Takeout/Employee Benefits: Homosexual Partners Now Insurable," *Crain's New York Business,* 6/19/95, p. 40.

12. See Richard Sandomir, "Louganis, Olympic Champion, Says He Has AIDS," *NYT,* 2/23/95, p. B11. Also, Greg Louganis, *Breaking the Surface* (New York: Random House, 1997).

13. Caryn James, "Comic Side of Sex in Age of AIDS," *NYT,* 8/4/95, p. C10; John Lahr, review of *Angels in America, The New Yorker,* 11/23/92.

14. Patrick Pacheco, "First Tony Kushner's 'Angels in America' Wins Every Theater Prize There Is. Then He Sits Down to Finish the Second Act," *Newsday,* 11/21/93, p. 10.

15. Daniel Harris, "Making Kitsch from AIDS," *Harper's Magazine,* 289:1730, 7/94, p. 55.

16. "Malice Toward Some," *The New Yorker,* 9/92, p. 6.

17. See Gerald Friedland, "Early Treatment for HIV: The Time Has Come," *NEJM,* 322:14, 4/5/90, pp. 1000–02.

18. Tom Bethell, "The Cure That Failed," *National Review,* 45:9, 5/10/93, pp. 33–37.

19. Laura Baenen, "Parents of HIV-Positive Girl Shun Drug AZT," *LAT,* 6/26/94, p. A15.

20. Joseph Palca, "New AIDS Drugs Take Careful Aim," *Science,* v. 246, 12/22/89, pp. 1660–61.

21. Alexander Dorozynski, "French Ban Immunotherapy Treatment," *Science,* v. 252, 6/21/91, p. 1608. Zagury was later accused of conducting unethical clinical trials, but was ultimately cleared.

22. See Anthony Fauci, "ddI: A Good Start, but Still Phase I," *NEJM,* 322:19, 5/10/90, pp. 1386–87.

23. Lawrence Altman, "Advances in Treatment Change Face of AIDS," *NIT,* 6/12/90, p. C1.

24. "The Changing Times," *The New Yorker,* 68:33, 10/5/92, 1992, p. 63.

25. For a good overview on the state of pharmaceutical development by 1991, see "Investment in AIDS Research by the Administration," 9/12/91, COS JS papers, AIDS: CF/OA 00470.

26. Geoffrey Cowley, "Bad News on Two AIDS Fronts," *Newsweek,* 122:5, 8/2/93, p. 62.

27. See A. C. Collier, R. W. Coombs, et al., "Treatment of Human Immunodeficiency Virus Infection with Saquinavir, Zidovudine, and Zalcitabine," *NEJM,* v. 334, 4/18/96, pp. 1011–18; also, Lawrence Corey, and King Holmes, "Therapy for Human Immunodeficiency Virus Infection—What Have We Learned?" *NEJM,* v. 335, 10/10/96, pp. 1142–44.

28. Quoted in Laurie Garrett, "AIDS: 'A Home Run,' " *Newsday,* 1/30/96, p. A5.

29. Quoted in Laurie Garrett, "New AIDS Hope: Drugs, Tests Seen as Way to Eradicate Virus from Body," *Newsday,* 6/14/96, p. A4.

30. Author's interview with Ho, 10/3/02.

31. Quoted in Laurie Garrett, "The Diamonds of AIDS Research," *Newsday,* 11/12/96, p. B21.

32. Ibid.

33. Ibid.

34. Author's interview with Ho, 10/3/02.

35. Philip Elmer-deWitt, "Man of the Year: Turning the Tide," *Time,* 148:29, 12/3/96, p. 52.

36. Here I quote correspondent Laurie Garrett, "The New AIDS Cocktails: What We Know," *Newsday,* 7/2/96, p. B19.

37. Paul Volberding and Steven Deeks, "Antiretroviral Therapy for HIV Infection: Promises and Problems," *JAMA,* v. 279, 5/6/98, p. 1343.

38. Quoted in Laurie Garrett, " 'A Home Run,' Detectable Traces of HIV Gone From Patients' Bodies in Short-Term Trials," *Newsday,* 1/30/96, p. A5.

39. Oren Cohen and Anthony Fauci, "HIV/AIDS in 1998—Gaining the Upper Hand," *JAMA,* v. 280, 7/1/98, p. 87.

40. Laurie Garrett, "A Turning Point: String of AIDS Discoveries Has Scientists Optimistic," *Newsday,* 7/1/96, p. A7.

41. Quoted in Daniel McGinn, "A 20-Year Toll," *Newsweek,* 137:24, 6/11/01, p. 48.

42. Quoted in David Dunlap, "New 'Miracle' Drugs: A Discussion," *NYT,* 2/2/97, p. D3.

43. Ibid.

44. Joe Nicholson and Dave Saltonstall, "AIDS: War's Not Over," *New York Daily News,* 2/2/97, p. 20.

45. Laurie Garrett, "Miracle Backlash: AIDS Advance Imperiled by Sexual License, Fears of Drug Resistance," *Newsday,* 12/17/96, A5.

46. See David Rose, "AIDS Drug Regimens That Are Worth Their Costs," *JAMA,* v. 279, 1/14/98, p. 160.

47. David Dunlap and Lawrence Fisher, "Drug Companies Turn Aggressive in Promoting New Drugs for AIDS," *NYT,* 7/5/96, p. A1.

48. Garrett, "A Turning Point," p. A7.

49. Daniel Haney, "Second Wind for AIDS Epidemic? Treatments Seen Failing," *AP,* as printed in *The Bergen Record,* 9/30/97, p. A13.

50. See Mark Wainberg and Gerald Friedland, "Public Health Implications of Antiretroviral Therapy and HIV Drug Resistance," *JAMA,* v. 279, 6/24/98, p. 1977.

51. Garrett, "Miracle Backlash," p. A5.

52. David Lewis, "They're Beating AIDS, and Now They Want Work, but Patients Face Many Hurdles," *New York Daily News,* 9/1/97, p. 4.

53. Dunlap, "New 'Miracle' Drugs: A Discussion," p. D3.

54. Ibid.

55. See Jon Cohen, "The HIV Vaccine Paradox," *Science,* v. 264, 5/20/94, pp. 1072–74.

56. J. Madeleine Nash, "An AIDS Mystery Solved: Eight Australian HIV Survivors Offer Hope for an Effective Vaccine," *Time,* 146:21, 11/20/95, p. 100.

57. Jay Levy, "Infection by Human Immunodeficiency Virus—CD4 Is Not Enough," *NEJM,* v. 335, 11/14/96, pp. 1528–30.

58. See David Ho, Joan Kaplan, et al., "Second Conserved Domain of gp120 is Important for HIV Infectivity and Antibody Neutralization," *Science,* v. 239, 2/26/88, pp. 1021–23; and Reginald Rhein Jr. and Resa King, "AIDS Vaccine: A Sliver of Hope?" *Business Week,* 8/31/87, p. 30.

59. D. Pendick, "NIH Advisers Endorse Disputed Vaccine Trial," *Science News,* v. 142, 12/12/92, p. 406. See also K. A. Fackelmann, "AIDS Vaccine Revs Up the Attack on HIV," *Science News,* v. 139, 6/15/91, p. 374.

60. C. Ezzell, "Two Strides Toward a Workable AIDS Vaccine," *Science News,* v. 141, 6/20/92 p. 405. See also K. A. Fackelmann, "Monkey Vaccine Prevents AIDS-Like Disease," *Science News,* v. 136, 8/19/89, p. 116.

61. Jon Cohen, "AIDS Vaccines: Is Older Better?" *Science,* v. 258, 12/18/92, p. 1881.

62. Christine Gorman, "Are Some People Immune to AIDS?" *Time,* 141:12, 3/22/93, p. 50.

See also David Baltimore, "Lessons from People with Nonprogressive HIV Infection," *NEJM*, v. 332, 1/26/95, pp. 259–60.

63. See Thomas Maugh II, "Studies Find Inborn HIV Resistance," *LAT Wire Services*, 8/9/96.

64. Rachel Nowak, "Are Researchers Racing Toward Success, or Crawling?" *Science*, v. 265, 9/2/94, p. 1373.

65. Lawrence Altman, "U.S. Reporting Sharp Decrease in AIDS Deaths," *NYT*, 2/28/97, p. A1.

66. Lawrence Altman, "Panel Offers Sharp Criticism of AIDS Research Projects," *NYT*, 4/14/96, p. A1; Robert Pear, "Clinton to Seek More Money to Help Pay for AIDS Drugs," *NYT*, 12/30/97, p. A14.

Chapter 12

1. Clyde Haberman, "Japan Plans to Deny Visas to Aliens with AIDS Virus," *NYT*, 4/1/87, p. A18.

2. Edward Gargan, "China Taking Stringent Steps to Prevent the Entry of AIDS," *NYT*, 12/22/87, p. A1.

3. Ibid.

4. Bill Keller, "New Soviet Law Makes AIDS Testing Mandatory," *NYT*, 8/27/87, p. B5.

5. See James Dearing, "Foreign Blood and Domestic Politics: The Issue of AIDS in Japan," in *AIDS: The Making of a Chronic Disease*, ed. Elizabeth Fee and Daniel Fox, (Berkeley: University of California Press, 1992), pp. 326–30.

6. Ibid., pp. 332–35.

7. Jonathan Mann, James Chin, Peter Piot, and Thomas Quinn, "The International Epidemiology of AIDS," *Scientific American*, 10/88, pp. 81–85.

8. Chris Beyrer, *War in the Blood: Sex, Politics, and AIDS in Southeast Asia* (London: Zed Books, Ltd., 1997), p. 21.

9. "The New Lepers," *Economist*, 316:7672, 9/15/90, p. 44.

10. Jonathan Mann and Daniel Tarantola, "Coming to Terms with the AIDS Pandemic," *Issues in Science and Technology*, 9:3, Spring 1993, pp. 41–49.

11. See, for example, Elena Yu, Qiyi Xie, et al., "HIV Infection and AIDS in China, 1985 Through 1994," *AJPH*, 86:8, 8/96, pp. 1116–23.

12. Andrew Ball, Sujata Rana, and Karl Dehne, "HIV Prevention Among Injection Drug Users: Responses in Developing and Transitional Countries," *PHR*, v. 113, 6/98, pp. 170–81.

13. See Bruce Weniger and Tim Brown, "The March of AIDS Through Asia," *NEJM*, v. 335, 8/1/96, pp 343–45.

14. Robert Steinbrook, "Dimensions of Asian AIDS Epidemic Cited," *LAT*, 6/18/91, p. A4.

15. Ball, Rana, and Dehne, "HIV Prevention Among Injection Drug Users," pp. 172–75. The authors report even worse conditions in Ukraine and Belarus, in which dealers might use human blood to dilute the communal solution.

16. For more details, see Ball, Rana, and Dehne, "HIV Prevention Among Injection Drug Users, pp. 170–81.

17. Rising heroin production rates in Burma were linked to political unrest and violence. Warring ethnic groups, barred from legitimate commodities, turned to opium production to fund arms purchases. See Beyrer, *War in the Blood*, p. 41.

18. Ba Thaung, Khin Maung Gyee, and Bo Kywe, "Rapid Assessment Study of Drug Abuse in Myanmar" (Myanmar Ministry of Health and UNDCP), cited in ibid.

19. See Beyrer, p. 43.

20. Quoted in ibid., p. 45.

21. Beyrer, p. 18.

22. Chris Lyttleton, *Endangered Relations: Negotiating Sex and AIDS in Thailand* (Amsterdam: Harwood Academic Publishers, 2000), p. 150.

23. Ibid, p. 156.

24. Cited in ibid., p. 154.

25. "Poor Man's Plague," *Economist*, 320:7725, 9/21/91, p. 21.

26. Ibid.

27. Philip Shenon, "Deadly Turning Point," *NYT,* 1/21/96, p. A1.

28. Lyttleton, *Endangered Relations*, p. 49.

29. Statistical reports vary on the success of the Thai condom campaign. The most optimistic data suggests that 90 percent of Thai prostitutes were using condoms by 1999, but other reports quote much lower rates of usage. See Joan Stephenson, "Swift Action Needed to Prevent Explosive HIV/AIDS Epidemics in Asia," *JAMA*, v. 286, 10/24/01, p. 1959.

30. Napaporn Havanon, Anthony Bennett, and John Knodel, "Sexual Networking in Provincial Thailand," *Studies in Family Planning*, 24:1, 1–2/93, pp. 1–17.

31. Shenon, "Deadly Turning Point."

32. Quoted in Matthew McAllester, "A Country in Denial/Lack of Care and Education Fuels Burma's AIDS Epidemic," *Newsday*, 1/6/98, p. C3.

33. "Myanmar's Secret Plague," *The Economist*, 344:8031, 8/23/97, p. 31.

34. Robert Horn, "Burma Ignores Its AIDS Crisis," *Time Atlantic*, 156:16, 10/16/00, p. 52.

35. Quoted in Shenon, "Deadly Turning Point."

36. Quoted in ibid.

37. Beyrer, p. 46.

38. Stephenson, "Swift Action Needed," p. 1959.

39. See UNAIDS, *A Scaled-Up Response to AIDS in Asia and the Pacific* (New York: 2005); as well as UNDP, *Thailand's Response to HIV/AIDS: Progress and Challenges* (New York: 2004), for statisticis on funds.

40. See Beyrer, pp. 63–65.

Chapter 13

1. Rita Delfiner, "U.S. AIDS Death Rate Drops by Nearly 50%," *New York Post*, 10/8/98, p. 4.

2. Marty Rosen, "AIDS Plunges Among IV Drug Users," *New York Post*, 2/19/99, p. 34; Raymond Hernandez, "In 1997, AIDS-Related Deaths in Prison Fell to 14-Year Low," *NYT,* 8/19/98, p. B5.

3. Cited in George Will, "An Epidemic's Evolution," *Newsweek*, 127:6, 2/5/96, p. 72.

4. Mike Mitka, "Slowing Decline in AIDS Deaths Prompts Concern," *JAMA*, v 282, 10/99, pp. 1216–17.

5. Quoted in "AIDS Infections Stop Declining, New Study Says," *NYT,* 8/31/99, p. A1.

6. Philip Rosenberg, "HIV in the Late 1990s: What We Don't Know May Hurt Us," *AJPH*, 91:7, 7/01, pp. 1016–18.

7. George Will, "An Epidemic's Evolution," p. 72.

8. "HIV and AIDS: United States, 1981–2000," *JAMA*, v. 285, 6/27/01, p. 3083.

9. Lisa Lee, John Karon, et al., "Survival After AIDS Diagnosis in Adolescents and Adults During the Treatment Era, United States, 1984–97," *JAMA*, v. 285, 3/14/01, p. 1308.

10. Quoted in Lawrence Altman, "AIDS Deaths Drop 48 Percent in New York," *NYT,* 2/3/98, p. A1.

11. Data from the Stop AIDS Project (San Francisco), reported in Erica Goode, "With Fears Fading, More Gays Spurn Old Preventive Message," *NYT,* 8/19/01 p. A1.

12. "AIDS Update—Bad News," *Time Atlantic,* 157:10, 3/12/01, p. 59.

13. Quoted in Kevin Sack, "HIV Peril and Rising Drug Use," *NYT,* 1/29/99, p. A10.

14. See Beth Harpaz, "Unsafe Sex Increases Among Gays as AIDS Crisis Matures," Associated Press, 2/1/99.

15. Ibid.

16. Alex Kellogg, " 'Safe Sex Fatigue' Grows Among Gay Students," *Chronicle of Higher Education,* 48:19, 1/18/02, p. A37.

17. Quoted in David Gelman, "The Young and the Reckless," *Newsweek,* 121:2, 1/11/93, p. 60.

18. From the CDC, reported in John Cloud, "AIDS at 20," *Time,* 157:23, 6/11/01, p. 83.

19. Anne Peterson, "High Rate of New HIV Infections Alarms Experts," *Dubuque Telegraph Herald* (AP), 7/1/00, p. A2.

20. Ibid.

21. Walt Odets, "The Fatal Mistake of AIDS Education," *Harper's,* 290:1740, 5/95, pp. 13–18.

22. Erica Goode, "With Fears Fading, More Gays Spurn Old Preventive Message," *NYT,* 8/19/01, p. A1.

23. Ibid.

24. Goode, "With Fears Fading," p. A1.

25. Marc Peyser, "A Deadly Dance," *Newsweek,* 130:13, 9/29/97, p. 76.

26. Charles Kaiser, "Overcoming a Death Wish," *NYT,* 11/30/92, p. A15.

27. Goode, "With Fears Fading," p. A1.

28. Yvonne Abraham, "AIDS Battle Facing Lethal Complacency," *BG,* 6/6/99, p. B1.

29. Stephen Joseph, "Keep Them Closed," *Newsday,* 9/22/92, p. 40

30. "Should Gay Bathhouses Reopen in San Francisco?" *San Francisco Chronicle,* 5/5/94, p. A27.

31. Phillip Matier and Andrew Ross, "Jordan Vows to Slam Door on Gay Bathhouse Plan," *San Francisco Chronicle,* 3/21/94, p. A15.

32. Quoted in David Kirp, "Love Among the Ruins," *The Nation,* 259:3, 7/18/94, p. 92.

33. Ibid., p. 93.

34. Andrew Sullivan, *Love Undetectable* (London: Chatto and Windus, 1998), p. 59.

35. See Gabriel Rotello, *Sexual Ecology: AIDS and the Destiny of Gay Men* (New York: Dutton, 1997).

36. Martin Duberman, "Review of *Sexual Ecology,*" *The Nation,* 264:17, 5/5/97, p. 27.

37. Quoted in Kirp, "Love Among the Ruins," p. 93.

38. Ibid.

39. Gabriel Rotello, "Creating a New Gay Culture," *The Nation,* 264:15, 4/21/97, pp. 11–16.

40. Ronald Bayer, "AIDS Prevention—Sexual Ethics and Responsibility," *NEJM,* v. 334, 6/6/96, p. 1541.

41. Dennis Rhodes, "There's a Way to Stop AIDS—And Yes, It's Responsibility," *New York Post,* 7/27/98, p. 26.

42. Harvey Fierstein, "The Culture of Disease," *NYT,* 7/31/03.

43. Sullivan, *Love Undetectable,* p. 65.

44. Jennifer Warren and Richard Paddock, "Randy Shilts, Chronicler of AIDS Epidemic, Dies at 42," *LAT,* 2/18/94, p. A1.

45. See Richard Goldstein, "The Real Andrew Sullivan," *The Village Voice,* 6/26/01, p. 51.

46. Kevin McDermott and Lisa Snedeker, "House Passes Bill to Make Clean Needles Accessible," *St. Louis Post-Dispatch,* 4/7/00, p. D4; Merrill Singer, Hans Baer, et al., "Pharmacy

Access to Syringes Among Injecting Drug Users: Follow-Up Findings from Hartford, Connecticut," *PHR,* v. 113 6/98, pp. 81–89; Joshua Weinstein, "Needle-Exchange Bill Signed into Maine Law," *Portland Press Herald,* 6/13/97, p. A1.

47. Michelle Ruess, "AIDS Advisory Council Backs Needle Exchange but Whitman Says Idea Might Foster Illicit Drug Use," *The Bergen Record,* 4/4/96, p. A3.

48. David Kocieniewski, "Hard Line on Needle Exchanges," *NYT,* 2/2/99, p. B1.

49. "Federal Funds for Clean Needles," *NYT,* 2/22/97, p. A20.

50. McDermott and Snedeker, "House Passes Bill to Make Clean Needles Accessible."

51. Katherine Seelye, "AMA Policy Group Backs Needle Exchanges," *NYT,* 6/27/97, p. A15.

52. Roel Coutinho, "Needle Exchange, Pragmatism, and Moralism," *AJPH,* 90:9, 9/00, pp. 1387–89.

53. A. R. Moss, "Epidemiology and the Politics of Needle Exchange," *AJPH,* 90:9, 9/00, pp. 1385–88.

54. Warren Leary, "Report Endorses Needle Exchanges as AIDS Strategy," *NYT,* 9/20/95 p. A1.

55. Coutinho, "Needle Exchange, Pragmatism, and Moralism," p. 1388.

56. Ibid.

57. Doug Ireland, "HIV Negatives," *The Village Voice,* 266:1, 1/5/98, p. 4.

58. Midge Decter, "Dying of the Light," *National Review,* 47:22, 11/27/95, p. 36.

59. Joseph Yuen, "How Not to Get AIDS: A Very Simple Cure," *New York Post,* 7/21/98 p. 26.

60. Ronald Eureka, "AIDS Cure? No Rush," *Cleveland Plain Dealer,* 7/12/00, p. B8.

61. Doug Ireland, "Remembering Herve," *The Nation,* 262:25, 6/24/96, p. 6.

62. Reprinted in "Fodor's the Born-Again," *Harper's Magazine,* 294:1763, 4/97, p. 18.

63. Dave Wedge, "Conservative Study Rips State Sex Ed Program," *Boston Herald,* 12/29/99, p. 24.

64. "Handle with Care," *The Economist,* 335:7920, 6/24/95, p. 27. *The Economist* suggested that perhaps it was Dornan who ought to be "handled with rubber gloves," referring to the embarrassing White House incident surrounding gay visitors.

65. Al Sunderland, "Homosexuality Is Aberrant," *Providence Journal-Bulletin,* 10/18/99, p. B8.

66. See Chandler Burr, "The AIDS Exception: Privacy Vs. Public Health," *Atlantic Monthly,* 279:6, 6/97, pp. 57–63.

67. Lawrence Gostin, "Mandatory Name Reporting in HIV Cases?" *New York Law Journal,* 3/9/98, p. 2.

68. For an example of the test-dissuasion argument, see M. Adams, C. Hanssens, and T. Lazarus, "Battling HIV on Many Fronts," *NEJM,* v. 338, 1/15/98, p. 198.

69. Quoted in Tom Precious, "State's HIV Confidentiality Policy May Change," *Buffalo News,* 11/1/97, p. A1.

70. Jessica Cordaro Depew, "People Spreading AIDS Don't Deserve Privacy," *Buffalo News,* 11/6/97, p. B3. See also ibid.

71. Loretta McLaughlin, "Poor Bear Sting of AIDS," *BG,* 7/3/98, p. A23.

72. Richard Wolitski, Ronald Valdiserri, et al., "Are We Headed for a Resurgence of the HIV Epidemic Among Men Who Have Sex with Men?" *AJPH,* 91:6, 6/01, pp. 883–85.

73. Bob Herbert, "In America, a Black Epidemic," *NYT,* 6/4/01, p. A17.

74. See Lawrence Altman, "Study in 6 Cities Finds HIV in 30 Percent of Young Black Gays," *NYT,* 2/6/01, p. A17.

75. Larry Grant, Will Green, et al., "HIV/AIDS and African Americans: Assumptions, Myths, and Realities," *Social Workers Speak Out on the HIV/AIDS Crisis,* ed. Larry Grant, Patricia Stewart, et al. (Westport, Conn.: Praeger, 1998), p. 3.

76. Quoted in John Yemma, "A Black Silence on AIDS Cited," *BG,* 10/23/96, p. A1.

77. Benoit Denizet-Lewis, "Double Lives on the Down Low," *New York Times Magazine,* 8/3/03, p. 30.

78. Quoted in Vivian Martin, "The Complex War on AIDS in the Black Community," *The Hartford Courant,* 6/14/01, p. A17.

79. Denizet-Lewis, "Double Lives on the Down Low," p. 31.

80. Barbara Kantrowitz, "From Hero to Crusader: Activists Debate What Magic Should Do Next," *Newsweek,* 118:21, 11/18/91, p. 69.

81. Sheryl Gay Stolberg, "Epidemic of Silence: A Special Report," *NYT,* 6/29/98, p. A1.

82. Ibid. Also, Rosalind Bentley, "Call and Response," *Minneapolis Star-Tribune,* 3/19/00, p. E1.

83. Steve Levin and Angela Agoawike, "AIDS Kills in Silence in Black Community," *Pittsburgh Post-Gazette,* 7/7/98, p. A1.

84. Quoted in Sara Neufeld, "Black Groups Turn Focus to AIDS Fight; Area Churches Deciding to Tackle Problem," *BG,* 8/23/99, p. A1.

85. See Martin Evans, "Black Clergy to Meet on Overcoming HIV Unease," *Newsday,* 10/26/99, p. A30.

86. Quoted in Erin McClam, "Dinkins' Group Urges Changes to Slow AIDS Spread Among Minorities," Associated Press, 6/8/01.

87. Richard Kim, "ACT UP Goes Global," *The Nation,* 273:2, 7/9/01, pp. 17–19. Numerous smaller, more local, black AIDS organizations worked to build awareness as well, notably Harlem United in New York City. See Willis Green, "The Challenges of an AIDS Service Organization Executive in Harlem," in *Social Workers Speak Out on the HIV/AIDS Crisis,* chapter 4.

88. Quoted in Jack White, "When Silence Is Sin," *Time,* 154:26, 12/27/99, p. 133.

89. Wil Haygood, "Rivers Urges Black Action on AIDS in Africa," *BG,* 12/8/99, p. A1.

90. Wil Haygood, "AIDS and Africa: Africans and Americans," *BG,* 10/13/99, p. A1.

91. Ibid.

92. Ibid.

93. Emma Sapong, "This Is a Crisis," *Buffalo News,* 8/20/01, p. A1.

94. Joey Pressley, "For 20 Years, the Scourge of AIDS," *NYT,* 6/6/01, p. A30.

95. Grant and Green, "HIV/AIDS and African Americans," p. 9.

96. Quoted in Denizet-Lewis, "Double Lives on the Down Low," p. 52.

97. Quoted in Katti Gray, "Living with HIV: People Infected with the Virus Go On with the Unfinished Business of Their Lives," *Newsday,* 6/12/01, p. B6.

98. David Morrow, "A Movable Epidemic: Makers of AIDS Drugs Struggle to Keep Up with Market," *NYT,* 9/9/99, p. C1.

99. Robert Steinbrook, "Caring for People with Human Immunodeficiency Virus Infection," *NEJM,* v. 339, 12/24/98, pp. 1926–28. Also, GAO, *HIV/AIDS Drugs: Funding Implications of New Combination Therapies for Federal and State Programs,* GAO/HEHS-99-2, 10/98, pp. 4–9.

100. Elizabeth Rosenthal, "1,000 Patients Lose Insurance to a Loophole," *NYT,* 1/20/96, p. A25.

101. Joan Stephenson, "Twenty Years After AIDS Emerges, HIV's Complexities Still Loom Large," *JAMA,* v. 285, 3/14/01, p. 1279.

102. Oren Cohen and Anthony Fauci, "Transmission of Multidrug-Resistant Human Immunodeficiency Virus—The Wake-Up Call," *NEJM,* v. 339, 7/30/98, pp. 341–43; C. Flexner, "Drug Therapy: HIV-Protease Inhibitors," *NEJM,* v. 338, 4/30/98, pp. 1281–93.

103. Raja Mishra, "Efficacy of AIDS Drugs Ebbing," *BG,* 12/19/01, p. A1.

104. S. A. Bozzette, S. H. Berry, et al., "The Care of HIV-Infected Adults in the United

States," *NEJM*, v. 339, 12/24/98, pp. 1897–1904. See also Paul Farnham, "Defining and Measuring the Costs of the HIV Epidemic to Business Firms," *PHR*, v. 109, 5–6/94, pp. 311–18.

Chapter 14

1. "WHO and UN: AIDS Not Losing Momentum," *PHR*, v. 115, 1–2/00, p. 7.
2. Kent Sepkowitz made this observation in a brief history of AIDS, which he published in 2001. See "AIDS—The First 20 Years," *NEJM*, 344:23, 6/7/01, p. 1764. For good comparative international fatality statistics in that year, see "The Spectre Stalking the Sub-Sahara," *The Economist*, 357:8199, 12/2/00, pp. 48–51.
3. See, for example, Mark Schoofs, "The Agony of Africa," *The Village Voice*, 11/9/99, p. 40.
4. Lawrence Altman, "Parts of Africa Showing HIV in 1 in 4 Adults," *NYT*, 6/24/98, p. A1.
5. Schoofs, "The Agony of Africa."
6. Michael Specter, "The Vaccine," *The New Yorker*, 2/3/03, p. 65.
7. Associated Press, "The Spread of AIDS in Caribbean Islands Is Causing Alarm," *St. Louis Post-Dispatch*, 2/26/00, p. 21.
8. Ibid.
9. See Rebecca Voelker, "HIV/AIDS in the Caribbean: Big Problems Among Small Islands," *JAMA*, v. 285, 6/20/01, p. 2961.
10. See Ellen Koenig, "AIDS in Paradise," *JAMA*, v. 282, 12/15/99, p. 2195. See also Voelker, "HIV/AIDS in the Caribbean."
11. Voelker, "HIV/AIDS in the Caribbean."
12. "The Global HIV and AIDS Epidemic," *JAMA*, v. 285, 6//27/01, p. 3081. Also, Andrew Purvis, "The Global Epidemic," *Time*, 148:29, 12/30/96, pp. 76–79.
13. "WHO and UN: AIDS Not Losing Momentum," *PHR*, v. 115, 1–2/00, p. 7.
14. Quoted in Marion Lloyd, "AIDS Crisis Spreads Across India," *BG*, 12/5/99, p. A27.
15. David Ho, "And Will We Ever Cure AIDS?" *Time*, 154:19, 11/8/99, p. 84.
16. See "A New AIDS Alert," *Newsweek*, 119:24, 6/15/92, p. 41.
17. United Nations AIDS data, reported in "AIDS Pandemic," *MacLean's*, 115:28, 7/22/02, p. 13. See also similar estimates in USAID, *HIV/AIDS in the Developing World* (Washington D.C.: GPO, 1999), WP/98–2, particularly tables 1 and 2.
18. "Tuberculosis Epidemic Worldwide Emergency," *PHR*, v. 111, 1–2/96, pp. 8–9.
19. "New TB Drugs Needed Alongside Antiretrovirals: Joint HIV-TB Approach a 'Must' As TB Is Number 1 Killer of AIDS Patients," *Ascribe Newswire*, 11/30/01.
20. "Tuberculosis, HIV Co-Epidemic to Multiply Sevenfold in Asia," *PHR*, v. 110, 1–2/95, pp. 108–9. See also Aisha Labi, "TB, a Killer's Return," *Time Atlantic*, 156:7, 8/14/00, pp. 22–23.
21. WHO figures, as reported in Jeffrey Bartholet, "The Plague Years," *Newsweek*, 135:3, 1/17/00, pp. 32–38.
22. See "Serial Killer at Large," *The Economist*, 346:8054, 2/7/98, p. 49. Also, "A Global Disaster," *The Economist*, 350:8100, 1/2/99, p. 42.
23. Johanna McGeary, "Death Stalks a Continent," *Time*, 157:6, 2/12/01, p. 44.
24. Simon Robinson, "Battle Ahead," *Time Atlantic*, 158:3, 7/16/01, p. 30.
25. From a joint NIH/Johns Hopkins University/Makerere University study. Reported in Marilynn Marchione, "Study Suggests Drug Treatment Might Slow Spread of AIDS," *Milwaukee Journal Sentinel*, 1/31/00, p. A3. See also R. A. Royce, A. Sentilde, and M. S. Cohen, "Current Concepts: Sexual Transmission of HIV," *NEJM*, v. 336, 4/10/97, pp. 1072–78.

26. Jon Cohen, "Is AIDS in Africa a Distinct Disease?" *Science,* 288:5474, 6/23/00, p. 2153.

27. Ibid.

28. Discussed in Kevin De Cock, Mary Glenn Fowler, et al., "Prevention of Mother-to-Child HIV Transmission in Resource-Poor Countries: Translating Research into Policy and Practice," *JAMA,* v. 283, 3/1/00, pp. 1175–82.

29. Cited in "A Global Disaster," *The Economist,* 350:8100, 1/2/99, pp. 42–45.

30. See "Serial Killer at Large," pp. 49–50.

31. Quoted in McGeary, "Death Stalks a Continent," p. 49.

32. Cited in "Silent Leaders Help the Virus to Spread," *The Economist,* 359:8228, 6/30/01, p. 42.

33. Quoted in Kurt Shillinger, "A Continent's Crisis," *BG,* 10/10/99, p. A1.

34. Cited in "Kurt Shillinger," "Couple Fights AIDS Virus, Taboos," *BG,* 10/12/99, p. A21.

35. From UNAIDS data, as reported in Lawrence Altman, "UN Issues Grim Report on the 11 Million Children Orphaned by AIDS," *NYT,* 12/2/99, p. A12.

36. Quoted in McGeary, "Death Stalks a Continent," p. 50.

37. See Rebecca Voelker, "Poor Nations Ravaged by AIDS Need the Right Resources Now," *JAMA,* v. 282, 12/1/99, p. 282.

38. Clare Nullis, "A Whole Generation Is Being Taken Out," *Chicago Sun-Times,* 6/28/00, p. 1.

39. Reported in "A Global Disaster," *The Economist,* 350:8100, 1/2/99, p. 42.

40. A vast literature exists on the economic consequences of the black death. Interested readers might wish to examine Lynn White, *Medieval Technology and Social Change* (New York: Oxford University Press, 1962).

41. See "The Cruelest Curse," *The Economist,* 358:8210, 2/24/01, p. 8.

42. "The Plague," *The Economist,* 358:8214, 3/24/01, p. 55.

43. Denise Gilgen, Catherine Campbell, Brian Williams, Dirk Taljaard, and Catherine MacPhail, *The Natural History of HIV/AIDS in South Africa: A Biomedical and Social Survey in Carletonville* (Braamfontein, South Africa: Council for Scientific and Industrial Research), p. 123.

44. Abt Associates, *The Impending Catastrophe,* as cited in Joan Stephenson, "AIDS in South Africa Takes Center Stage," *JAMA,* v. 284, 7/12/00, p. 165.

45. See Mark Mathabane, *African Women: Three Generations* (New York: HarperCollins, 1994), excerpted in Mark Mathabane, "Tradition Dooms African Women," *Cleveland Plain Dealer,* 3/28/00, p. B9. Also, Suzanne Daley, "A Post-Apartheid Agony: AIDS on the March," *NYT,* 7/23/98, p. A1.

46. Kurt Shillinger, "Most Leaders Won't Confront the Epidemic," *BG,* 10/12/99, p. A1. Also Wil Haygood, "Rape Victim: I Felt Myself Drowning," *BG,* 10/11/99, p. A25.

47. Tom Nevin, a reporter for *African Business,* observed, "Under the old South Africa, prostitution and pornography were so heavily policed that even taking a peep at a girlie magazine could land you in jail." From "South Africa's Booming Sex Industry," 12/98, p. 15.

48. George Will, "AIDS Crushes a Continent," *Newsweek,* 135:2, 1/10/00, p. 64.

49. Quoted in Wil Haygood, "Prostitution Plays Key Role in Fueling Africa's AIDS Crisis," *BG,* 10/11/99, p. A25.

50. Nevin, "South Africa's Booming Sex Industry," *African Business,* 12/98, p. 15.

51. See "South Africa's President and the Plague," *The Economist,* 355:8172, 5/27/00, pp. 45–46.

52. Quoted in Helen Epstein, "AIDS in South Africa: The Invisible Cure," *New York Review of Books,* 7/17/03, p. 44.

53. Quoted in Samantha Power, "The AIDS Rebel," *The New Yorker,* 5/19/03, p. 56.

54. Quoted in "Heads in the Sand," *The Economist,* 360:8241, 9/29/01, p. 51. At least part of the problem stemmed from legislative blocks. Although the country was technically a

representative democracy by 2000, in reality the parliament served largely to passively endorse government policy. R. W. Johnson noted in a 1996 article that members of the minority Democratic Party, while holding only 2 percent of seats in parliament, asked 40 percent of all parliamentary questions. "No other African state has had a party like the DP to ventilate the political system, though all have needed one," Johnson wrote. See "The New South Africa," *National Review,* 48:25, 12/31/96, pp. 48–51.

55. Katherine Floyd, Alasdair Reid, et al., "Admission Trends in a Rural South African Hospital During the Early Years of the HIV Epidemic," *JAMA,* v. 282, 9/15/99, p. 1087.

56. Donald McNeil, "A Lonely Crusade Warning Africans of AIDS," *NYT,* 11/28/01, p. A1.

57. "The Worst Way to Lose Talent," *The Economist,* 358:8208, 2/10/01, pp. 65–67.

58. Kurt Shillinger, "Officials Prodded on Discrimination," *BG,* 10/12/99, p. A20.

59. Barings Investment Bank concurred in its own estimates. See "The Cruelest Curse," *The Economist,* 358:8210, 2/24/01, pp. 8–11.

60. See Joan Stephenson, "AIDS in South Africa Takes Center Stage, *JAMA,* v. 284, 7/12/00, p. 165–67.

61. See Samantha Power, "The AIDS Rebel," *The New Yorker,* 5/19/03, pp. 54–67.

62. See Epstein, "AIDS in South Africa: The Invisible Cure," p. 47.

63. See Samson Mulugeta, "AIDS Drug Ordered in South Africa," *Newsday,* 12/15/01. Also, Kurt Shillinger, "Officials Prodded on Discrimination," *BG,* 10/12/99.

64. Ginger Thompson, "In Grip of AIDS, South African Cries for Equity," *NYT,* 5/10/03.

65. See "UC San Francisco AIDS Research Institute Launches International Program to Focus on Global HIV/AIDS Issues," *Ascribe Newswire,* 4/25/00.

66. Laurie Garrett, "AIDS-Defeat Cost Put at $9.2B a Year," *Newsday,* 6/22/01, p. A24; GAO, *HIV/AIDS: USAID and U.N. Response to the Epidemic in the Developing World,* GAO/NSIAD-98-202, 7/98; GAO, *Global Health: Joint U.N. Programme on HIV/AIDS Needs to Strengthen Country-Level Efforts and Measure Results,* GAO-01-625, 5/01, p. 12.

67. Donald McNeil Jr., "Faulty Condoms Thwart AIDS Fight in Africa," *NYT,* 12/27/98, p. A1.

68. James Brooke, "In Deception and Denial, an Epidemic Looms," *NYT,* 1/25/93, p. A1.

69. See, for example, Anthony Faiola, "Macho Brazil's Denial of the AIDS Epidemic: Women Face Especially Difficult Challenges," *Newsday,* 10/14/01, p. A20.

70. Cited in James Inciardi, Hilary Surratt, and Paulo Telles, *Sex, Drugs, and HIV/AIDS in Brazil* (Boulder, Colo.: Westview, 2000), p. 109.

71. One study found that even within the highly vulnerable prostitutes of the nonindustrialized world, those who engaged in anal sex were more likely to contract AIDS than those who did not. Salim Abdool Karim and Gita Ramjee, "Anal Sex and HIV Transmission in Women," *AJPH,* 88:8, 8/98, pp. 1265–66.

72. "The Battle with AIDS," *The Economist,* 356:8179, 7/15/00, p. 17.

73. Robert Horn, "Back to No Future," *Time Atlantic,* 156:16, 10/16/00, pp. 50–52;

74. Brooke, "In Deception and Denial."

75. Arthur Allen, "Sex Change," *The New Republic,* 5/27/02, p. 14. Also, Global AIDS Program, National Center for HIV, STD, and TB Prevention, CDC, "The Global HIV and AIDS Epidemic, 2001," *JAMA,* v. 285, 6/27/01, p. 3081.

76. See Napaporn Havanon, Anthony Bennett, and John Knodel, "Sexual Networking in Provincial Thailand," *Studies in Family Planning,* 24:1, 1–2/93, pp. 1–17.

77. Tina Rosenberg, "Look at Brazil," *New York Times Magazine,* 1/28/01, p. 26.

78. Melody Petersen and Donald McNeil Jr., "Maker Yielding Patent in Africa for AIDS Drug," *NYT,* 3/15/01, p. A1.

79. Associated Press, "Plan to Cut Cost of AIDS Drugs in Africa Will Have Little Effect on Most," *St. Louis Post-Dispatch,* 5/14/00, p. A2. Also, S. A. Bozzette, G. Joyce, et al., "Ex-

penditures for the Care of HIV-Infected Patients in the Era of Highly Active Antiretroviral Therapy," *NEJM*, v. 344, 3/15/01, pp. 817–23.

80. R. Steinbrook and J. M. Drazen, "AIDS—Will the Next 20 Years Be Different?" *NEJM*, v. 344, 6/7/01, pp. 1781–82.

81. Sheryl Gay Stolberg, "Africa's AIDS War," *NYT*, 3/10/01, p. A1.

82. One striking statistic speaking to Rosenberg's argument was the efficacy of preventing maternal-child transmissions through the use of combination therapy. Without the therapy, the rate was 25 percent for infected women; with the therapy the transmission rate dropped to 1.4 percent. See John Sullivan and Katherine Luzuriaga, "The Changing Face of Pediatric HIV-1 Infection," *NEJM*, v. 345, 11/22/01, pp. 1568–69.

83. A well-articulated moral and theological argument for violating patent protections of AIDS drugs can be found in Kevin O'Brien and Peter Clark, "Drug Companies and AIDS in South Africa," *America*, 187:17, 11/25/02, pp. 8–11.

84. Andrew Sullivan, "Profit of Doom?" *New Republic*, 224:13, 3/26/01, p. 6.

85. "The AIDS Initiative," *Wall Street Journal*, 2/7/03, p. A10. Also, "The Rip-Off Merchants of Drug Patents," *Wall Street Journal*, 2/18/03.

86. Rachel Swarns, "Free AIDS Drugs in Africa Offer Dose of Life," *NYT*, 2/8/03, p. A1. Also, Laurie Garrett, "AIDS at 20," *Newsday*, 6/24/01, p. A8.

87. Jonathan Cohn, "Brasilia Diarist: Sexual Healing," *The New Republic*, 6/30/03, p. 38.

88. Sullivan, "Profit of Doom?"

89. See "United Against AIDS?" *The Economist*, 359:8228, 6/30/01, pp. 73–74.

90. GAO, *U.S. Agency for International Development Fights AIDS in Africa, but Better Data Needed to Measure Impact,* GAO-01-449, 3/01, p. 3.

91. Joan Stephenson, "UN Conference Endorses Battle Plan for HIV/AIDS," *JAMA*, v. 286, 7/25/01, p. 405.

92. For this stark contrast, I am grateful to *Boston Globe* reporter Kurt Shillinger. See "Most Leaders Won't Confront the Epidemic," *BG*, 10/12/99, p. A1.

93. Robert Borosage, "Unparalleled Plague Fails to Attract Needed U.S Attention," *Milwaukee Journal Sentinel,* 7/23/00, p. J1.

94. Solomon Benatar, "AIDS in the 21st Century," *JAMA*, v. 342, 2/17/00, pp. 515–17.

95. Shillinger, "Most Leaders Won't Confront the Epidemic."

96. Benatar, "AIDS in the 21st Century."

97. "Terrorism Is Not the Only Scourge," *The Economist*, 361:8253, 12/22/01, p. 10.

98. Sheryl Gay Stolberg, "Getting Religion on AIDS," *NYT*, 2/2/03, p. D1.

99. Amy Waldman, "Gates Offers India $100 Million to Fight AIDS," *NYT*, 11/12/02, p. A8.

100. Donald McNeil Jr., "One by One, Charities Attack the AIDS Juggernaut," *NYT*, 11/18/02, p. A1.

101. Ibid, p. A26.

102. "Bill and Melinda Gates Foundation Give 25 Million to Harvard School of Public Health for AIDS Prevention in Nigeria," *Ascribe Newswire*, 11/13/00.

103. Cesar Chelala, "AIDS Epidemic Assails Another Front," *BG*, 4/29/01, p. D5.

104. Amy Waldman, "As AIDS Spreads, India Is Still Struggling for a Workable Strategy," *NYT*, 11/11/02, p. A7.

105. Kong-lai Zhang, "Epidemiology of HIV in China," *British Medical Journal*, 324:7341, 4/6/02, pp. 803–4.

106. M. J. Friedrich, "Chinese and US Health Care Leaders Discuss Challenges of the 21st Century," *JAMA*, v. 286, 8/8/01, p. 659.

107. Elizabeth Rosenthal, "With Ignorance as the Fuel, AIDS Spreads Across China," *NYT*, 12/30/01, p. A1.

108. Laurie Garrett, "Report Shows Surges of HIV," *Newsday*, 11/29/01, p. A12. See also Zhang, "Epidemiology of HIV in China."

109. Geoffrey Cowley, Michael Laris, and Mary Hager, "From Freedom to Fear: When AIDS Hits China," *Newsweek*, 127:14, 4/1/96, p. 49.

110. "Confession Time: A Very Serious Epidemic," *The Economist*, 360:8237, 9/1/01, pp. 36–37. Also Associated Press, "China Reveals That 118 Villagers Got AIDS Through Sale of Blood," *The Bergen Record*, 10/12/01, p. A20.

111. Christopher Williams, *AIDS in Post-Communist Russia and Its Successor States* (Brookefield, Vt.: Avebury Books, 1995), p. 28.

112. Andrew Meier, "The Death of a Nation," *Time Atlantic*, 157:3, 1/22/01, p. 28.

113. Joan Stephenson, "AIDS in Eastern Europe," *JAMA*, v. 287, 1/9/02, p. 180. Also, Stephenson, "HIV/AIDS Surge in Eastern Europe," *JAMA*, v. 284, 12/27/00, p. 3113.

114. See Leon Aron, "Russia's Revolution," *Commentary*, 11/02, pp. 22–30.

115. See John Curtis, "On Russia's AIDS Front," *Yale Medicine*, Spring 2003, pp. 28–35.

116. Ibid., p. 33.

117. "Downfall of the Iron City, *The Economist*, 349:8099, 12/19/98, p. 48. Also, Associated Press, "HIV Cases on Rapid Increase, Group Says," *BG*, 11/25/99, p. A60; Michael Wines, "Needle Use Sets Off HIV Explosion in Russia," *NYT*, 11/24/99, p. A10.

118. Quoted in Laurie Garrett, "Crumbled Empire, Shattered Health," part II, *Newsday*, 11/2/97, p. A6.

119. Cited in Laurie Garrett, "Crumbled Empire, Shattered Health," part I, 10/26/97, p. A5.

120. Masha Gessen, "Mental Health," *The New Republic*, 223:9/10, 8/28/00, p. 16.

121. Matthew Kaminski, Kim Palchikoff, and Bill Powell, "The Crisis to Come," *Newsweek*, 129:15, 4/14/97, p. 44. Also, Joan Stephenson, "Researchers Wrestle with Spread and Control of Emerging Infections," *JAMA*, v. 287, 4/24/02, p. 2061.

122. Quoted in Kaminski, Palchikoff, and Powell, "The Crisis to Come."

123. Elizabeth Rosenthal, "Poorly Prepared Asian Countries Warned of AIDS Epidemic," *NYT*, 10/5/01, p. A14.

124. "HIV Infection: The Growing Scourge of India," *The AIDS Crisis: A Documentary History*, Feldman and Wang Miller, eds., (Westport, CT: Greenwood, 1998) p. 129. The going rate for intercourse with roadside prostitutes in India was as low as 28 cents.

125. C. M. F. Antunes, "Sex, Drugs, and HIV/AIDS in Brazil" (book review), *NEJM*, v. 344, 4/19/01, pp. 1257–58.

126. Eloise Salholz, Theresa Waldrop, and Ruth Marshall, "Watching the Babies Die," *Newsweek*, 115:8, 2/19/90, p. 63.

127. NIH data from Brian Vastag, "HIV Vaccine Efforts Inch Forward," *JAMA*, v. 286, 10/17/01, p. 1826.

128. Recognizing these disincentives, Senator John Kerry (D-Mass.) proposed special tax rebates for research in AIDS vaccines, along with malaria and tuberculosis, in 2001. See Anthony Shadid, "Fighting Scourges with Funds Once Almost Ignored, Malaria, TB Research See Flood of Cash," *BG*, 5/30/01, p. C4.

129. See Gary Taubes, "Antibody Drug Revival," *Technology Review*, 7–8/02, pp. 59–65.

130. Joan Stephenson, "AIDS Vaccine Moves into Phase 3 Trials," *JAMA*, v. 280, 7/1/98, p. 7.

131. See Geoffrey Cowley, "Is AIDS Forever?" *Newsweek*, 132:1, 7/6/98, p. 60.

132. See Barry Schoub, "The Quest for the HIV Vaccine," in Barry Schoub, ed., *HIV and AIDS in Perspective*, 2nd ed. (New York: Cambridge University Press, 1994), pp. 185–203.

133. See Daniel Haney, "Vaccine Said Unlikely to Protect from AIDS," Associated Press, 2/12/03.

134. Quoted in H. R. Shepherd, "World Needs an AIDS Vaccine—and Fast," *Newsday*, 7/23/97, p. A42.

135. See James Jones, *Bad Blood* (New York: The Free Press, 1981).

136. Michael Specter, "The Vaccine," *The New Yorker*, 2/3/03, p. 59.

ACKNOWLEDGMENTS

Thank you to Robert Guinsler of Sterling Lord Literistic and to Elisabeth Dyssegaard of Smithsonian Books for shepherding the book through the acquisitions process, to Amy Vreeland of HarperCollins for supervising the production, and to Barbara Ward of Seton Hall's Walsh Library for all of her work on interlibrary loan requests. Steve and Dale Sonnenberg hosted me in my Texas research sojourns, as did Bruce Ellman and Michelle Missaghieh in Los Angeles. Adwoa Owusu-Acheampong took care of my microfilm work; Rita Esteves and Nadine Behrens kept the family running smoothly. My wife, Roz, made it all fun.

INDEX

CDC, *see* Centers for Disease Control

Ceaucescu, Nicolai, 317

Cedars-Sinai Hospital, 242

Centers for Disease Control (CDC), 31, 35, 58, 69, 105, 112, 175, 184, 267–68; AIDS hotline of, 190; AIDS myths and, 195, 198; Atlanta headquarters of, 101, 110; blood transfusions and, 34; first AIDS reports and, 5–8, 22, 76; funding of, 77, 175, 179, 180, 185, 189, 192; homophobia at, 20

Center for Population Options, 85

Central African Republic, 51

cervical fluid, 33

cervix, 32, 203

charity, 43, 115–17, 186, 236; *see also specific groups*

Charlton Research, 75

Cheeks, Kwabena Rainey, 284

Chesley, Robert, 119

Chicago, Ill., 104, 165, 181*n*

children, 132, 259, 292; in Africa, 223, 227–30, 286, 295, 296, 298, 300; AIDS in, 8, 40–41, 80, 115–16, 128, 148, 149, 160, 164, 172–74, 212, 223, 296; black, 148, 160, 173; excluded from testing, 134; Hispanic, 160, 164, 173; HIV in, 26, 183; orphans, 223, 229–30, 286, 298, 317; as prostitutes, 149, 153, 305, 326; runaway, 149; treatment of, 128, 131, 134, 183

China, 255, 257, 260, 293, 313–14, 319, 324

Chirac, Jacques, 60

Chirimuuta, Richard, 208

Chirimuuta, Rosalind, 208

chlamydia, 220

cholera, 35, 96

Chow, Yung-Kang, 240

Christian-Christiansen, Donna, 285

Christianity, 46, 47, 70, 120–23; in Africa, 222–23, 297; *see also* Protestantism; Roman Catholicism

Cipla, 309

circumcision: female, 213–14; male, 203–4, 219–21, 295

civil libertarians, 37, 41, 46–47, 95, 281, 282

civil rights, 72–75, 88, 92, 95, 100, 111, 182, 184, 322

Clark, Eugene, 70

Clark, Hilton, 156

Clinton, Bill, 192, 233–34, 252, 277–80, 312–13

CMV retinitis, 139–40

COBRA, 185, 247

cocaine, 33, 151, 152–53

Colgate, Stirling, 194

college campuses, 26, 70, 194

College of Physicians, Reagan's speech to, 102

Colorado, 89, 281

combination therapy, 239–40, 253, 263, 302, 303, 319, 324; backsliding and, 268, 272, 286–89; cost of, 246, 247–48, 253, 292, 308–11; drawbacks of, 245–46; reactions to, 246–49

Combivir, 309

Commentary, 197

Community Program for Clinical Research on AIDS (CO-CRA), 143

"Compound Q," 128

condoloma, 34

condoms, 16, 18, 29, 81–87, 144, 206, 256, 305–7; in Africa, 212, 214–17, 222, 223, 297–98, 302; in Asia, 261–62, 293; backsliding and, 269–71, 278, 283; black community and, 148, 161, 163–64; Catholic view of, 120, 121, 158; distribution of, 38–39, 40, 80, 89, 134, 171, 172, 194, 223, 231, 261; Hispanic community and, 148, 164–65, 166; prostitutes and, 34, 157, 215, 216, 305, 306; risk profile and, 204

confidentiality, 90, 100, 169, 182

Confronting AIDS (IOM document), 101

Congo, 51, 296

Congo, Belgian, 2, 3, 50, 51

Congress, U.S., 35, 74, 76, 99, 110, 134, 137, 183, 234, 279; AIDS-related funding and, 21, 69, 77, 102, 109, 116, 144, 180–81, 192; drug safety and, 132–33; *see also* House of Representatives, U.S.; Senate, U.S.

Congressional Black Caucus, 285

Congressional Office of Technology Assessment, 177

Connecticut, 177, 276

conservatives: backlash of, 69–102, 323; backsliding and, 278–82

conspiracy theories, 19–23, 205–10, 224

contact, casual, 35, 53, 82, 87

Cooper, Ellen, 138, 139

Cosmopolitan, 196

cost of AIDS, 6–7, 42, 149, 155, 175–82; in Africa, 228–30, 292, 298–300, 303; AZT and, 110, 130, 131, 230, 292;

HIV (*continued*)
use and, 152, 156; military testing and,
148–49, 196; mutation of, 61–62, 64–65,
235, 243, 250, 251, 288–89; natural
immunity to, 251; in prisons, 167–71,
184; ramifications of discovery of,
63–66; as retrovirus, 60, 61, 64, 67, 205;
in Russia, 314–16; subtype E of, 262,
264; treatment of, 128, 129, 130, 244–45,
247, 248; tuberculosis and, 294; vaccines
and, 249–52
HIV-2, 62, 212
Ho, David, 241–43, *241*, 247, 248, 293–94
Hoffman, William, 119
Hoffmann–La Roche, 128, 240, 243–44, 309
holistic, organic, and alternative healers,
44, 208, 209
Hollander, Harry, 44
Holleran, Andrew, 17
Hollywood, Calif., 117, 118, 119, 190, 236,
242
homeless people, 149–50, 185–86, 187, 298
homophobia, 20, 22, 23, 53, 78, 114,
242; in Africa, 214; backlash and,
44–49, 69–75, 80, 82, 93, 102; of black
Americans, 112–13, 160–61, 283–85
homosexuals, 69–78, 87, 193, 233–36,
321–24; in Africa, 214, 215; in Asia,
263; backsliding and, 268–75, 278–82,
318–19; black American, 112–13, 160,
282–86; in Caribbean, 292–93;
conspiracy theories and, 19–23, 208;
genetics and, 238; in Haiti, 9, 50,
53; information clearinghouses and
educational resource centers of, 103–5;
leveling off of AIDS among, 29, 39, 48,
95–96, 233–35; lifestyle of, 8, 11–19,
235–38, *237*; number of, 199; number
of sex partners of, 7, 16, 71, 96, 198,
270, 323; political lobbying and activism
of, 103, 109–12; public health response
and, 36–40; religious views on, 70,
113, 120–23, 157, 160–61, 284–85; as
risk group, 6, 28, 39, 47, 87, 194; sex
education and, 84, 85; stigma feared by,
37–38, 89–90; tourism of, 9, 25, 50, 53
Hooks, Benjamin, 161
Hooper, Edward, 50, 51
hospitals, 42, 149, 150, 176–79, 184, 186,
187, 246; in Africa, 225, 226, 227, 302; in
Asia, 263; inpatient resources and, 105–8
House of Representatives, U.S., 234, 279
housing, 185–89, 268–69, 279

Housing and Urban Development (HUD),
188–89
Housing Opportunities for Persons with
AIDS program, 188
Howard Brown Memorial Clinic, 104
HPA-23 (antimonotungstate), 43–44, 128
HPV, 9
Hudson, Rock, 26, *27*, 43–44, 70
human T cell leukemia virus, 9–10
human t-lymphotropic virus (HTLV); I
and II, 55–58; III, 58–59, 62
Hutchinson, Earl Ofari, 284
hymka, 316

IAF Biochem International, 240
Illinois, 276
immigrants, 184, 196
Immigration and Naturalization Service
(INS), 93
immune system, 35, 55, 239, 251,
294, 296; collapse of, 2, 3, 7–9, 30,
56; lymphocytes and, 8–9, 56, 60;
macrophages and, 65; of monkeys, 60,
207; strengthening of, 128
immuthiol (sodium
diethyldithiocarbamate), 128
Imperial College, 48
imunovir, 128
"Incredible Shrinking AIDS Epidemic,
The" (Fumento), 197
India, 257, 264, 293, 309, 312, 319, 324–25;
prostitutes in, 313, 316
Indiana, 85
Indian Health Service, 189
Indonesia, 262, 316
infanticide, 223
infants: AIDS in, 8, 40–41, 153, 172–73,
223, 227, 235, 296; crack-addicted,
276–77; testing of, 234
information clearinghouses, 103–5
Inkanyezi project, 303
inpatient resources, 105–8
insects, 25, 33, 66–67, 87, 169
Institute of Medicine (IOM), 101, 155, 191
Institut Merieux, 128
interferon, 55
interferon alpha, 44, 128, 129
Interleukin-2, 137
international aid, 305, 311–13; in Africa,
230–31; in Asia, 263, 264–65
International AIDS Trust, 313
intravenous (IV) drug users, 8, 25, 31–34,
47, 49, 72, 100, 117, 193, 198, 256,